Beyond Health, Beyond Choice

Critical Issues in Health and Medicine

Edited by Rima D. Apple, University of Wisconsin–Madison,
and Janet Golden, Rutgers University, Camden

Growing criticism of the U.S. health care system is coming from consumers,
politicians, the media, activists, and health care professionals. Critical Issues in
Health and Medicine is a collection of books that explores these contemporary
dilemmas from a variety of perspectives, among them political, legal, historical,
sociological, and comparative, and with attention to crucial dimensions such as
race, gender, ethnicity, sexuality, and culture.

For a list of titles in the series, see the last page of the book.

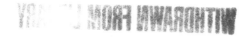

Beyond Health, Beyond Choice

Breastfeeding Constraints and Realities

Edited by
Paige Hall Smith
Bernice L. Hausman
Miriam Labbok

Rutgers University Press
New Brunswick, New Jersey, and London

Library of Congress Cataloging-in-Publication Data

Beyond health, beyond choice : breastfeeding constraints and realities / edited by Paige Hall Smith, Bernice L. Hausman, Miriam Labbok.
   p. ; cm. — (Critical issues in health and medicine)
  Includes bibliographical references and index.
  ISBN 978-0-8135-5303-0 (hardcover : alk. paper) — ISBN 978-0-8135-5304-7
(pbk. : alk. paper) — ISBN 978-0-8135-5316-0 (e-book)
  I. Smith, Paige Hall. II. Hausman, Bernice L. III. Labbok, Miriam H. IV. Series: Critical issues in health and medicine.
  [DNLM: 1. Breast Feeding. 2. Feminism. 3. Public Policy. WS 125]
  649'.33—dc23

                              2011037583

A British Cataloging-in-Publication record for this book is available from the British Library.

Visit our Web site: http://rutgerspress.rutgers.edu

Manufactured in the United States of America

To our mothers

In memory of Chris Mulford:
mother, feminist, and activist for breastfeeding

Contents

Preface and Acknowledgments   xi

Introduction: Breastfeeding Constraints and Realities   1
Bernice L. Hausman, Paige Hall Smith, and
Miriam Labbok

Part I   Frames

Chapter 1   Feminism and Breastfeeding: Rhetoric, Ideology,
             and the Material Realities of Women's Lives   15
             Bernice L. Hausman

Chapter 2   Breastfeeding Promotion through Gender Equity:
             A Theoretical Perspective for Public Health Practice 25
             Paige Hall Smith

Chapter 3   Breastfeeding in Public Health: What Is Needed for
             Policy and Program Action?   36
             Miriam Labbok

Part II   Studying Breastfeeding across Race,
               Class, and Culture

Chapter 4   Breastfeeding across Cultures: Dealing with Difference 53
             Penny Van Esterik

Chapter 5   The Dangers of Baring the Breast: Structural Violence
             and Formula-Feeding among Low-Income Women   64
             Nancy Chin and Ann Dozier

Chapter 6   Racism, Race, and Disparities in Breastfeeding   74
             Joan E. Dodgson

Part III   Medical Institutions and Health Education

Chapter 7   Pediatrics, Obstetrics, and Shrinking Maternal Authority 87
             Jacqueline H. Wolf

Chapter 8   New Professions and Old Practices: Lactation Consulting
             and the Medicalization of Breastfeeding   98
             Aimee R. Eden

Chapter 9   Preparing Women to Breastfeed: Teaching Breastfeeding
             in Prenatal Classes in the United Kingdom   110
             Abigail Locke

Part IV   Roles and Realities

Chapter 10   "Are We There Yet?" Breastfeeding as a Gauge of
             Carework by Mothers   123
             Chris Mulford

Chapter 11   Breastfeeding and the Gendering of Infant Care   133
             Phyllis L. F. Rippeyoung and Mary C. Noonan

Chapter 12   Working out Work: Race, Employment, and Public Policy   144
             Jennifer C. Lucas and Deborah McCarter-Spaulding

Chapter 13   The Impact of Workplace Practices on Breastfeeding
             Experiences and Disparities among Women   157
             Amanda Marie Lubold and Louise Marie Roth

Part V   Making and Marketing Mothers' Milk

Chapter 14   Marketing Mothers' Milk: The Markets for Human Milk
             and Infant Formula   169
             Linda C. Fentiman

Chapter 15   Empowerment or Regulation? Women's Perspectives on
             Expressing Milk   180
             Sally Johnson, Dawn Leeming, Steven Lyttle, and
             Iain Williamson

Part VI   Morality and Guilt

Chapter 16   Feminist Breastfeeding Promotion and the Problem
             of Guilt   193
             Erin N. Taylor and Lora Ebert Wallace

Chapter 17   Breastfeeding in the Margins: Navigating through the
             Conflicts of Social and Moral Order   203
             Danielle Groleau and Lindiwe Sibeko

Part VII Media and Popular Culture

Chapter 18   Reinstating Pleasure in Reality: Promoting Breastfeeding
             through *Ars Erotica*   215
             Fiona Giles

Chapter 19   Breastfeeding in the "Baby Block": Using Reality
             Television to Effectively Promote Breastfeeding   226
             Katherine A. Foss

Chapter 20   Rethinking the Importance of Social Class: How Mass
             Market Magazines Portray Infant Feeding   236
             N. Danielle Duckett

Part VIII Sexuality and Women's Bodies

Chapter 21   Breastfeeding in Public: Women's Bodies, Women's Milk   249
             Sally Dowling, Jennie Naidoo, and David Pontin

Chapter 22   Sexual or Maternal Breasts? A Feminist View of the
             Contested Right to Breastfeed Publicly   259
             Carol Grace Hurst

Chapter 23   Intersections: Child Sexual Abuse and Breastfeeding   269
             Emily C. Taylor

             Conclusion: Beyond Health, Beyond Choice:
             New Ways Forward in Public Health   281
             Paige Hall Smith, Bernice L. Hausman, and
             Miriam Labbok

             Bibliography   287

             Notes on Contributors   327

             Index   333

Preface and Acknowledgments

As industrialization takes hold, women are
less and less free to suckle their infants on
demand. As Western notions of glamour
and the role of wife as sex object take over,
the effects of prolonged lactation on the
breast are found to be unacceptable. As
Western marketing pushes the idea of
super babes fed on superhuman formula,
breastfeeding falls into disuse. As husbands
learn from the West that a husband takes
precedence over his children in enjoying
access to his wife's body, the practice of
postpartum abstinence is seen as primitive.

Germaine Greer, *Sex and Destiny:
The Politics of Human Fertility*, 1984

This collected volume results from presentations at the fifth Breastfeeding and
Feminism Symposium held March 20, 2010, at the Weatherspoon Art Gallery
on the campus of University of North Carolina at Greensboro (UNCG), cohosted
by the University's Center for Women's Health and Wellness and the Carolina
Global Breastfeeding Institute at UNC Chapel Hill. Since 2005 this symposium
has brought together academic scholars, practitioners, activists, and policy
makers from the United States and abroad who are interested in considering
feminist perspectives to address breastfeeding as a health priority for women
and children. Since 2005 the six Breastfeeding and Feminism Symposia have
stimulated a growth in public discourse and scholarship on the sociocultural,
economic, and political constraints on women's infant feeding choices. In addition, the symposia have focused attention on how public health approaches to
breastfeeding must go beyond promoting health to include serious consideration of the realities of women's lives, which are complicated by structural
inequities that feminists investigate through gender, race, and class analysis.

Although arguments about motherhood, work, and gender differences have
been central to feminist thought, historically feminists have had little to say

about breastfeeding. Throughout the 1970s and 1980s, contemporary feminist scholarship was concerned with understanding how women might achieve social, economic, and political equality with men. Strategies generally thought essential to that end included increasing women's employment and decreasing the primacy of the mothering role. Consequently, while feminist policy initiatives did attempt to address how pregnancy and childbirth should be handled by workplaces and employers, continuing breastfeeding after women returned to work was not considered an issue of commensurate importance.

Public health and policy interest in breastfeeding has exceeded feminist thought and action. In 1998 Representative Carolyn Maloney (D-NY) introduced into the U.S. Congress the New Mothers' Breastfeeding Promotion and Protection Bill (HR 3531). This bill would have amended the Pregnancy Discrimination Act of 1978 to include breastfeeding as a protected behavior under civil rights law, as well as the Family and Medical Leave Act of 1993 to make mothers eligible for a one-hour unpaid nursing break. It also offered tax credits to encourage employers to provide lactation rooms and equipment and outlined the need to develop minimum standards for breast pumps. Although this legislation did not pass, it is noteworthy that the National Organization for Women, historically an ardent supporter of gender-neutral strategies, supported this legislation, signaling a significant change in their philosophy. The ideas outlined by Representative Maloney's 1998 bill have just now come to fruition as part of the Obama administration's 2010 Patient Protection and Affordable Care Act.

One consequence of the relative absence of a public feminist voice in support of breastfeeding mothers is that much of the policy and programmatic development has occurred independent of a feminist perspective, being shaped instead by medical, capitalist, and maternalist interests and values. Partly as a result of feminism's own lack of interest in breastfeeding, we now have a situation in which the public health call for women to breastfeed exclusively for six months, in conjunction with recommendations to continue breastfeeding for at least a year or longer, has not been accompanied by systematic attempts to reduce the constraints to breastfeeding imposed by the complicated realities of women's lives. Ironically, there is now a surge of feminist voices that are antibreastfeeding. This surge is based on the perceived public pressure to breastfeed, thought to induce women to breastfeed as a way of entrapping them in the maternal role. This may also be a response to the fact that breastfeeding initiation, exclusivity, and duration are slowly but surely on the rise, threatening the perception of formula-feeding as normative and "normal." While seeking social change in specific arenas, this group of feminists clings to the earlier conceptualizations of formula use as freedom. Rather than seeing constraints to breastfeeding as part of a larger pattern of sex discrimination excluding mothers from employment and public spaces, these feminists point to breastfeeding itself as a problem that limits women's freedom.

The chapters in this book present an alternative feminist voice, one that seeks improvements in both breastfeeding *and* women's economic, social, and political status. We are beginning to partner with other organizations, movements, and individuals who share this view. In our estimation, dominant feminist responses to the "breast-bottle" controversy are mired in the equality versus difference debate, which has limited feminist politics concerning mothering. This situation is compounded by the fact that the United States, which is the single largest purchaser of commercial infant formula for its Women, Infants, and Children supplemental nutrition program (WIC), remains the only industrialized country that does not guarantee paid maternity leave. As a result, U.S. women find themselves constrained by tensions between work and family, and they seem to choose a side—work *or* family—that is articulated in public debates about breastfeeding. The tensions between feminist interpretations of the breast-bottle debate mirror the so-called Mommy Wars pervading the public sphere.

In our view, breastfeeding, as a part of women's reproductive life cycle, should be protected and supported in equal measure to women's other reproductive experiences. Women must be valued for the full range of productive and reproductive roles they play in modern societies. Mothering and paid employment are forms of labor that are valuable and honorable and should be supported as such by civil society. Our volume reflects this perspective as a way of transforming the disabling dichotomies currently defining feminist research in this area.

In 2004 Paige Hall Smith was awarded the Linda Arnold Carlisle Professorship in Women's and Gender Studies at UNCG. As part of her professorship Smith organized the first Breastfeeding and Feminism Symposium at UNCG in 2005, where Bernice Hausman was the keynote speaker. At the second symposium, in 2006, Miriam Labbok, on the heels of taking up her position as director of the Carolina Global Breastfeeding Institute at UNC Chapel Hill, was an invited speaker. Since that time the Center for Women's Health and Wellness at UNCG and the Carolina Global Breastfeeding Institute at UNC Chapel Hill have cosponsored the Breastfeeding and Feminism Symposium Series. This book would not have happened without this symposium and without conversations provided by the many speakers and participants who, over the years, have engaged in spirited transdisciplinary debate about the critical challenges facing breastfeeding mothers, and how we, as concerned feminists, mothers, policy makers, practitioners, and academics, should position our scholarship and action to best support them.

We extend our appreciation to the Office on Women's Health in the U.S. Department of Health and Human Services for providing funding for the symposium in 2008, 2009, and 2010. We are also indebted to our authors, whose contributions to this volume and to the contentious public debates about infant feeding are brave attempts to reorient both feminist thinking and public health approaches to breastfeeding. In addition, we would like to thank the College of Liberal Arts and Human Sciences at Virginia Tech, which awarded Bernice L. Hausman a Niles Faculty Fellowship in 2010–2011. The funds from this fellowship paid a subvention to Rutgers University Press to enable the publication of this manuscript, as well as providing for three graduate assistants from the Virginia Tech English department to support the complex editorial needs of the book. Brian Gogan, Libby Anthony, and Amy Reed did the lion's share of work formatting the manuscript and communicating with authors about citations, and we are grateful for their dedicated attention to detail.

Over the years graduate students at the Center for Women's Health and Wellness and the Carolina Global Breastfeeding Institute have contributed significantly to the success of the symposia, including Sheryl Coley, Laura Beth Haymore, Treva Curtis, Donna Duffy, Erin Reifstat, Sheryl Abrahams, Pam Dardess, Leslie Echerd, and Hannah Pollet. Jen Porter, a Virginia Tech undergraduate, also provided logistical support. Finally, we would like to thank UNC Chapel Hill and the Carolina Global Breastfeeding Institute for the heartfelt support of Mary Rose Tully for the first four years of the series, and to note that over the past four years the Symposium Series has relied on the intellect, dedication, and energy of Emily Taylor. Without all of their dedicated efforts, the symposia could not have occurred. We continue to be inspired by an emerging cadre of young feminist scholars breaking new ground in this field, and we are excited to include many of them in this volume.

Finally, to all of you who have participated, supported, and shared in the Breastfeeding and Feminism Symposium Series, we extend our heartfelt appreciation for your ongoing support for women and their decision to breastfeed.

Beyond Health, Beyond Choice

Bernice L. Hausman, Paige Hall Smith,
and Miriam Labbok

Introduction

Breastfeeding Constraints and Realities

Recently there has been an explosion of feminist attention to breastfeeding, in addition to increased activity in public health and medical research. Our collected volume, *Beyond Health, Beyond Choice: Breastfeeding Constraints and Realities*, contributes to this diverse field of research, policy, and practice by drawing on women's voices, feminist theory, public health, and novel inter-disciplinary conceptualizations. Our aim is to expand the understanding of women's experiences of breastfeeding and to provide insight for public health policy and planning.

Our title indicates the main elements of our approach. Current public health promotion of breastfeeding *per force* relies heavily on health messaging and individual behavior change, often failing to take into account the myriad constraints on women's choices and practices. The result is a perceived pres-sure on women to breastfeed without necessary social and cultural support. The reality of women's lives is diverse and constrained by structural factors outside of their personal control. Our volume focuses attention on the multi-ple contexts that affect women's behaviors, beliefs, and practices, exploring ways to refocus public debate about infant feeding decisions in the United States and elsewhere.

Beyond Health, Beyond Choice is a unique contribution to the burgeoning field of breastfeeding studies. Contributing authors hail from various disci-plines and countries, and include social scientists, humanities scholars, health workers, and public health activists and policy makers. We focus attention not only on describing the problem but also on strategies and approaches that inform policy, programming, and practices in health care and public health, basing our analyses in feminist practice and theory. Our commitments to feminism and to public health define the basic framework of our analysis. Our interest is in developing public health approaches to breastfeeding promotion, advocacy, and support that are embedded within a distinctly feminist perspective.

Beyond Choice: Feminist Standpoints and Women's Experiences

Feminism is diverse and changing. Feminism has never been and never will be one thing. As a result, our authors demonstrate varied feminist commitments. However, feminism as a general framework does suggest several basic principles that guide our understanding and inform our research.

First and foremost, feminism values women's experiences and the perspectives that they develop from those experiences. Standpoint feminism is one approach that seeks to honor women's perspectives on their own experiences. It is a specific version of what Donna Haraway has called *situated knowledge.*[1] Both standpoint feminism and the notion of situated knowledge suggest that because women's experiences often result from their lower status in society vis-à-vis men, these experiences offer an important window through which everyone can see new truths and possibilities. That does not mean that women's experiences in and of themselves represent unquestioned sources of knowledge or truth. It does mean, however, that the ideological and material contexts of women's lives are a critically important part of the reality that needs to be identified and taken seriously in the development of public health polices.[2]

The experience of breastfeeding seems to engender divergent and contentious responses. Many women express anger at perceived pressure to breastfeed. Contemporary blogs about infant feeding contain emotionally charged discussions about how pressure to breastfeed from medical professionals or breastfeeding supporters can lead to feelings of maternal failure or anger at biological insufficiency. Some women face censure for public breastfeeding, which, when publicized, can motivate widespread "lactivism" in support of breastfeeding women's rights. U.S. feminist labor activists bemoan medical recommendations to breastfeed that are thought to increase feelings of maternal guilt among working women while seeming to ignore the fact that the United States lags behind the rest of the industrialized world in providing maternity leave. Meanwhile, feminist breastfeeding advocates and supporters identify pitfalls in a health care system that seems to deny mothers accurate information of the contributions that breastfeeding makes to maternal and infant health. These varied responses to breastfeeding, breastfeeding promotion, and perceptions of breastfeeding support or censure offer important openings for feminist analysis of the politics of motherhood and infant feeding.

At this point in time, much feminist analysis of breastfeeding has focused on breastfeeding promotion that is unaccompanied by real support, identifying it as a factor contributing to women's continuing cultural and political subordination. Notably, this is the approach taken by feminist political scientist Joan Wolf in her recent book *Is Breast Best?* and others, such as Hanna Rosin, author of "The Case Against Breastfeeding" in the April 2009 *Atlantic Monthly*.[3] It is our view that this response is wrongheaded, as it places blame on breastfeeding as a source of women's inequality rather than on the political, economic, and sociocultural constraints in women's lives that make breastfeeding difficult. These constraints, in fact, not only affect breastfeeding but also reduce women's economic, political, and social status.

The approach we take in this book is that such constraints—for example, the lack of social support, the lack of paid maternity leave, the difficulty in meshing paid labor with breastfeeding, the limitation of practical support to the medical profession, the sexualization of women's bodies as the property of men—are more appropriately viewed as the problem. We look to the difficulties women experience with breastfeeding as symptomatic of the problems that breastfeeding poses to modern societies—the difficulty of integrating women fully into the public sphere, women's role as health managers for their families and the stress that this role entails, the reproductive burdens of childbirth and child rearing that women continue to bear disproportionately to men, a marketing climate that creates demand for industrial products by linking identity with consumption, and the economic inequality that is based, at least in part, on women's commitments to family well-being over career and individual self-advancement. Thus, when *we* honor women's experiences we investigate the meanings of maternal anger and regret in the context of a full analysis of medical evidence, public health goals, structural constraints, signifying practices, and the realities of women's lives. We want to know why one dominant response to contemporary breastfeeding promotion seems to be anger at the public health establishment and breastfeeding supporters, rather than a focus on the social circumstances that inhibit women's breastfeeding success in the context of increasing evidence from health care and public health sectors that breastfeeding contributes significantly to health and well-being.

We begin with the premise that women's perceptions of their own experience are enmeshed in social contexts that are ideologically influenced.[4] To value women's experience means that we must analyze the contexts that give rise to the stories that they tell about those experiences. Many women are angry that they did not or could not breastfeed after being told that breastfeeding is best for their infants and that not breastfeeding can lead to ill health and cognitive deficits. In their anger, many women writing about their experiences of breastfeeding failure suggest that breastfeeding promotion is too forceful because breastfeeding itself is not important as a public health measure. It is noteworthy that the predominant public story about breastfeeding is one of failure that is followed by a diatribe against public health promotion of breastfeeding. Another target for this critique is the overly zealous exhortation by people identified as "breastfeeding Nazis."

As feminist breastfeeding promoters, supporters, researchers, and advocates, we are pained by a public feminist response to this situation that blames other women (the so-called breastfeeding Nazis) rather than identifying a set of negative social, commercial, and economic circumstances as the problem to be addressed. This volume explores these structural constraints and identifies specific impacts that they have on breastfeeding practice and success, paying attention to economic constraints and commercial pressures, workplace rules and support, the constraints of women's social roles, the changing context of public policy and law, the influence of race and racism, the importance of social class, the effects of medicalization, the complex interplay of discourse and practice, the significance of institutional history, the meaning of women's exposed bodies in public, and the liberatory possibilities offered by new media and popular culture. Readers will see how shifting the lens of analysis toward the constraints of the social sphere changes the way we understand women's experiences and their negotiation of motherhood. Such a shift also suggests new ways of influencing public health thinking and action.

Beyond Gender: Integrating Race and Class

Public health promotion efforts at times may be, in feminist terms, ideologically objectionable because they can contribute to certain forms of gender subordination, especially when they manipulate expectations of women as responsible mothers.[5] Yet public health practice exists within a complex economic, political, and ideological system that is set up to favor capitalistic practices like feeding with formula. The domain of infant feeding debate is rife with varied and conflicting forces, which we examine in this book, paying special attention to how women are particularly vulnerable as they traverse this difficult geography. To a significant extent, we are trying to influence public health assumptions about how to go about promoting and supporting breastfeeding by focusing on the social, cultural, economic, commercial, and familial contexts that impact breastfeeding decisions and practices. Feminist theory helps us to identify the salient contexts to investigate and teaches us to consider gender in relation to other socially stratifying identities and structures.

Feminist insights have also considered race and class as contributing factors to women's subordination. Intersectional approaches understand gender, race, and class—as well as other categories of identity and stratification, like disability, nationality, or sexual orientation, to name only a few—to be inextricably intertwined in their effect on women's lives. The characteristic triumvirate "gender, race, and class" has become, in some circles, a casual reference to this theoretical insight, but serious feminist analysis never forgets that gender does not operate as a singular social and cultural force. Breastfeeding, while reminding us of women's biological capacities as female mammals, is also, and perhaps predominantly, a social activity that is practiced in contexts saturated with racial meanings and class impacts. Current statistics that disaggregate breastfeeding rates according to racial and class categories demonstrate the significant impact of these forces in the United States, and elsewhere, today.

In the United States and most of the global north, black women and poor women continue to lag behind wealthier white women in rates of breastfeeding initiation and duration. Educational attainment continues to be an important indicator of breastfeeding initiation and success, tracking racial and class categories. In order to understand *how* race and class impact breastfeeding rates, our authors have addressed the contexts within which women mother, identifying ways in which women in different racial and class categories experience, for example, breastfeeding in public, expressing milk at work, and managing on public assistance. Race and class are not simply categories of identity—they indicate possibilities that are open to women, systems of care and companionship, and structural impediments to change, as well as cultural and historic commonalities. In the United States, racism and poverty are also associated with violence, both in terms of individual risk and the structural violence engendered by punitive laws and institutional limitations that burden people's lives.

The focus on choice in public health promotion of breastfeeding, a focus created by educational messaging concerning the health contributions of breastfeeding without attention to the differing and difficult contexts that define women's lives, does little to acknowledge how race and class dynamics affect maternal infant feeding decisions. Choice paradigms tend to lump all women together in one category and define good or bad decisions according to their alignment with public health goals. Such paradigms thus imagine women as having significant control over their surroundings and relationships, a laudable goal of feminism but certainly not the reality that exists for many (or most) women today. Choice paradigms, in other words, implicitly imagine women as white and middle class, with the typical resources available to realize individual goals. (That white, middle-class women in the United States do not themselves breastfeed much beyond six months, when the recommendation is to continue for a year at least, suggests that even resources and will are not enough to comply with medical guidelines.)

Our focus on social, cultural, and economic constraints on breastfeeding demonstrates concrete effects of race, racism, and class on mothers' behaviors and experiences. In understanding how women's experiences are always constructed in the complex intersections of these social forces—which have both ideological and material impacts—we offer more than lip service to the meaning of race and class in women's lives. We are especially disappointed in previous feminist approaches to this topic that, in their attempts to understand poor and black women's lack of breastfeeding success, fail to adequately criticize the structures that limit these women's practices and constrain their maternal behaviors.[6] We do not assume that all women will ever want to breastfeed, but we do believe that sympathetic analysis of mothers' experiences with breastfeeding should include the frank assessment of the inequalities that construct the horizon of possibility in their lives. Breastfeeding success is not only a matter of belief or ideology—although both are crucial contributors—it is also a result of concrete material circumstances and the resources that any given woman has under her own control.

Beyond Health: Breastfeeding, Medicine, and Public Health

Infant feeding is both public and private. Its public health dimensions are measured across populations, although many women breastfeed because of the individual health benefits they seek for their own children. Breastfeeding has not been a main focus of public health, although the population-wide effects of not breastfeeding were evident when women began to abandon breastfeeding in the nineteenth century. However, breastfeeding in particular and infant feeding more generally have been a preoccupation within the medicalization of family life that French philosopher Michel Foucault argues emerged in the eighteenth century in Europe.[7] Medicalization of infant feeding has put profound pressure on mothers to feed their infants in an optimal manner, assuring not only survival but also health and well-being, often without adequate nutritional support themselves.

Pushing against breastfeeding as an ideal or optimal mode of infant feeding are cultural norms, which for a half century, at least in the United States, have favored replacement feeding. The *bottle-feeding culture* is how breast-feeding advocates and promoters identify these norms. We agree with this assessment and believe that these norms are supported by social and economic structures, as well as marketing paradigms, to such an extent that they no longer register as norms but are experienced as natural. Because of this, we have no interest in using this introduction to demonstrate or defend the health contributions of breastfeeding; such a defense is an element of the breast-bottle controversy that favors replacement feeding through its polarizing framework. All of the authors writing in this volume believe in breastfeeding and its contributions to health, although not all of us have breastfed all of our children in a manner that we may have wanted or planned. But focusing on this element of the public debate about infant feeding limits conversations about breastfeeding to its individual, and individualizing, aspects as a health maximizing practice. Instead, we treat the health contributions of breastfeeding and human milk as premises that underlie each chapter.[8]

Public health relies on various frameworks for understanding and assessing public health problems and planning interventions. Within the field of public health, the Social-Ecological Model (SEM) provides a theoretical framework for considering social influences that closely correlates with our observations about the constraints on breastfeeding and limitations to current efforts to promote breastfeeding. The Social-Ecological Model draws attention to "the importance of social influences on health and disease" and, significantly, highlights the relationships between various registers of social life in developing health promotion efforts.[9] For many of our authors, the Social-Ecological Model offers a valuable framework upon which to build feminist approaches to breastfeeding, capturing the feminist impulse to situate women's experiences in their full sociocultural and economic contexts. But the Social-Ecological Model does not specifically address how gender interweaves throughout these levels to shape women's behavior, including breastfeeding.

Social marketing through health messaging has been a key strategy of U.S. efforts to promote breastfeeding. This is an interpersonal-level strategy designed to change mothers' knowledge, beliefs, and attitudes about breastfeeding. An example of the messaging approach to alter attitudes and behavior is the U.S. National Breastfeeding Awareness Campaign, which ran from 2004 to 2006. The campaign had a number of different interventions, but focused on video and radio public service announcements and poster advertisements targeted to convince readers, viewers, and listeners of the health risks of not breastfeeding. While it is true that attitudinal changes are necessary to broader cultural shifts, it also seems clear that healthy behavior is complicated by social structure;

telling people how to behave in a healthful manner, especially when such behavior goes against cultural norms, is not sufficient to lead to widespread population-level change in infant feeding practices. The message "breast is best" had been shown to serve little useful purpose as early as the 1980s. It was known even then that the need was for substantive advice concerning how to overcome obstacles. The promulgation of more complex versions of this same message has no more likelihood of impact than did the original. Today, public health messaging in support of breastfeeding emphasizes what is needed for success (for example, the Business Case for Breastfeeding), but still rarely considers the complex environment facing contemporary mothers.

In January 2011, as we write this introduction, U.S. Surgeon General Regina M. Benjamin has just unveiled a new "Call to Action to Support Breast-feeding." Focusing on removing obstacles to breastfeeding at the personal, community, institutional, economic, and national levels, the "Call to Action" seeks to create an environment that will support women and "make breast-feeding easier."[10] Other recent strategies include institutional changes in the way the U.S. Department of Agriculture's (USDA) Women, Infants, and Children (WIC) program promotes and supports breastfeeding, the Department of Health and Human Service's (DHHS) campaign to improve workplace supports for breastfeeding, and the recent legal requirements in the federal 2010 Patient Protection and Affordable Care Act concerning lactation breaks for breastfeeding workers. It remains to be seen whether these strategies will have the desired effects to increase rates of breastfeeding initiation and dura-tion, but we applaud these developments in national-level planning and law to support breastfeeding, as their focus on identifying and removing constraints on women's breastfeeding intentions matches the analysis provided here.

Targeting a public health audience interested in breastfeeding and (per-haps) less familiar with feminism, this volume is intended to offer public health professionals new insights that may influence emerging strategies to address suboptimal breastfeeding, especially by moving beyond the standard and simplistic injunction to breastfeed due to its health benefits. *Beyond Health, Beyond Choice: Breastfeeding Constraints and Realities* offers public health practitioners original and provocative ways of thinking about and addressing the issues that they face every day in counseling, institution building, social marketing, capacity building, policy making, and community organizing.

Conclusion

The organization of the volume reflects the varied nature of constraints on breastfeeding, dividing chapters topically rather than by theoretical approach or method. We begin with chapters by the editors to make explicit the ideas that guide our scholarly work in this area. "Frames" demonstrates our own disciplinary commitments and scholarly backgrounds, but it also sets out the broader frameworks of the volume's collaborative analysis. These include feminist theories within cultural studies approaches, focusing on the role of ideology and discourse in constructing individuals' life worlds; sociological emphases on women's status and the structures of gendered power in the context of women's multiple roles; and breastfeeding in the context of public health planning and policy, focusing on health outcomes, medical evidence, and population-level strategies. In this section we lay out an argument for looking at constraints to breastfeeding rather than breastfeeding as a constraint; define and describe the impact of ideology on maternal behavior; and discuss women's roles in the context of an analysis of gender and power. We also identify the difficulties of studying breastfeeding and understanding its health impacts in the context of public health planning, programming, and policy making that have not made it a focus of their endeavors.

"Studying Breastfeeding across Race, Class, and Culture" initiates a consideration of constraints that are associated with cultural differences, poverty, and race. Significantly, the three chapters that make up this section demonstrate the importance of anthropological approaches to breastfeeding variability and the meanings of culture as an influence on behavior. In addition, the final chapter in this section challenges readers to consider how racism as a structural element of discrimination is at play in breastfeeding disparities.

"Medical Institutions and Health Education" focuses on how varied health professions—medical specialization of obstetrics and pediatrics, the new allied health profession of lactation consultants, and prenatal educators—influence breastfeeding. Methodologically, the approaches in this chapter are varied, ranging from qualitative social science to history to interdisciplinary anthropology and cultural studies. This section as a whole examines the impacts of institutionalized aspects of breastfeeding—how it is included in medical care during gestation, its role within pediatrics, how prenatal educators deal with it, and how lactation consulting (as an emerging profession) has been involved with its medicalization—demonstrating how breastfeeding as an intimate practice of mother and baby is framed by and constructed through institutional contexts and the implicit rules and expectations of those contexts.

"Roles and Realities" follows the theoretical elaboration of role theory in "Frames," focusing on the two roles most often in contention in infant feeding debates: domestic and waged labor. Here the authors argue for a consideration of breastfeeding as productive labor, explore the impact of breastfeeding on the distribution of domestic labor, identify the elements of workplace practices that make breastfeeding success possible for employed women, and analyze the relation of race to employment as a way of understanding suboptimal breastfeeding among African American women. The next section, "Making and Marketing Mothers' Milk," shifts this focus on roles to the meanings of human milk when it is extracted from the mother's body, examining the potential of explicit markets in human milk and the experiences of milk expression as a practice of mothering.

The final three sections of the volume, "Morality and Guilt," "Media and Popular Culture," and "Sexuality and Women's Bodies," focus on the cultural contexts of breastfeeding, breastfeeding promotion, and the possibilities of breastfeeding support through alternative media uses and transformed media messaging. We know that public health messaging concerning breastfeeding has involved troublesome ideas about good mothering; two of our chapters here investigate the moral dimensions of women's responses to breastfeeding success and failure, in the context of discursive connections between good mothering and breastfeeding. Other chapters examine the implications of mothers breastfeeding in public, in contexts of social disapproval and censure. Two of our authors imagine alternative uses of media to reinstate pleasure in public health messaging about breastfeeding or to offer more realistic depictions of breastfeeding to television audiences. Another chapter demonstrates that messages about breastfeeding in popular magazines make implicit assumptions about class that limit working-class women's access to information about breastfeeding. And one chapter boldly challenges received wisdom about the breastfeeding behaviors, beliefs, and experiences of adult survivors of childhood sexual abuse, identifying breastfeeding as a potentially redemptive, rather than predictably traumatic, practice for these women.

Taken together, these chapters that make up *Beyond Health, Beyond Choice: Breastfeeding Constraints and Realities* seek to inaugurate a new relationship between public health, feminism, and breastfeeding—one that develops a productive dialogue about women's experiences of breastfeeding in a culture of constraints. It is our hope that readers see new ways forward for themselves in this volume—to continue a line of research, to reflect on personal experience, to reframe their own practice, to rethink received ideas. Both feminism and public health are oriented toward social action and social justice— practices to improve human experience and end inequalities that contribute to health disparities—and we hope that this volume, like the many conversations it has engendered in the course of its development, will continue to spur its readers forward in their efforts toward an egalitarian and healthy future.

Notes

1. Haraway, "Situated Knowledges."
2. For a definition and discussion of ideology, see Hausman, this volume.
3. See Hausman, this volume, for further citations in this genre.
4. Teresa de Lauretis, in the first chapter of *Technologies of Gender*, has a particularly useful discussion of the effects of ideology on experience.
5. See Hausman, *Viral Mothers*, 72–87, for a discussion of this issue with respect to the U.S. National Breastfeeding Awareness Campaign.
6. For example, Blum, *At the Breast*.
7. Foucault, "The Politics of Health."
8. Chapter 3 does discuss the health contributions of breastfeeding as understood in current literature in order to outline current thinking on the matter and its significance within public health.
9. McLeroy et al., "An Ecological Perspective," 351, 354–355. This perspective is developed with further discussion in chapter 3.
10. U.S. Department of Health and Human Services, News Release, January 20, 2011. See also U.S. Department of Health and Human Services, *The Surgeon General's Call to Action to Support Breastfeeding*.

Part I

Frames

Feminism and Breastfeeding

Rhetoric, Ideology, and the Material Realities of Women's Lives

The current popular feminist critique of breastfeeding advocacy and promotion is unhelpful at best and destructive at worst. Its overall effect is to anger breastfeeding supporters rather than to encourage them to different approaches, and it puts feminism in an antagonistic, rather than collaborative, relation with public health. Yet feminism has much to contribute to an improved and more effective public health approach to breastfeeding.[1]

My aim in this chapter is to demonstrate how feminist analysis could be used to improve public health approaches to breastfeeding, infant health, and maternal health, by focusing on three core feminist issues that, with respect to breastfeeding, translate as the importance of a rights framework for conceptualizing breastfeeding as a maternal practice; an emphasis on social constraints, rather than biological inadequacies, as contributors to breastfeeding failure or cessation; and an analysis of the ideology of the good mother as a primary strategy to promote breastfeeding. Attention to breastfeeding as a woman's right and to structural and ideological constraints on breastfeeding as maternal practice constitute mechanisms to reframe public health policy and action in this area.

Feminist Rhetoric and Medical Evidence

Feminist criticism of breastfeeding promotion efforts—most recently exemplified by Joan Wolf's *Is Breast Best?*, Hanna Rosin's "The Case Against Breastfeeding," and Julie Artis's "Breastfeed at Your Own Risk"—argues that such efforts ignore the material realities of women's lives. These critics also challenge the scientific evidence supporting public health measures to increase rates of maternal nursing. This trend has been evident in feminist writing since the mid-1990s. Pam Carter's *Feminism, Breasts, and Breast-Feeding*, Jules Law's "The Politics of Breastfeeding," and Linda Blum's *At the Breast* all hedge their arguments about the relative benefits of breastfeeding over formula-feeding, suggesting that existing evidence—while perhaps valid in poorer areas of the world—is just not strong enough to support vigorous public health campaigns in the United States to improve rates of breastfeeding initiation and duration.[2]

The argument that breastfeeding promotion is based on ambiguous scientific evidence only motivates health care professionals and public health policy makers to reaffirm the health benefits of breastfeeding. This response, in turn, further angers feminist critics, because the argument for the evidence suggests that health benefits outweigh material difficulties and social circumstances—in other words, that women's experiences are beside the point.

Thus, the continuing public debate between breastfeeding advocates and promoters and feminists has produced a stalemate that continues to emphasize medical evidence yet is divided over its meanings. The debate fails to address feminist concerns about women's experiences, as the focus on the value of the medical evidence hinders productive exchange about the other potent issues raised by feminist scholars and popular writers: how breastfeeding affects the sexual division of labor at home, whether breastfeeding is a drag on women's professional success, and how not breastfeeding might be a strategic response to current and historical social circumstances.[3] Addressing this stalemated situation as rhetorical—that is, as an effect of the particular staging of the debate—offers a salutary opportunity to engage other, more productive questions raised by feminist analysis—namely, attention to social constraints, women's rights, and the power of ideology to enforce behavioral norms.[4]

A rhetorical analysis of public debate over infant feeding may feel uncomfortable to those who believe that medical evidence should be the last word. Yet from feminist perspectives, scientific evidence has long been used to circumscribe women's freedom. In the nineteenth century, this came in the form of recommendations that women not pursue higher education on the theory that intense intellectual endeavors during late adolescence would cause atrophy of their reproductive organs.[5] Because feminists are sensitive to the ways that medical advice and information continues to implicitly limit women's life choices—by suggesting that nonparturient women over thirty have a higher risk of breast cancer, for example—perceived pressure to breastfeed in order to ensure infant health can be identified as part of a larger cultural project to maintain patterns of female domesticity and subjugation.

Breastfeeding promotion campaigns like the National Breastfeeding Awareness Campaign (NBAC) explicitly use rhetorical tools to persuade women of the risks of not breastfeeding. Because public health efforts are themselves steeped in sophisticated rhetorical projects, we cannot suggest that unvarnished or bare medical evidence is itself sufficient to promote awareness of breastfeeding as an important, or imperative, component of infant nutrition and care. And, of course, awareness itself is not the goal of breastfeeding promotion: improvements in the rates of breastfeeding initiation and duration are. Rhetoric—in this case, the effective and persuasive use of language—is crucial to breastfeeding promotion efforts, and the presentation of scientific evidence is as rhetorical as other elements of these efforts.

Feminists have drawn attention to the rhetorical elements of these campaigns and objected to various aspects of their address to women.[6] But rhetorical criticism cuts both ways. Setting aside or challenging medical evidence concerning breastfeeding's contributions to health allows feminists to draw attention to the social and cultural constraints *of* breastfeeding as a maternal practice, targeting breastfeeding and the discourses supporting it as limitations on women's freedom. It seems to me, however, that limitations on women's freedom and ongoing unequal relations between the sexes negatively affect women's ability to breastfeed.

Social Constraints on Breastfeeding

Leaving aside the question of medical evidence allows us to consider the social and cultural constraints *on* breastfeeding, rather than breastfeeding itself as a constraint, including ideological impacts and the question of women's rights. When we shift our focus we find that there exists a significant body of research concerning the constraints on breastfeeding success. For example, we know that inadequate lactation management is a significant problem, that return to work poses almost insurmountable barriers for many mothers, and that other cultural constraints, including difficulties breastfeeding in public and lack of familial support, influence mothers' decisions not to breastfeed or to wean early. We also know that demographic factors place infants at risk for not being breastfed—race, socioeconomic status, education level of the mother. Some of these constraints involve issues of self-efficacy that can be addressed by attention to personal decision making, but most are structural or large-scale cultural issues that need approaches not directed to women or mothers per se but to material contexts, the law, and public perceptions.[7] Promotional campaigns that attempt to educate mothers and focus on decision making and self-efficacy will often do so without attention to how individual action is

framed by structural constraints, including community expectations and interpersonal relationships.

For example, the public service announcements in the NBAC, which
portrayed visibly pregnant women engaged in log-rolling contests or riding a
mechanical bull in a bar, rendered bad pregnant mothers as isolated in their
decision making, even though the activity took place within a crowd of people.
Neither PSA showed the women with an identified partner (who may have
encouraged or demanded the dangerous behavior) or portrayed the activity as
anything but willful behavior on the part of the mother. Such representations
deny existing limitations on many women's daily behaviors, especially if they
are involved in abusive relationships, and place the viewer in the position of
judging critic. The posters accompanying the NBAC focused solely on medical
evidence concerning risks of not breastfeeding, suggesting that the decision to
breastfeed could be based entirely on medical information rather than other
complicating social or familial factors.

Educating mothers without addressing constraints leads to experiences of
maternal failure and consequent guilt and anger. It is out of these feelings that
the feminist critique emerges.[8] After all, intentions that are met with obstacles
that demand heroic self-sacrifice or significant personal and financial resources
will not be achievable for most women. It is time we address these constraints
on breastfeeding as public health problems themselves, insofar as sociocultural and economic constraints block women from achieving what public health
officials have determined to be an important health-promoting practice.[9]
A rights framework, rather than a choice framework, would better facilitate
this endeavor.[10] A rights framework can identify broad social constraints on
women's capacity to realize their rights. A choice framework, in neoliberal
contexts, tends to individualize both decision making and practice, rather than
see both as embedded in a nexus of sociocultural expectations and structures
that limit the achievement of personal intentions or desires.[11]

In addition, focusing on constraints inhibiting the realization of rights
clarifies the role of ideology in women's experiences of breastfeeding. Ideology
shapes women's experiences of their bodies, obscuring the social impacts on
breastfeeding. Dominant ideologies focus women's attention on their own
bodies as lacking rather than on social systems that fail to support their
practices and goals. For example, inadequate milk supply is the most common
reason given for early weaning.[12] Women perceive low milk supply to be a
biological failure of their bodies, yet it is most often the effect of poor lactation
management, which is itself a social constraint in a cultural context unfamil-
iar with the demands of breastfeeding. Biological capacities are thus shaped by

external social forces, but ideology naturalizes lactation failure as both individual and common. Furthermore, specific ideologies that help to maintain women's subordination often surface in public health campaigns to promote breastfeeding. Recurrent images—the good mother and pure breast milk—are used to encourage women that breastfeeding is better than alternative modes of infant feeding, but also work to moralize infant feeding and serve as implicit evaluations of mothers' fitness.

The Rights Framework for Breastfeeding

The World Health Organization (WHO) includes health as a basic human right in its initial principles, and breastfeeding is supported in several United Nations rights documents.[13] However, this international understanding is not readily apparent in the U.S. context, which has tended to ignore international agreements concerning breastfeeding in favor of business-oriented policies. Historically, American feminists have been concerned about any rights provision claiming that being breastfed is the right of a child, given that such a universal claim would make specific, unalterable demands on mothers. Yet to understand breastfeeding as a woman's right transforms the demand from one made on women's bodies to one made on the political and social context, focusing attention on her ability to realize her rights.[14] Thus, a women's rights framework reorients the debate from one focused on the medical evidence thought to influence mothers' choices (and thus from the "educating mothers" paradigm) to one focused on obstacles to the realization of those rights. This approach suggests a powerful political understanding of how social contexts frame expectations about public health strategies.

Fundamentally, a rights perspective transforms public health from a focus on the individual to the social contexts that inform and structure personal experience. If one major problem with improving breastfeeding duration is return to work, then individualized attention to mothers' specific plans (Can you pump at work? How many breaks do you have during the day? Can your caregiver bring the baby to you at midday?) will only be successful with mothers who have a significant amount of control over their time during the workday and resources to sustain the inconvenience of being away from a breastfeeding baby. Mothers with personal resources, either familial or financial, may succeed, but given the broad structural constraints, such success will demand significant determination and forcefulness that many women— subject to gendered expectations of behavior since infancy—are not able to muster. Rights frameworks point us toward the structural elements influencing personal decisions and practices, and they assume that individual intention, will, and fortitude are insufficient to address such constraints. Public health achieved many of its most important and life-changing gains in the early twentieth century through broad-based infrastructure changes. The rights framework suggests a return to these priorities, a goal sought by many in public health.[15]

Because rights are impinged upon not only by explicit social and economic structures, but by more insidious and ambiguous cultural forces, a rights approach to breastfeeding must also involve a critique of how dominant ideologies of mothering impact breastfeeding. Ideologies support the economic system through the force of community norms and expectations. It is difficult to disregard or disable ideological influences precisely because ideology functions below the level of consciousness. But belief systems are crucial elements of constraint; this is apparent when the majority of women accept lactation failure as a normal event and fault of their own bodies' incapacity. Public health approaches to breastfeeding must attend to ideological constructions of motherhood that feminists have identified as detrimental to women's full citizenship.

Ideology: The Good Mother

Ideology is the name given to cultural forces that function to make people identify with the given structures and meanings of their social contexts. Dominant ideologies are those sets of ideas that make the contradictory experiences of everyday life seem cohesive. Their function is to block inquiry into aspects of the existing social system that perpetuate inequities and disadvantages to most ordinary people. Ideologies in the classic sense obscure the realities of existence from people who come to identify with social systems that operate against their best interests.

Ideologies are transmitted through mainstream discourses permeating the culture—television programs, popular literature, and advice books, for example—as well as common everyday experiences like washing oneself or putting on clothing. As a term, then, *ideology* refers to the dominant meanings that are conveyed through practices and social structures; it represents an external constraint on behavior that becomes a part of who people are and how they experience reality. No one escapes ideological influence, although some people can teach themselves how to notice and interpret ideologies at work and thus begin to counteract their more insidious effects on human behavior. Most of us not only live in compliance with the dominant ideologies of our culture, but also transmit these ideologies to others, mutually reinforcing the status quo and supporting those who benefit from it.

Feminists have adopted various forms of ideological analysis in order to understand women's experiences in male-dominated societies, and especially to ascertain why most women are complicit with social systems that oppress them.[16] A case in point is the good mother. Historians Molly Ladd-Taylor and Lauri Umansky point out that the idea of a good mother is a "relatively recent invention," perhaps only two centuries old. The "new maternal ideal," as they put it, emerged in concert with modern changes to the organization of work that divided public and private spheres and gendered them.[17] The figure of the good mother haunts breastfeeding support literature. Initially, La Leche League's motto was "Better Mothering through Breastfeeding," then quickly changed to "Good Mothering through Breastfeeding," eventually settling on "Mothering through Breastfeeding" to get rid of the evaluative assumption.[18] Pregnancy and infant care advice manuals insist that women who do not breastfeed are still good mothers, a negative assertion demonstrating ambivalence about the issue. Public health education materials concerning infant feeding moralize breastfeeding and consequently promote the idea that breastfeeding makes one a better mother or is evidence that one is a good mother.[19] The good breastfeeding mother was implied in the public service announcements in the NBAC, as the obverse of the pregnant women riding mechanical bulls or participating in log-rolling contests.

The idea of the good mother operates as an ideology circumscribing women's behaviors: as the NBAC public service announcement shows, mothers are persuaded to breastfeed because they don't want to be bad mothers. As Ladd-Taylor and Umansky note, it's not that ideas about good mothering are all bad, it's that they tend to define a narrow set of behaviors that end up doing more to confine than to liberate women. They point out that even feminist use of ideas about good mothering has itself functioned historically to intensify criticism of "mothers deemed to be bad."[20] Foucaultian-oriented scholars extend this kind of analysis by demonstrating how individuals respond to ideologies of mothering by incorporating them into their own practices and self-concepts. Disciplining the self according to the ideals of good mothering is, in this view, a kind of "quiet coercion" that meets the state's need for "self-regulating subjects."[21]

The reiteration of health benefits associated with breastfeeding in the context of a society permeated with ideologies of good mothering tends to reinforce an implicit connection between breastfeeding and the good mother. Religious iconography of the Madonna breastfeeding Jesus contributes to this tendency to see breastfeeding as a practice of dutiful mothers.[22] Religious iconography also promotes the idea of pure breast milk, which is an explicit element of breastfeeding promotion and an aspect of its moralizing rhetoric.[23] Because ideology permeates belief systems and the material practices that sustain them, promotion campaigns that focus on education tend to reinforce dominant ideologies.

As an alternative, public health can disrupt its own complicity with ideologies of good mothering and endorse alternative models of mothering behavior in relation to breastfeeding. As part of this project, public health needs to rethink its focus on risk messaging. The NBAC, with its negative risk message, ran from 2004 to 2006, but it does not seem to have made a significant difference in the breastfeeding practices of mothers giving birth during that period.[24] Instead of risk messaging, public health efforts with respect to breastfeeding should target institutions, structures, environments, and belief systems. This reframing constitutes a rhetorical shift, a political charge for public health activity concerning breastfeeding, and a return to public health roots in broad-based social reform.

Conclusion

As feminists we cannot turn a blind eye to material conditions in our desire to promote breastfeeding as a healthful mode of infant feeding. Nor should anger at the popular feminist critique of the medical evidence supporting breastfeeding obscure the real contribution that feminism can make to public health efforts at promoting breastfeeding.

Arguing against the medical evidence provides feminist critics with a way to fight what they see as the ideologically troublesome effects of breastfeeding promotion—guilt for mothers who cannot breastfeed or decide against it for a variety of reasons, inattention to the real needs of mothers and children, and the inappropriate shaming of women by the use of the bad mother image to educate them about the importance of breastfeeding.[25] Yet evidence never speaks for itself—it must be argued into existence as meaningful through a variety of rhetorical styles. Medical research may be especially prone to this difficulty, as confounding factors are hard to isolate and bracket from the focus of any given study. Infant feeding in particular may present special problems in this regard. The randomized controlled trial, the "gold standard" of evidenced-based medicine, is not a viable method to explore most questions about the health effects of various modes of infant feeding. In addition, it may be impossible to separate effects of human milk from the act of breastfeeding, or from the other behaviors that seem to follow from breastfeeding, such as extended holding of the infant and more physical contact between mother and baby.[26] The cohort and quasi-experimental design necessary to address many public health questions may not adequately isolate the impact of feeding alone.

Rhetorical analysis demonstrates that when evidence is the focus of debates about breastfeeding, effective communication stalls and issues concerning sex inequity and its contribution to constraints on mothers' practices are neglected. Yet if public health policy makers and practitioners shift their attention from mothers and their individual decisions to social and economic structures that constrain mothers' actions, and ideologies that contribute to and enforce particular beliefs and practices, they will go a long way toward enabling women's right to breastfeed. Breastfeeding advocates in the United States idolize Scandinavian countries for their high rates of breastfeeding initiation and duration, but we must acknowledge the correlation between those statistics and sociocultural choices for enhanced gender equality, as well as legislative efforts to promote social welfare.[27] We cannot pretend that individual practices will make up for a sociocultural context inimical to breastfeeding, because our expectation that mothers can supersede their material and ideological realities contributes to the very constraints on breastfeeding that we want to change.

Notes

1. Not all feminists are against breastfeeding promotion and/or breastfeeding. The feminist antibreastfeeding promotion position simply takes up a lot of public space in debates about infant feeding that surface periodically in academic and popular venues. Examples of academic feminists who come to breastfeeding studies through a supportive approach include Bartlett, *Breastwork*; Smyth, "Intimate Citizenship"; Wolf, "What Feminists Can Do"; and McCaughey, "Got Milk?"

2. For a discussion of Law, Carter, and Blum, see Hausman, *Mother's Milk*, 196–207. Kukla also uses this strategy in her article "Ethics and Ideology," as do Rosin, "Case Against Breastfeeding," and Wolf, "Is Breast Really Best?" and *Is Breast Best?*

3. These issues are addressed, respectively, by Law, "Politics of Breastfeeding"; Rosin, "Case Against Breastfeeding"; Blum, *At the Breast*. The last point is also raised by Lee, "Infant Feeding in Risk Society," who discusses women's "pragmatic" responses to infant feeding choice.

4. For current medical assessments of breastfeeding's contributions to infant and maternal health, see Ip et al., *Breastfeeding and Maternal and Infant Health Outcomes*; Chen and Rogan, "Breastfeeding and the Risk of Postneonatal Death"; Bartick and Reinhold, "Burden of Suboptimal Breastfeeding."

5. See Russett, *Sexual Science*.

6. Kukla, "Ethics and Ideology"; Artis, "Breastfeed at Your Own Risk"; Joan Wolf, "Is Breast Really Best?"; Jacqueline Wolf, "What Feminists Can Do."

7. For a discussion of return to work and breastfeeding, see Calnen, "Paid Maternity Leave"; see also Li et al., "Breastfeeding Rates," for rates of breastfeeding initiation and duration comparing various demographic factors. Milligan et al., "Breastfeeding Duration," treats factors associated with low rates of breastfeeding and early

weaning among low-income women. Van Esterik and Greiner, "Breastfeeding and Women's Work," provides a theoretical discussion. Li, Fridinger, and Grummer-Strawn, "Public Perceptions," reveals public views that affect breastfeeding duration and weaning. Taylor, *Constraints to Exclusive Breastfeeding*, provides a synopsis of material and cultural constraints.

8. Hausman, "Motherhood and Inequality."
9. The new *Surgeon General's 2011 Call to Action to Support Breastfeeding* does highlight obstacles, including social constraints, to breastfeeding, which is an important step forward. See U.S. Department of Health and Human Services, *The Surgeon General's Call.*
10. Hausman, "Women's Liberation." See also Hausman, *Mother's Milk*, 153. See Smyth, "Intimate Citizenship," for a discussion of the right to breastfeed in relation to intimate citizenship.
11. Neoliberalism is a perspective on political economy that explains social relationships through market metaphors, such that individuals are seen as autonomous and rational decision makers. See Ong, *Neoliberalism as Exception.*
12. Jacqueline Wolf, pers. comm. with author, July 5, 2010.
13. World Health Organization, "Constitution."
14. See Labbok, "Breastfeeding."
15. Alcabes, "Epidemiologists Need to Shatter."
16. See de Lauretis, *Technologies of Gender*, especially the first chapter, "The Technology of Gender."
17. Ladd-Taylor and Umansky, "Introduction," 6–7.
18. Cahill, *Seven Voices*, 56. Many critics contend that LLL still holds onto breastfeeding as a practice that leads to good mothering.
19. See Wall, "Moral Constructions of Mothers," and Lee, "Infant Feeding."
20. Ladd-Taylor and Umansky, "Introduction," 7, 11.
21. Murphy, "Expertise and Forms of Knowledge," 432–433, plus discussion 434–437; see also Lee, "Infant Feeding"; and Wall, "Moral Constructions of Mothers."
22. Giles has made this point in a number of lectures—for example, "Reimagining Breastfeeding."
23. See Hausman, *Viral Mothers*, 98–129, for a discussion of purity and breast milk.
24. U.S. Department of Health and Human Services, "Breastfeeding among U.S. Children."
25. Artis, "Breastfeed at Your Own Risk"; Kukla, "Ethics and Ideology."
26. The 2007 AHRQ study is careful to mention only "associations" between breastfeeding and improved infant and maternal health outcomes. See Ip et al., *Breastfeeding and Maternal and Infant Health Outcomes.*
27. Bennhold, "In Sweden." This article does not discuss breastfeeding. However, it does demonstrate Sweden's commitment to gender equality. Sweden boasts almost 100 percent breastfeeding initiation, with around 98 percent of babies "ever breastfed" in 2006 (World Health Organization, "Infant and Young Child Feeding Data").

Breastfeeding Promotion through Gender Equity

A Theoretical Perspective for Public Health Practice

The connection between gender inequality and women's breastfeeding practice has been recognized since the early days of the breastfeeding movement. Numerous documents produced or endorsed by the breastfeeding movement have articulated the link between women's status and breastfeeding practice. Breastfeeding advocate Ted Greiner, for example, parallels the desired agendas of the breastfeeding movement with those of the women's movement: "improved working conditions and maternity benefits for working women; help with the burdens of child care and household tasks, especially during the first weeks after delivery; health care that is more sensitive to the needs of women; the opportunity to space babies as they choose; and freedom from the fear and suffering caused by poverty and malnutrition."[1]

Most health behavior change interventions have focused attention on how to change critical factors at the individual, interpersonal, community, or organizational level, but rarely do public health interventions focus directly on reducing gender inequality; this neglect may be because we do not know enough about how to reduce the structures that sustain inequality. This chapter outlines a theoretical perspective on how gender inequality affects the maternal practice of breastfeeding, ultimately articulating some principles for breastfeeding protection, promotion, and support that may improve breastfeeding through gender equity.

A theory of gender is critical to breaking down the monolithic and one-dimensional terms *gender inequality* and *women's status* in ways that allow us to understand and study how gender inequality arises and is sustained. For purposes here, *gender inequality* refers to the difference in economic, political, and social status between men and women. My framework interweaves theories of gender developed by Christine Oppong and R. W. Connell to understand, study, and document how women's roles and status affect their breastfeeding practices.[2]

Setting the Stage: Gender Role Differentiation

Over twenty years ago, Christine Oppong, then a senior scientist with the International Labor Organization, developed a theoretical framework to further the understanding of women's status in society, their roles and productive contributions, and how these affect demographic changes and economic development. According to Oppong, status has three dimensions: economic, political, and social. She proposes that women's status is configured through the activities, expectations, resources, and authority associated with seven different roles: occupational, domestic, partner, parent, community member, kinship and family, and individual.

As daughters (kinship) we are often accountable to our parents' values, and we often must care for them as they age. If we are part of a couple (partner) we engage in reciprocal care, support, love, and sex. As a mother (parent) we must help feed and raise our children, and if we have a home we usually have to maintain it (domestic). In addition, we may wish or need to enter the paid labor force (occupational) and contribute to the life of our community through volunteer service and participation in the public life (community). Last, and often least, we may want to engage in activities that improve our own mind and body or that are just good fun (individual).

Each role comes with its own unique set of expectations, constraints, and stressors. The more roles we take on, the more responsibilities we have and the greater the constraints on our time. However, each role also provides unique opportunities, benefits, and resources, expands our social network, exposes us to new ideas, and provides opportunities for joy and love. For each of us, then, life involves a series of decisions and turning points about how to best allocate our resources—our time, our money, our possessions, our energy, our bodies—across our different roles over time so that we obtain what we need for a meaningful and secure life.

Oppong highlights four noteworthy aspects to women's roles. First, women's multiple roles and their characteristics combine to shape women's economic, political, and social status. Economic status is affected by the activities we perform in the roles, social norms, values, legal protections, perceptions of our work performance, whether and how we acquire the knowledge and skills needed to perform well in the roles, and the extent of our acquisition of financial and nonfinancial resources. Political status, or personal power, is affected by the control and authority we have over resources, opportunities, and decisions that require action by others. Social status, or prestige, is affected by the relationships we have with others, particularly the degree to which we acquire positive attention, admiration, deference, and imitation.

The second important point is that sex and gender matter. The roles available to women and men, as well as the resources, opportunities, authority, support, and admiration women and men receive for their roles, are different. Oppong writes, "Women's productive activities are, first, never-ending and they absorb far more of their working hours than those of their male counterparts; second women by and large do the work in the home which is unpaid; and third, women's work both outside and inside the home remains to a large extent unremunerated and invisible."[3] As a result, men continue to acquire more wealth than women, do less child care and housework than women with no loss of social status, and own or have control over more resources and institutions.

Third, an examination of all these roles provides an understanding of how and why woman's economic, political, and social statuses are dissimilar across different roles. For instance, women's main source of economic status may be their occupational role (with respect to which they may have little power), while their major sphere of influence may be the domestic role (which is not a source of economic reward). Such a configuration of statuses, in which economic and power statuses do not coincide, may be associated with lack of ability to respond to opportunities or initiate change.[4]

Fourth, the demands and expectations of one role are often at odds with the demands and expectations of another, leading to role strain (the lack of time or material resources needed to fulfill role expectations) and/or role conflict (tensions or struggles produced by competing expectations for a person's time, energy, resources, or loyalties). Many women are presented with the dilemma of how to be employed and still provide for and/or allocate sufficient time and money to ensure the health and well-being of family member's.[5] However, it is not the activities of the roles per se that lead to role strain and conflict, but other role characteristics, such as personal and social values and role expectations; resource acquisition and control; role agency; social, family, and community support; and social role position. Role conflict and strain, in turn, lead to behavioral choices that may stem more from time and resource constraints than from personal preferences. With respect to infant feeding, in times of scarce resources or famine, infant formula may be seen as the easier choice for some women.[6]

Institutionalizing Status Inequities: Gendered Social Structures

While Oppong's theory helps us understand how societies' construction of role activities, expectations, supports, and rewards sets the stage for gender inequities, sociologist and gender scholar R. W. Connell has constructed a theory describing how social structures sustain and carry forward gender differences in opportunities, resources, and constraints. Connell outlines three structures at the societal level that affect economic, political, and social status: the sexual division of labor, which affects economic status; the sexual division of power, which affects political status; and the sexual division of social relationships, which affects social status.

Economic Status through the Sexual Division of Labor

The sexual division of labor refers not just to the allocation of women's and men's labor across the different roles, but also to how work is organized and how the rewards of work are distributed.[7] The sexual division of labor, which typically allocates carework to women and paid work to men, results in important differences in the resources, opportunities, constraints, and stressors that accrue to men and women. The gendered division of labor does not occur by accident nor do biological constraints or natural forces sustain it. Rather, this division is sustained by two principles: the "gendered logic of accumulation," meaning that economic wealth accumulates gains in one direction and losses in another; and the "political economy of masculinity," meaning both that those with more economic clout (that is, men) are able to make the choices that sustain the current division of labor and that masculinity itself becomes an economic resource.[8]

A variety of social, cultural, and legal mechanisms support these principles, including lack of maternity leave and affordable quality child care; the way work is organized (expectations for overtime, mobility, and travel; tolerance for sexual harassment and discrimination); availability of flexible work opportunities; opportunities for wealth accrual (pay equity, access to credit, and access to health insurance)—as well as practices that promote gender solidarity (labor force segregation into "pink" and "blue" collar work, gendering of work-oriented social activities, and sex discrimination in hiring and promotion).

Joan Williams, a feminist legal scholar, observes that much sexual division of labor stems from the ways that societies separate role activities, opportunities, and rewards into an unequal dichotomy separating the public world of work and community from the private world of home and family. This public-private dichotomy has two defining characteristics. The first is the organization of public, economically remunerative work around the ideal of a full-time worker who is available for overtime work and takes little or no time off for childbearing or rearing. The second characteristic is that our social system of providing care for children and the sick is privatized and unpaid, and it marginalizes the caregivers, cutting them off from most of the social roles that offer responsibility and authority.[9] This analysis illustrates how, as Connell proposes, the design and organization of work makes it difficult for mothers to perform as ideal workers, which constrains their ability to secure greater income and wealth.

As with most dichotomies, one side is more privileged than the other. The distinction between public and private is often thought of as natural, not socially constructed. Joyce Fletcher, feminist scholar in management, observes that the activities done in the public world of work (occupational role) are associated with doing masculinity while those done in the caregiver roles (for example, domestic, kin, and parental roles) are associated with doing femininity. These distinctions, in turn, help define what is considered good work in each role.[10] As with all dichotomies, this construction serves to maintain and continually re-create the separation. As a consequence, work done in occupational roles is seen as masculine and is perceived as superior, receiving better remuneration regardless of whether the worker is a man or woman. Similarly, work done in caregiver roles is seen as feminine even if done by men. This public-private dichotomy contributes to the consistent allocation of carework to women and to gender solidarity.[11]

Breastfeeding is an activity associated with the private world of mothering, not the public world of paid work. It is an unpaid activity mothers do "because we want to" and out of love; a maternal behavior that involves women's time, energy, body, and emotions; a 24/7 activity with an ambiguous time frame, involving both day- and nighttime work. Women need both mothering and breastfeeding to be more flexible to accommodate their personal and social expectations across multiple roles, yet this need butts up against the rigidity of the gendered nature of labor and the continuing organization of labor-related norms, values, perceptions, resources, opportunities, and decision-making authority around the lives the men, as well as the biological constraints of lactation.

Political Status and the Sexual Division of Power

In Connell's view the sexual division of power refers to the "deep-rooted gendered imbalance of social power in advantage or an inequality of resources in a workplace, community, household or relationship."[12] This is consistent with

Oppong's view that gender differences in political status stem from differences in men's and women's ability to acquire and control financial and nonfinancial resources and opportunities and the power to make decisions that require others to act.

As with the sexual division of labor, there are social, cultural, and legal mechanisms that support male power advantages. Particularly important are the social laws, norms, and ideologies that govern the use of force, including establishing who has power and authority to use force, to enforce a definition on a situation, to set the terms within which events are discussed and understood, or to formulate ideals and define morality. Male supremacy is one ideology that frames our construction and perception of the use of force and authority.[13] The sexual division of power is sustained or disrupted by social organizations that have power to uphold or counter the ideology of male supremacy, including religious institutions, courts, and the mass media. Connell describes two principles that systematically uphold the ideology of male supremacy and the sexual division of power: the ideology of masculinity and the gendered logic of power.

Connell argues that the ideology of masculinity leads society to exaggerate the importance of biological sex differences (for example, reproduction, pregnancy, and lactation) in order to continually justify masculine power structures, since these differences make it more difficult for women to fit within the authoritative norm. However, not paying attention to the biological needs of mothers does not necessarily lead to equity. Negating the needs of the maternal body serves to exaggerate the differences between men and women by making it more difficult for women to perform as ideal workers. Indeed, a practice of discounting the reality of the needs of pregnant and lactating mothers reinforces workplace norms that work against the need for maternity leave, child care, flex time, and breastfeeding support. By negating the body we do not empower mothers; we simply transform the distribution of gender inequities, thereby resulting in greater equity for women who can function as men do and less equity for those who cannot, which may explain some of the race, class, and educational differences we see in breastfeeding rates.

The second principle of inequality, the "gendered logic of power concentration," results in hierarchies of authority by gender within institutions and across roles. Connell argues that we can envision a core within the power structure that is tightly guarded by men and a periphery where gendered power is more contested or diffuse. The periphery is where women generally have more power; it typically includes those arenas that involve carework or those areas that have few opportunities for financial resource accumulation, such as the family and kinship roles, and, to a certain extent, volunteer community work. This sexual division of labor allows men and women to accumulate sex-specific bodies of knowledge that, in turn, enhance and reinforce sex-specific arenas of power.

Accordingly, power over infants should reside with mothers. However, many have observed that various social institutions of power, including medicine, tend to meddle in infant feeding. Indeed, the history of infant feeding and breastfeeding is littered with examples of how largely male-dominated social institutions have sought to devalue women's common knowledge of breastfeeding in favor of new scientific knowledge held by experts. These institutions redirect power over infant feeding away from mothers and women's kinship networks toward social institutions and direct attention toward human milk as product and away from breastfeeding as process.[14]

Social efforts to control infant feeding can be seen as a systematic use of the sexual division of power to increase men's power in infant feeding markets, authority, and decisions. These efforts systematically undermine what is the main benefit to women of the sexual division of labor—namely, the accumulation of a female-owned body of common knowledge—and contribute to women's alienation from their lactating bodies and poor breastfeeding practice. Such efforts also reinforce gender inequality by reducing the power that women enjoy in their traditional parental and kinship roles. These efforts ultimately pit the needs and security of mothers against those of their children, induce women to breastfeed out of a sense of maternal obligation with no concomitant provision of social supports, and deny employed or vulnerable mothers the opportunity to breastfeed.

Social Status and the Sexual Division of Social Relationships

Oppong recognizes social status, or prestige, as the degree to which a person is an object of admiration, an object of deference, an object of imitation, a source of suggestion, and a center of attraction. To assess status, Oppong recommends looking at the types of relationships women have, including their emotional ties and social support. The gendered social structure that affects social status is what Connell calls *cathexis,* or the norms governing sexuality and emotion in social relationships. In this he includes the myriad relationships we develop across our roles. From this perspective, sexuality and emotion in social relationships, like power and labor, are socially constructed, not biologically based. Emotional attachment may be hostile as well as affectionate or ambivalent.

Cathexis is supported by social and cultural norms and laws that prohibit certain types of relationships while romanticizing and inciting others.

Connell observes that we become most aware of cathexis when we bump up against social taboos; for example, if we engage in actions that violate laws or conventions about incest, rape, prostitution, bigamy, age of consent, and homosexuality. These prohibitions, which vary across cultures and religions, include customs and conventions regarding the proper relationships.

One of the principles of inequality that helps organize cathexis is "the gendered logic of coupling." This principle refers to the fact that coupling is based on a role reciprocity formed by the sexual divisions of labor and power. The dowry that men and women bring to their partnership is that which is promised by their future roles and position (that is, she will be a good mother; he will be a good provider); hence, what men and women bring is structurally unequal in terms of wealth, power, and prestige.

However, in the United States it is marriage, or heterosexual coupling, that protects women against the "feminization of poverty" that comes from a sexual division of labor that assigns to women those roles that pay less and from which accrue relatively lower levels of wealth and power. Marriage allows some women the opportunity to remain out of the paid labor force to breast-feed or raise children and to participate in the paid labor force that remains structured around the ideal worker and continues to underpay them—all without being plunged into poverty. However, single motherhood, divorce, and widowhood, as well as male disability and unemployment, all complicate the package and increase the poverty of women and children and the complications women experience in combining paid work with motherhood.

We may also bump up against cathexis when we experience emotions—particularly of the sexual, erotic, or sensual nature—that fall outside of heterosexual adult coupling or outside of what is allowed in maternal-child or peer relationships. The constructions of emotional attachments are governed by the second principle of inequality, which I call *primacy of masculinity*. Connell writes that "objects of desire are generally defined by the dichotomy and opposition of masculine and feminine. . . . The process of sexualizing women as objects of heterosexual desire involves a standardizing of feminine appeal."[15] The sexualization of women's bodies and their breasts has been implicated as a factor contributing to concerns women have about breastfeeding outside the home.[16]

Since both the gendered logic of coupling and the primacy of masculinity establish the parental couple as the location for erotic or sexual expression and fashion women's bodies for male pleasure, it seems reasonable to theorize that the experience of eroticism or other supposedly nonmaternal emotions in the mother-child relationship fall into the prohibited category. Hence, norms that limit women's sexual feelings and expression in this way could have direct effects on how women's male partners, or others, feel about women using their breasts for the benefit of children or enjoying breastfeeding as a sensual experience. These ideas may also be why most breastfeeding promotion emphasizes the product (milk), not the means (breasts), framing breastfeeding as work of the *good mother*, the "best food," and the "natural way" while ignoring the playful, sensual or erotic, or pleasurable aspects of breastfeeding.[17]

Cathexis places myriad constraints on how women and men experience and express their sexuality and emotions across a variety of important relationships. These constraints create contradictory norms and expectations that affect breastfeeding. Because of the sexualization of women's bodies and breasts, women who breastfeed at work bring their sexuality into the workplace. They may be legitimately concerned about how breastfeeding or pumping may affect their relationships with their colleagues or superiors, or how breastfeeding might affect the admiration and respect others have for them (that is, social status at work). They may also be concerned about, or actually experience, sexual harassment. In other situations, women have reported that male partners believe that their breasts belong to them (that is, the men) and are not for the baby.[18]

Implications for Public Health Approaches to Breastfeeding Promotion and Support

This chapter proposes that public health efforts to protect, promote, and support breastfeeding need to ask two critical questions: to what extent, and how, do our efforts to promote breastfeeding reinforce, reproduce, or reduce gender inequality; and to what extent will efforts to reduce gender inequality improve breastfeeding outcomes? The theoretical perspective outlined here illuminates how women's decisions about the ways they allocate their body, time, resources, and energy arise from the complex intersection of social forces that construct their experiences across their multiple roles, and the way these experiences converge to form their economic, political, and social status. Women's challenges to gender inequality have too often negated the female body, which has probably made it easier for women to break into the labor force, but has also made it more difficult for women, especially those with pregnant and lactating bodies, or those who mother, to succeed there. One reason why we have the demographic pattern of breastfeeding that we see today is that women who are able to function effectively within the existing structures do better, and women who have more control over their body, time, and space are able to breastfeed longer with better quality than women who have less control.

We also see that the breast pump has become a normalized part of women's breastfeeding practice in the United States: our social solutions have emphasized the value of human milk as a product over the breastfeeding process, as well as the value of the dyadic relationship, and offered lactation rooms rather than maternity leave and child care at work.[19]

We must challenge the systems that sustain forces that undergird the sexual divisions of labor, power, and social relationships. Rather than negate the needs of women's bodies and maternal needs, we must find strategies that challenge the ideology of masculinity without defining women's essence by their bodily abilities. We need to find ways that reclaim women's historical power in the infant care arena without abandoning their power in public spaces. We need strategies that equate power with femininity alongside masculinity. We need to envision an economy that allows caregivers to accumulate wealth without limiting women's opportunities for wealth in the public world of work and which allows single or singled women and mothers to remain economically self-sufficient. We need to find ways to counter the dehumanizing sexual objectification of women without reducing women and mothers to asexual beings whose breasts are just human feeding tubes. We need programs, policies, and other strategies that empower women in their multiple roles. We need to promote role expectations that are realistic in today's world and provide social, community, and workplace supports that reduce the role strain and conflict that working mothers experience while enhancing women's role agency and actualization.

Notes

1. Greiner, "Ideas for Action," 64–65. See also WHO/UNICEF, "Innocenti Declaration"; ILCA et al., "Women's Human Rights"; Amin, "Brief History."
2. R. W. Connell, *Gender and Power*; Oppong, "Synopsis of Seven Roles."
3. Oppong, "Synopsis of Seven Roles," 5.
4. Oppong and Abu, *Handbook for Data Collection*, 5.
5. Bianchi, Casper, and King, "Complex Connections."
6. Turner, "Significance of Employment"; Jabs and Devine, "Time Scarcity"; Glynn et al., "Association between Role Overload"; Lewis and Ridge, "Mothers Reframing Physical Activity."
7. Connell, *Gender and Power*, 102.
8. Ibid., 105–106.
9. Williams, *Unbending Gender*, 1.
10. Fletcher, "Gender Perspectives."
11. Williams, *Unbending Gender*.
12. Connell, *Gender and Power*, 107.
13. Other ideologies that can frame our construction of force are racism and capitalism.
14. Whitaker, *Measuring Mamma's Milk*. See also Wolf, this volume.

15. Connell, *Gender and Power*, 113. See also the American Psychological Association, *Report of the APA Task Force on the Sexualization of Girls.*
16. See Hurst, this volume.
17. See Giles, this volume; Dorfman and Gehlert, *Talking about Breastfeeding.*
18. Smith et al., "Choosing Feeding."
19. Labiner-Wolfe et al., "Prevalence of Breast Milk Expression."

Breastfeeding in Public Health

What Is Needed for Policy and Program Action?

Breastfeeding, especially exclusive breastfeeding, has been shown to be the most important infant and child survival intervention in terms of its potential impact on mortality. Increased exclusive breastfeeding could prevent about 13 percent of all preventable child deaths worldwide, including at least nine hundred infant deaths annually in the United States, and reduce the rate of many infectious and chronic diseases in both industrialized and developing country settings.[1] However, active support for breastfeeding is rarely a central component in public health programming.

Concerns about alternative feeding filled the health literature in the nineteenth century, and the response was to try to improve human milk substitutes.[2] The concept that increasing breastfeeding might be the best response, rather than fine-tuning the substitutes, has been considered worthy of public health research support only recently. This new support for breastfeeding may have resulted from the increase in mainstream medical recognition of the negative health possibilities with commercial formula use, consumer interest in breastfeeding in the 1970s and thereafter, the global women's and children's rights agenda in the 1980s and 1990s, in concert with the recognition and evolution of "child survival" as a major global health and development measure. However, no one sector has stepped to the fore; contributions from multiple sectors have been necessary to create this interest. Concurrently, another sector—the evolving commercial market and the marketing of supplements and complementary foods—is expanding and offers a reliable ongoing source of resources to use *against* the perceived competition of increasing support for breastfeeding.

The global public health sector, represented by the World Health Organization (WHO) and the United Nations Children's Fund (UNICEF), records its support for breastfeeding as a vitally important practice for health and survival.[3] In addition, the European Union, the U.S. Department of Health and Human Services (DHHS), and virtually all health professional organizations now agree that the data support the need for improved breastfeeding for public health. Nonetheless, given ongoing discourses in the media, encouraged by the commercial sector, it would seem that the importance of breastfeeding for maternal, child, and intergenerational health remains controversial. Media headlines, at least one corporate blog, and recent feminist popular and academic literature bombard us with the argument that there is no defensible science supporting the health impacts of breastfeeding—arguments often rendered by persons with little breastfeeding research expertise—and that the practice of breastfeeding is a barrier to women's rights.[4] Other media emphasize that breastfeeding is simply a replacement for formula, one that places a heavy burden on the mother. In fact, global rights documents support breastfeeding as both a woman's and child's right. The challenge to the evidence published over the last few decades is a result of the fact that we cannot ethically randomize women to feed exactly as we dictate. The randomized controlled trial, the "gold standard" of evidence-based medical research, is not possible with this population. The study of breastfeeding demands large groups, or cohorts, and careful control for factors such as social class or education that might influence both the decision to breastfeed, success in breastfeeding, and the health outcomes of both mothers and infants.

Despite increasing medical evidence, programming to support or promote breastfeeding is poorly funded compared to the other global child health programs, such as HIV/AIDS, clean water, vitamin A, and immunization. Further, where intervention programs exist, they often include only breastfeeding promotion—that is, mention of its importance—but do not provide active or skilled support or protection for breastfeeding in light of the onslaught of polished commercial messages for formula. Such promotion-only programs can, indeed, place the entire burden on the mother, without offering any social or clinical support.

For women to consider breastfeeding positively, to decide to exclusively breastfeed, and to succeed in optimal breastfeeding, appropriate social, educational, health care, and economic support must be readily and freely available and accessible, and the messages must be clear and complementary.

This chapter explores how we might create momentum and increase support for breastfeeding policy and programming in public health. While breastfeeding could be supported by a variety of sectors and disciplines, it is becoming increasingly clear that change has been catalyzed only when there is interdisciplinary and cross-sectoral support, partnerships across the social-ecological spectrum, and active collaboration in concert with recognition of the perspective of and impact on the mother, who is, with her child, the central figure in breastfeeding decisions and action.

What Is Breastfeeding?

Breastfeeding is the act of direct milk transfer from the mother's breast to baby through a mutual dyadic physiological process. Breastfeeding, often assumed to be a "natural" and therefore easy and instinctual practice, becomes a complex practice in modern society, where outside pressures work against the mother and child to act as a biological and behavioral dyad. Breastfeeding is an interactive physiological process and feedback system that includes neuro-endocrine, mammary, placental, and ovarian activity. Prolactin, the hormone that supports milk production, is present before birth but suppressed. After birth, the baby, placed on the mom, skin to skin, will massage the breast with face and hands, provoking oxytocin release, which in turn causes the muscles around the alveolus (the groupings of cells that secrete milk) and the milk ducts to tighten, forcing milk out toward the nipples and beyond. As the baby suckles, emptying the breast, prolactin increases, and more milk is produced. In sum, the more the infant massages and empties the breast, the more milk is produced. If milk builds up in the breast, it can create negative feedback and cause the breast to slow its milk production, so frequent feeding is a must. This physiology also contributes to a reliable birth spacing method: the Lactational Amenorrhea Method. If a mother is amenorrheic, is fully or nearly fully breastfeeding, and the baby is less than six months old, her risk of pregnancy is between 1 and 2 percent, similar to the risk with oral contraceptive use.[5]

Breastfeeding also delivers baby's food in a manner that allows the infant to act on satiety. The initial milk is more like a sweet and salty broth, and the final, or hind, milk is rich with fats, much like a meal is planned worldwide: from a soup (to satisfy immediate thirst and electrolyte needs) to dessert (to ensure satiety). Parental support of the infant's satiety, demonstrated in her stopping suckling when full, may help prevent obesity later in life. All in all, the process of breastfeeding and the milk itself, together, create the many health benefits of this practice.

The outcome of successful breastfeeding is improved survival, health, and well-being for both mother and child. Formula use, or lack of optimal breastfeeding, is associated with short- and long-term health risks for mother and child.[6] Carefully controlled observational research has shown that formula use, or less than optimal breastfeeding, is associated with an increase in the risks for the child to experience nonspecific gastroenteritis (that is, diarrhea and vomiting); asthma where there is no family history; obesity and overweight; type 1 diabetes; type 2 diabetes; childhood leukemia; nearly twice the risk of sudden infant death syndrome (SIDS); severe lower respiratory tract infections, with about 60 percent more hospitalizations; about twice the incidence of otitis media (inner ear infections); atopic dermatitis; hypertension (high blood pressure); high cholesterol; lower intelligence and scholastic performance; and, among prematures, significantly more NEC (necrotizing enterocolitis), a deadly but all too common infliction in this group of infants.[7] Mothers who do not breastfeed have an increased chance of experiencing type 1 diabetes; type 2 diabetes; breast cancer; ovarian cancer; hypertension; slower uterine involution; increased blood loss; increased maternal stress; decreased efficiency in nutrient metabolism, with modified calcium metabolism; and earlier fertility return.[8]

Breastfeeding has social implications and is, in turn, impacted by social contexts. Societal norms inform health thinking, and, since the middle of the twentieth century, artificial feeding has been the social and medical norm in the United States and much of the global north. The practice of formula-feeding was bolstered by a call for women in the workplace during World War II, a women's movement largely centered on worksite equity and reproductive freedom, and an onslaught of advertising by formula companies reassuring them by emphasizing that formula-feeding is safe, clean, neat, easy, and a modern "mother's helper." Hence, women came to understand breastfeeding as unsafe, dirty, messy, difficult, antiquated, and antiwoman. While lactation is a biological response to childbirth, ongoing breastfeeding success in the global north is often dependent on medical support for mother/baby togetherness as well as family and community knowledge of breastfeeding skills. Often the skills to support the biology are lost, and adequate common community knowledge for breastfeeding support and problem solving can be forgotten within one to three generations.

In sum, breastfeeding may be seen as a public health priority through its impact on nutrition, reproductive health, women's issues, or economic development. Given the complex social and physiological issues involved, public health support for breastfeeding must look well beyond direct health care and offer a comprehensive approach to enable and re-create sustainable behavior change in social, cultural, and health system contexts.

What Is Public Health?

While the goal of public health is to improve lives through the prevention and treatment of disease, one of the major issues we face in exploring

"breastfeeding" and "public health" is that both terms have multiple definitions, are used differently by multiple sectors of interest, and must be applied
in multiple cultural settings where women play a wide variety of roles.

Developing a common understanding of each term is a challenge. It may
be a surprise that even the term "health" is not consistently defined; while the
World Health Organization defines health as "a state of complete physical,
mental and social well-being and not merely the absence of disease or
infirmity," there are other definitions and many constructs that contextualize
what "health" is and define its determinants.[9]

So, what is "public health"? Nearly a century ago, public health was
defined as the science and art of preventing disease, prolonging life, and
promoting health through organized effort for sanitation, control of com-
municable disease, organization of health services for prevention and early
diagnosis, education for personal health, and the development of the "social
machinery" to assure a standard of living adequate for health.[10] The dictionary
definition states that public health is the general health of a community and the
practice and study of ways to preserve and improve it. Public health includes
health education, sanitation, control of diseases, and regulation of pollution.
Today, the Association of Schools of Public Health defines it as the science
and art of protecting and improving the health of communities through
education, promotion of healthy lifestyles, and research for disease and injury
prevention. It is concerned with threats to the overall health of a community
based on population health analyses. The population in question can be as
small as a handful of people or as large as all the inhabitants of several
continents.

There are two distinct characteristics of public health: it generally deals
with preventive rather than curative aspects of health and with population-
level rather than individual-level health issues. Preventive measures may be
further considered primary prevention, which is the reduction or control of
causative factors for a health problem and includes reducing risk and environmental exposures; secondary prevention, which includes early detection and
treatment of the problem, or lessening the impact; and tertiary prevention,
which includes appropriate supportive and rehabilitative services to minimize
morbidity and maximize quality of life.[11]

Where Does Breastfeeding Fit in Basic Public Health
Rhetoric, Policy, and Program Frameworks?

Because researchers have identified breastfeeding as having the potential to
significantly reduce neonatal, infant, and child mortality, to contribute to child

health and development, and to reduce maternal illness (both postpartum and lifelong), it fits within public health as a primary preventive practice with significant individual, community, and population level outcomes. However, it is important that we also note that breastfeeding is not directly addressed in any of these definitions, and that in addressing preventive, population-level, and health service infrastructure, we are removed from the intimate support of the mother/baby dyad. Further, none of these definitions specifically note the importance of nutrition, reproductive health, women's issues, or economic development as central areas in public health thinking. The result is that breastfeeding has no clearly defined home in any one public health or preventive construct, but rather is a subset of many. What are the risks and benefits of having many homes?

In traditional settings, breastfeeding is viewed as a nutrition issue, a reproductive health issue, a women's work issue, and an economic issue. Translation into public health constructs necessitates examination of the home and role of nutrition, reproductive health, women's roles, women's economic contribution, and the role breastfeeding plays in each.

Breastfeeding and Nutrition

By definition nutrition is the provision of the materials necessary (in the form of food) to support life. Other definitions add that it should support proper function as well. Therefore, the nutrition community has a primary interest in food and its nutrient composition and the quantities of nutrients consumed. In this field, support for breastfeeding can be problematic, as it is difficult to quantify and its consumption is only for a short duration in the lifespan; therefore, it is not generally a primary focus of the nutrition sector.

Breastfeeding and Reproductive Health

In nature, reproduction is the production of a viable next generation. Reproductive health, or sexual health and hygiene, addresses the reproductive processes, functions, and system at all stages of life. Implicit in this area is often the right of access to appropriate health care that will enable women to proceed safely through pregnancy and childbirth, and provide couples with the best chance of having a healthy infant.

Breastfeeding contributes both to timing of pregnancies and the health of the infant, but in this field, support for breastfeeding can be problematic in that the primary interests are generally the timing of conception, the decisions surrounding the pregnancy, and the birth of a healthy infant, rather than the ability of that infant to reach the age of reproduction.

Breastfeeding and Women's Issues

The U.S. Office of Global Women's Issues works for the political, economic, and social empowerment of women, for the most part supporting the global definitions offered by the Convention on the Elimination of All Forms of Discrimination Against Women (CEDAW). Support for breastfeeding can be problematic when the economic and empowering roles of women are defined only in terms of their role in formal employment. When elimination of discrimination means it is the right of women to be empowered to be equal to men, concerns that are biologically unique to females are often not addressed.

Breastfeeding and Economic Growth and Development

Economic growth is based on monetary issues, while economic development often is broadened to include issues such as quality of life, health, and well-being. Economic development depends on an effective and educated workforce, so in this field breastfeeding may be viewed as problematic, as it might keep a woman out of formal education (depending on when she has her children) and also out of the formal employment sector. If, however, breastfeeding is accounted for as a contribution to the gross national product, it may be possible to increase interest in breastfeeding in this sector.

In sum, breastfeeding may be viewed as incidental to many sectors, but a priority of none. Nonetheless, there are global and local breastfeeding policies. In the United States, the Healthy People 2010 goals for breastfeeding have been updated in the 2020 goals. The earlier goal of 75 percent of mothers breastfeeding in the early postpartum was achieved, and the new goal, based on projections, is 81.9 percent. The other 2010 goals for exclusivity and continuation of breastfeeding, which in the long run would have a major impact on health, were not reached. The previous goals were to have 50 percent of mothers still breastfeeding at six months (increased to 60.6 percent in the 2020 goals), and 25 percent at one year (increased to 34.1 percent), as well as 40 percent (increased to 46.2 percent) and 17 percent (increased to 25.5 percent) exclusively breastfeeding at three and six months respectively.[12] In order to achieve these targets, action is needed. While there are many public health constructs in various sectors, the goal must be to find approaches that support breastfeeding in a comprehensive manner so that nutrition, reproductive health, women's concerns, and economic realities are all addressed.

Public health planning demands that we fit breastfeeding into accepted constructs. Let us start by excluding the disease-based constructs that try to eliminate poor health, one disease at a time. In general, the public health response in this model is disease-specific, such as immunization campaigns or vaccine development, but may also include generally accepted behavioral change interventions, such as hand washing or, on occasion, breastfeeding. Unfortunately, this construct leaves little room for interventions that prevent or impact on more than one disease.

There are other models that are solid but abstract, such as the Assess, Act, and Adapt Model that calls for practitioners to assess, act, and adapt, then start again, with assessment, and so on, in a cyclic approach. While this model defines an excellent process for any programmatic enterprise, and therefore should be applied generally, it does not call for action on specific issues.

Systems and infrastructural models call for a balance and order in program and policy design and implementation. One such model may support breast-feeding: the Maternal and Child Health Pyramid and related constructs.[13] The pyramid of care emphasizes the need in public health thinking for a great deal of attention to evaluation, planning, and building of infrastructure, rather than individual care, prioritizing population-based interventions, such as screening and health information dissemination.

A corollary to this approach considers the development of program systems as the primary act: the belief is that "if you build it—they will come." These constructs assume that a well-developed, well-maintained health care infrastructure will lead to improved health outcomes. Alternatively, models have been developed that provide lists of essential components. One such model is the Ten Essential Public Health Services, which includes steps that identify the problem, diagnose the source, and develop interventions, evaluations, and further research. The approach of listing essential services targeting the population, like the Pyramid, emphasizes program and infrastructure rather than the individual.

There are additional models that are more cross-cutting, addressing either time or social differences that impact a health issue. For this reason, they may be more applicable to breastfeeding intervention, where it is necessary to create change in the entire social and health fabric of women's lives. For example, the Lifecycle Reproductive Health Model provides the public health decision maker with a set of intergenerational entry points for planning preventive interventions that need not be temporally related to the potential outcome. An intervention to impact infant nutrition should, therefore, be initiated as early as possible during the life of the mother—or the life of her mother before her! The timing of the intervention may have no obvious connection to the problem or disease.

Social and behavioral based constructs that are most commonly used to support breastfeeding include the Determinants of Health Models and the derivative Nutrition Model, as well as the Social-Ecological framework, which provides a planning landscape for these constructs.[14] These models are based on the recognition of causally interacting systems. While they illustrate the many systems that impact health, their contribution to program planning is more at the theoretical level. The Nutrition Model was designed and used by UNICEF in program development for more than two decades. It remains an excellent framework for consideration of the factors that influence nutritional outcomes. While it clearly includes the levels that must be considered in support of breastfeeding, it would be necessary to modify it to meet the intensive behavioral change expected of women in order to achieve exclusive breast-feeding. The Social-Ecological Model (SEM) provides the planning landscape for complex behavioral change that is called for in the social and behavioral based constructs. Currently, SEM may be the most frequently cited base of thinking for public health planning, and it supports the complex array of changes needed to support breastfeeding.

The CDC and WHO promote a five-level version of the SEM to guide research and practice related to effective programs and policies. This model considers the complex interplay between individual, relationship, community, and societal factors.

Individual: The first level identifies biological and personal history factors that increase the likelihood of breastfeeding or impact breastfeeding behavior. Some of these factors are age, education, income, family structure, beliefs, values, opportunities, resources, and stressors.

Interpersonal: Relationship, or interpersonal, includes those factors that increase the risk of not breastfeeding or the likelihood of breastfeeding due to relationships with intimate partners, family members, friends and peers, or children, and interactions with health care providers and community members.

Community: The third level explores the settings, such as schools, workplaces, health care settings, and neighborhoods, in which social relationships occur, and seeks to identify the characteristics of these settings that are associated with breastfeeding.

Societal: The fourth level looks at the broad societal factors that help create a climate that encourages breastfeeding or inhibits it. These factors include social and cultural norms, as well as the health, economic, educational, and social policies that help to maintain economic, social, gender, or racial inequalities between groups in society.

Civil Society/Government: These terms are more often used in international parlance, where the responsibility for ensuring the rights and health of the individual rest more clearly with national leadership, whether reflective of the civil society or otherwise in place. In the rights framework, this level is the ultimate duty-bearer.

An Alternative Construct for Reproductive Health and Breastfeeding

The SEM and the Lifecycle Model—addressing social, economic, and political strata and entry points in time—comprise two dimensions of public health. These models encourage us to consider the full environment, or space, of each individual and to consider the entry points, or times, when one might intervene. I would like to raise a very important third construct—how we intervene.

Public health thinking certainly attends to place (where we act) and time (when we act). We must add the third dimension—how we act. And how we act for the health of the public includes maintenance of both preventive and medical modalities. What do we consider at the time and place of intervention? Do we consider both the long- and short-term impact? Do we consider the mother's interests and desires? Do we consider the consequences for both mother and baby, and how do we balance that decision? In considering breastfeeding in this new three-dimensional construct (that is, where, when, and how we intervene) we must consider the role and evolution of medical support for reproduction. Pregnancy, birth, and breastfeeding are all female-specific experiences, and the fact that our species survived for millennia without medical intervention in these three uniquely female considerations speaks to the robustness of life. Part of the definition of life is the ability to reproduce. However, as humans, we consistently strive to improve our lives through technologies, and we increasingly rely on technologies for work and play. Reproductive health is not exempt from technological advances either. Obstetrical technologies have helped save the lives of many women and infants who would have died or been severely compromised without such interventions. However, overuse of technologies, when respect for normal biology and psychology are lost, can be dangerous. The physiological and interactive hormonal feedback cascade that occurs within the mother/baby dyad during the mother's transition from pregnancy to motherhood is a delicate balance. Intervention during this period can be life-saving for both mother and baby, but it also can upset this cascade, leading to additional problems and even death. Increasing technological interventions may provide momentary solutions to specific perceived crises, but the field of public health takes a longer-term view.

The normal physiological cascade with ongoing interaction and feedback between the mother/baby dyad during labor and delivery and the immediate postpartum period changes the fetus into an infant. It is this cascade—including hormones, instinctual behaviors, and seemingly automatic responses—that facilitates breastfeeding. However, medical sciences have artificially separated this dyad in the name of improved medical technologies and so-called hygienic practices. This separation, increased by the growth of both the separate surgical specialty of obstetrics for mothers and the pediatric nutrition specialty for infants, has created significant problems in initiating and managing breastfeeding in the immediate postnatal period.

In terms of birth itself, we have progressed to the stage that modern medicine intervenes in nearly all births. Intervention, *per force*, disrupts the physiological cascade, often leading to another cascade—the cascade of obstetric interventions that leads to Cesarean births:

1. Medical care providers wish to avoid crises, and perhaps the concomitant lawsuits, and therefore place a monitor on every woman and keep an intravenous line open for medications, in case of an emergency.
2. Intravenous lines and continuous electronic monitoring of the fetus lead to limitation of mobility and activity for the mother and concomitant discomfort. In addition, minor changes and false positive monitor readings lead to anxiety, disrupting the hormonal cascade and slowing labor.
3. Attempts to speed labor, such as artificial rupture of the membranes and use of artificial hormones (pitocin), lead to substantially increased pain for the mother.
4. Pain medications and anesthesia can lead to abnormal fetal heart patterns and may also slow labor further, initiating an intervention to address detected fetal distress or stalled labor.
5. Vacuum extraction or forceps use or, increasingly, Cesarean section, is the result of this medico-technological cascade, changing the mother-baby postpartum recovery into maternal surgical recovery and isolating the baby in a foreign, nonmaternal environment.

As a result, the other outcome of the disruption of the normal cascade of events is often great difficulty in establishing breastfeeding, both due to the disruption of the intimate hormonal interactions, as well as the pain of surgery and the creation of a sleepy, anesthetized infant.

What is the answer to this conundrum? The Coalition for Improving Maternity Services (CIMS) and the International MotherBaby Childbirth Organization (IMBCO) propose less invasive supportive care during labor and delivery.[15] They argue that less invasive care would both reduce growing Cesarean rates and provide support for the hormonal cascade that culminates in breastfeeding—the fourth stage of labor—and normal, rapid maternal recovery. They propose special sets of ten steps to address both obstetric practices and breastfeeding, known as the Ten Steps of the Mother-Friendly Childbirth Initiative in the United States, and internationally as the Ten Steps to Optimal MotherBaby Maternity Services. Such a change would marry clinical and preventive medicine, taking into account not only the time and place of events, but also how that time and place fits into the rest of the life of the individual.

Currently, obstetric technologies are utilized to avert crises as though they had no long-lasting effects on mothers and babies. This "just in case" thinking can lead to a cascade of problems that lie at the root of difficult initiation of breastfeeding in the United States and elsewhere, leading to maternal frustration and negative feelings about breastfeeding. The three-dimensional model forces us to consider how actions that are medically sound for the rare case might damage future relationships or practices for the vast majority. From the public health perspective, the best outcomes for the majority should be the central consideration. The three-dimensional model focuses on when we act (when in the intergenerational life cycle do we intervene or not?), where we act (where in the Social-Ecological framework do we intervene or not?), and how we act (how do we best support the mother/child dyad as we intervene or not?) and recognizes that both the mother and the child must be considered in reproductive health, including breastfeeding support. But we still must consider what is necessary to create the momentum for any action at all.

What Has Catalyzed Action on Breastfeeding Policy and Programs Support in the Public Health Arena?

Given that none of the existing public health interest areas or constructs specifically support breastfeeding, it is amazing that breastfeeding is supported at all within global public health policy and programming. The fact that there is support is a testimony to hard work by dedicated individuals in each of these sectors, as well as a bit of serendipity. In the 1980s a small group of midlevel social science and health professionals reached across sectors to hold a series of meetings to address breastfeeding definitions, as well as its role in health services, the workplace, women's issues, nutrition, and other sectors. While the hope of this group was to have some impact on global policy, it happened that at the exact time that this effort was going forward, a parallel and highly supported effort based on the new Convention on the Rights of the Child pressed UNICEF to display a new action in this regard. UNICEF then offered its Innocenti Research Centre in Florence as a home for a high-level ministerial meeting to support breastfeeding as both a mother's and a child's right. Seen in this new context—as a right—policy for action on breastfeeding emerged in the 1990 Innocenti Declaration. This declaration constituted the first global recognition of need for action on this issue and spelled out four pillars for action to achieve protection, promotion, and support for breastfeeding. (In the context of international guidelines and policies, *protection* refers to freedom from false and misleading advertising to health care workers or to the public; *promotion* refers to the need for social marketing and health counseling; and *support* refers to direct clinical and social support.) In order to protect, promote, and support breastfeeding, the four Innocenti operational targets are civil commitment and policy, health system quality and health worker training, protection against false and misleading advertising through implementation of the International Code of Marketing of Breast-milk Substitutes, and maternity protection including paid maternity leave and breaks, worksite child care, and improved maternity practices. All of these are to be sustained by a building base of consumer demand.

Today these four operational targets remain to support the right of every child to the best start in life and the right of every parent to be knowledgeable and successful with breastfeeding. With the publication of the Global Strategy for Infant and Young Child Feeding and the Innocenti Declaration + 15, breastfeeding supportive policy is on the books in the global arena. The current global health and development policy that should be supporting breastfeeding is the Millennium Development Project and its goals for improving maternal and child health, which include gender equity and reproductive justice as underlying needs.

In the United States, the 2011 Surgeon General's *Call to Action to Support Breastfeeding* similarly evolved from a group of technical staff in various agencies representing women's issues and reproductive health and nutrition, as well as preventive health, and across government and private agencies and organizations, inspired at least in part by the Innocenti Declaration. These individuals took the 2000 *Breastfeeding: HHS Blueprint for Action* to a new level and revitalized action on breastfeeding through a coordinated interagency and cross-sectoral set of sessions, including public in-person and electronic forums and expert advisories. The surgeon general reviewed every recommendation and fully endorsed the effort.

Conclusion: What Is Needed to Create Viable and Effective Breastfeeding Programs in the Public Health Arena?

To overcome malaise and to create action on breastfeeding, various individuals and groups—across sectors, disciplines, and professions—must identify the means to work together for sustainable change; we need to go beyond time and place to intervene, and we must also consider how we intervene. Breastfeeding has an important, but generally minimally supported, role in many public health interest areas: nutrition, reproductive health, women's issues, economic development, and human rights. However, breastfeeding tends to sit squarely at the bottom of the priority programming listings in each sector, if it is there at all. This lack of a strong home within current public health constructs is compounded by two other deficits: the lack of a strong donor base and the lack of a well-funded private sector partner.

To achieve action in support of breastfeeding, we must be clever. The synergy created when individuals reach across sectors and work for mutual support can provoke innovative and creative programming. Examples of policy and program actions in support of breastfeeding that have been achieved through coalitions of support include the following:

1. National and governmental multi-sectoral commitment, which has come into effect through coalitions that include women's and children's rights and health as arguments for change.
2. Health training and services improvement necessitating cooperation and partnership among state health departments, health professional associations, accrediting organizations, and academic faculties.
3. Provision of evidence-based, unbiased information at the family and community level, a level that has natural allies in organizations that support birth spacing and safe motherhood, especially when complementary messaging is involved.
4. Legislation and policy for maternity protection and paid leave, health insurance coverage, freedom to breastfeed as children need, and protection against aggressive advertising of infant formula.[16]

Creating the demand among families and consumers for adequate support for breastfeeding across sectors may be the sole key to creating programs and other forms of support, especially when an issue is a priority for none. This book explores current thinking on breastfeeding from many viewpoints. Perhaps those who read these chapters will find new ways to find mutuality of purpose and synergy in programming so that women everywhere will find the support they need to succeed in a biologically sound practice within the social, economic, and political pressures of their lives.

Notes

1. Jones et al., "How Many Child Deaths"; Black, Morris, and Bryce, "Where and Why"; Martines et al., "Neonatal Survival"; Black et al., "Maternal and Child Under-nutrition"; Bartick and Reinhold, "The Burden"; Ip et al., *Breastfeeding and Maternal and Infant Health Outcomes*; Horta et al., "Evidence on the Long-term Effects."
2. As described in Wolf, this volume.
3. Jones et al., "How Many Child Deaths"; WHO/UNICEF, "Global Strategy."
4. Gottlieb, "When Population-Wide Politics." See also Wolf, this volume.
5. Labbok et al., "Lactational Amenorrhea Method."
6. See the systematic reviews of Ip et al., *Breastfeeding and Maternal Infant Health Outcomes*; McNiel, Labbok, and Abrahams, "What Are the Risks."
7. Horta et al., "Evidence on the Long-Term Effects."
8. Jonas et al., "Short- and Long-Term Decrease"; Negishi et al., "Changes in Uterine Size"; Irons et al., "Simple Alternative"; Bullough, Msuku, and Karonde, "Early Suckling"; Mezzacappa, Kelsey, and Katkin, "Breast Feeding"; Ward, Adams, and Mughal, "Bone Status"; Chantry et al., "Lactation among Adolescent Mothers."
9. World Health Organization, "Definition of Health."
10. Winslow, "Untilled Fields."
11. U.S. Department of Health and Human Services, "A Framework for Assessing the Effectiveness."
12. U.S. Department of Health and Human Services, *Healthy People 2010* and *Healthy People 2020 Summary of Objectives.*
13. "Maternal and Child Health Pyramid of Health Services."
14. U.S. Department of Health and Human Services, "A Systematic Approach to Health."
15. The International MotherBaby Childbirth Initiative, "Ten Steps to Optimal MotherBaby Maternity Services"; Coalition for Improving Maternity Services, "Ten Steps of the Mother-Friendly Childbirth Initiative."
16. Labbok, "Transdisciplinary Breastfeeding Support."

Part II

Studying Breastfeeding across Race, Class, and Culture

Breastfeeding across Cultures

Dealing with Difference

Feminism refers to theories and actions that reduce (and ultimately eliminate) inequality and discrimination on the basis of gender, race, class, and ethnicity. As with all "isms," feminisms have histories. In South Asia, local feminism emerged out of nationalist fights against colonial imperialism. Western feminisms began not with a demand for national independence, but with a concern for discrimination against women. More recently, Western feminists have acknowledged that gender cannot be separated from other dimensions like race, ethnicity, class, or sexual orientation, for example. Queer theory forced feminist theory to grapple with the relation between sex and gender to add a more nuanced measure of how sexual orientation intersects with other differences, including differing abilities. Feminism emerges not just from feminist theory but also from feminist practice, from social movements that struggle with what is politically necessary to change local systems of gender inequality, often in concert with other social movements. This chapter is a feminist and anthropological argument about how a serious, methodologically rich examination of difference could enrich understanding of breastfeeding and motivate innovative approaches to its support and promotion.

Feminism, Social Science, and Breastfeeding

Newer approaches in feminist social science draw attention to both oppression and empowerment (and the connections between them), by emphasizing women's agency, as well as the complexity of gender dynamics, and the importance of revaluing women's knowledge. The male bias of many ethnographers and cultural systems often pushes this women's knowledge underground, devaluing it, and in many parts of the world, women's knowledge of nurture has been replaced with biomedical expert knowledge of infant care and feeding established through evidence-based medical research.

The social sciences and some health sciences have embraced feminist methods, including gender analysis, to understand differences in definitions of masculinity, femininity, and local gender ideologies; the sexual division of labor; positionality, or the importance of a writer's standpoint; and the value of women's stories as experiential embedded narratives, not as frivolous anecdotes. These approaches have all found their way into community-based health research.

As a feminist anthropologist, I take from feminism the argument that the personal is political, that theory cannot be separated from practical action or praxis, that everyday life is an important reference point for grounding theory, and that there are dangers lurking in dualistic thinking that opposes minds and bodies, public and private, nature and culture. Feminist theory requires us to embrace both/and, not either/or explanations. As an anthropologist, I often find myself playing the culture card, always arguing for context and looking for ways to get beyond Euro-American approaches to infant feeding. As a breastfeeding advocate, I rely more on my feminist politics, but I enjoy the challenge of having clearly defined opponents, such as aggressive marketing of infant formula or inappropriate hospital practices.

Many years ago, I began to use the terms *breastfeeding style* and *infant feeding style* to refer to the systematic manner of feeding an infant characteristic of an individual, a time, and a place. While working on a study of infant feeding practices in Bangkok, Semarang (Java), Bogota, and Nairobi, I found that the statistical results generated from the large cross-sectional surveys carried out by public health researchers did not capture the differences in the way that breastfeeding as a holistic activity was embedded in local practices. Breastfeeding style as a conceptual tool is useful for addressing patterned variation within traditions. Breastfeeding and infant feeding styles are personally and culturally constructed and reconstructed on a shared primate physiological base shaped by local regimens. Childbirth educator and leader in the alternative birth movement Sheila Kitzinger refers to these individual differences as lactational signatures, referring to breastfeeding in Euro-American contexts.

Lactation specialists Jan Riordan and Kathleen Auerbach, in their influential textbook, *Breastfeeding and Human Lactation*, refer to the concept of breastfeeding style and use it to address how cultural factors influence infant feeding practices, including the distinctions between breastfeeding as a process and breast milk as a product, a basic distinction included in breastfeeding style.

But when breastfeeding style is used in a public health context, it is often reduced to factors such as the frequency and length of time spent breastfeeding.[1]

Feminism and Public Health

Feminism as a social movement has much in common with public health. Both are modern social movements determined to make changes in the world, part of a modernist discourse of reform and progress. Unlike contemporary anthropology, which is ambivalent about making claims about the betterment of society, both feminism and public health want to improve, reform, and make progress in an imperfect world. Women instigated the public health movement in North American cities in the late nineteenth century to improve conditions, particularly for poor immigrants. In cities like New York, Chicago, and Montreal at the turn of the twentieth century, public health workers assumed that immigrants needed reforming. In actuality, poor immigrants were probably making better use of available foods, cultivating gardens, retaining culinary skills, and breastfeeding more successfully than nonimmigrants. In Canada, where departments of public health were established by 1882, immigrants were found to have longer breastfeeding durations.[2]

Public health is mandated to protect and improve the health of communities—both local subgroups and national populations. But public health professionals cannot improve health until they know more about people's living conditions. This is where detailed descriptive ethnographies may be useful.

Ethnography and Public Health

An ethnography is a written analysis and description of a community or institution based on intensive, long-term participant observation. Ethnography is more concerned with descriptions of the human condition generated from explicit theory and method than it is with trying to fix anything. Ethnographic cases substitute for scientific experimentation that cannot be done without affecting the social relations we seek to understand. Consider, for example, the ethical complexities of assigning infants to different feeding regimes when one mode of feeding—exclusive breastfeeding—is already known to be superior. Ethnographers cannot control variables, but they can contrast cases.

Ethnographies always expand and entangle, while public health and epidemiology must reduce and untangle. In looking for causes and health consequences, public health must simplify the complexity that ethnographies reveal. On the other hand, public health professionals must be accountable in ways that NGOs and feminist academics are not. Public health relies on epidemiology

and quantitative surveys of health indicators to get at evidence-based outcomes. Differences must be measurable in order for public health initiatives
to be effective. Measurement in public health programs and research requires
bounded categories and must remove confounding variables. But what public
health calls confounding variables, ethnographers call thick description.
Public health is heir to the biomedical factory analogy of the individual as a
discrete bounded body. When breastfeeding is treated as a kind of factory production in need of regulation in order to increase initiation or duration rates,
the subjective and experiential process is easily lost. In the development of
breastfeeding targets for national guidelines, public health employs a
discourse of mastery. Targets and numerical objectives are a part of this
discourse.[3]

In short, public health must oversimplify in order to act. Part of this oversimplification involves the boxification of culture, the reduction of cultural
differences to measurable traits. These fixed categories can be represented as
checklists of features that capture differences. In *Breastfeeding and Human
Lactation*, Riordan and Auerbach provide a chart to show how "possible cultural beliefs and practices" affect breastfeeding among Asian, African American,
and Hispanic-Chicano mothers. The dimensions of difference on the chart
include beliefs about health, the support person for a new mother, infant
feeding, family and parenting, and infant care. The intention of the section is
to sensitize health workers to the fact that cultural differences can have an
enormous impact on the way an infant is fed. The problem is that the chart
creates stereotypes and suggests that some differences matter more than other
differences. For example, income, housing arrangements, religion, or experience
of abuse may be much more important influences on breastfeeding than culture
or ethnic identity. The chart, while intending to help health professionals be
sensitive to cultural differences, misses the fluidity of ethnic identity and
essentializes large segments of the population without providing information
that could help lactation consultants support mothers from these communities.[4] More often, cultural differences are used to define risk groups in need of
short-term clinical intervention. Instead of addressing issues of power between
groups, community empowerment as a vague ideal becomes the way to deal
with health disparities.

Ethnographic Evidence One

Feminist social science, critical medical anthropology, and public health all
approach breastfeeding and cultural differences from distinct perspectives. We
are missing the best that different disciplinary approaches bring to breastfeeding

programs not because feminist social science and public health have different goals but because they employ different metaphors and work from distinct theoretical paradigms.

What feminist social science brings to the table is a way to address the fluidity of categories, rather than the bounded categories necessary for biomedical discourse—a way to unpack fixed identities of gender, ethnicity, race, ability—and even the difference between breastfeeding moms and bottle-feeding moms. Ethnographies, public culture, and women's stories alert us to the movement between categories, the back-and-forth compromises of everyday life. For example, a Canadian breastfeeding mother was angry when people contrasted breastfeeding and bottle-feeding mothers, since she considered herself a breastfeeding mother but fed expressed breast milk to her infant in a bottle; a Thai mother considered herself a breastfeeding mother, although her friend bottle-fed her infant for a week while the mother traveled up-country for her father's funeral (infants in Thai culture represent new life and should be kept physically and conceptually apart from death). In the process of remembering, women construct and reconstruct their own personal narratives about their breastfeeding experiences as part of the "moral work" of breastfeeding.[5]

The fluidity of self-defined categories is a disaster for epidemiologists who need to be able to show the impact of exclusive breastfeeding on specific populations. But individual autonomous discrete bodies, body parts, and bounded categories work for research and operations on kidneys but not for lactating breasts or for breastfeeding as a biosocial process.

To understand breastfeeding as a process, we must look to feminist and ethnographic work on embodiment, agency, and intersubjective relational discourses. Individually based theories can do little to explain or understand intersubjective processes like breastfeeding. Breastfeeding is, after all, about creating social relationships.

Ethnographies highlight differences and are rich in context. Not all ethnographies are feminist; many have ignored women. Few ethnographies focus on infancy, and fewer on infant feeding. Ethnographies on child rearing are rarely free of Western theoretical bias. But they work against the boxification of culture that results from reducing difference to single variables like ethnicity or race. Like style and stories, they expose local worlds that are difficult to reduce and simplify.

Public health policy makers often use ethnographic examples to learn how health messages and interventions are likely to be received. This knowledge increases compliance to national and global policy. Ignoring so-called cultural factors often accounts for the mismatch between global policy and local practice.

Some public health programs have made good use of cultural information in designing their programs.

A project in Bolivia worked with differences between local and national approaches to neonatal and maternal morbidity. Bolivian women were unresponsive to public health messages about immediate breastfeeding after birth but were very concerned about retained placentas. The project focused on the fact that breastfeeding immediately postpartum increases uterine contractions, helping the placenta to be delivered more rapidly. As a result, women no longer waited two to three days for the good milk to come in but began breastfeeding in order to expel their placentas. This example illustrates the value of putting women's concerns first, as well as the holism characteristic of the continuum of care in reproductive work.

But knowledge and application of cultural context can also have unintentional negative consequences. Two Japanese American women living in the United States advised La Leche League members about how to counsel Japanese mothers, explaining that Japanese women are respectful of authority. In an effort to promote breastfeeding in Japan, traditional Japanese breast massage was reintroduced to increase milk production, but in the process it was medicalized. An unanticipated result is that now Japanese women feel they need breast massage to produce adequate milk. A traditional cultural trait becomes embedded in a new context, where the practice is understood as necessary to produce adequate milk. This case may provide suggestions for how health professionals might deal with women of Japanese heritage. It also provides a clue to help us think through what happens when traditional practices become medicalized.[6]

Ethnographic Evidence Two

Breastfeeding is a holistic activity that is embedded in local practices in complex and patterned ways. When we examine how breastfeeding is embedded in different cultures, it is much harder to isolate cultural factors. Isolating cultural traits and taking them out of context changes their meaning in unanticipated ways. How can public health make the best use of ethnographic examples and get beyond the so-called cultural factors listed in breastfeeding manuals? What other kinds of evidence can be found in ethnographies concerning local solutions to the universal problem of how to nurture and feed a newborn?

Breastfeeding in Buddhist Thailand thrives in the essentially pre-Buddhist system, dominated by spirits, where individuals struggle to nurture rice as well as infants and fear the death of a pregnant woman, knowing her capacity to produce the most feared and dangerous ghosts. Mothers drink warming soups to increase their breast milk and rest by a heat source to dry out the uterus. During this period, they rest and often give their newborns to a trusted relative or friend who nurtures well to help develop good breastfeeding habits in the newborn. Thus, the newborn moves immediately into a broader social group. The Thai local regimen adapts Thai infants into Thai society through the nurturing practices of the household they are born into.

Long after ghosts have been relegated to premodern superstition, and modernity has relegated customs to traditional tourist theme parks, the older cultural logic that supported breastfeeding is still visible in remnants of household rituals. Ordination ceremonies and wedding ceremonies still begin by reference to paying mothers back for their milk. Yet modern Thai women quickly learned that resting by a heat source is old-fashioned and that clinic births are safer. If these changes come with too many Cesarean sections and infant formula, at least more children survive, which makes mothers, the national health service, and the World Health Organization happy. Along with lying by the fire, the postpartum rest has also disappeared.

Some of the best ethnographic work on children was done by Margaret Mead and Gregory Bateson in the late 1930s. Their photographic analysis of *Balinese Character* set standards not only in visual anthropology, but also in the analysis of infant and child development. While the culture and personality framework is dated, the photographic record illustrates elements of a distinctive infant feeding style recognizable seventy years later.

Bateson and Mead are among the rare ethnographers who linked infant and child feeding to emotion and adult eating. Building from the psychological assumptions of their day, they analyzed thousands of photographs and observations to argue that eating meals and defecating (accompanied by shame) was conceptually distinct from eating snacks, drinking, and urinating (accompanied by no shame); they suggested that eating prechewed food (by infants) is the prototype for eating meals (by adults), while breastfeeding is the prototype for casual snacking and drinking among adults. This hypothesis was developed through detailed observations about the casualness of breastfeeding, often accomplished by turning the nipple upward into the baby's mouth, instead of the downward motion of pushing prechewed food into the infant's mouth, replicated in adults by tipping the head back and hunching over food while eating their normal meals. With breastfeeding, the baby is unconstrained and takes the initiative to breastfeed at will, having free access to the breast when it is carried next to the mother's body in a sling. The child's body, held against the mother's body is curved, relaxed, as it adapts to the mother's postures. The photographs also suggest that breastfeeding is associated with fun and pleasure, not coercion, pressure, or shame. The example of Balinese infant feeding style shows how groups like the Balinese seek balance between autonomy and connectedness, between the living and the dead. Through breast-feeding and eating, Balinese infants develop constitutions that strain to control emotions. Breastfeeding is key to setting this pattern linking bodily functions like eating and emotion throughout the lifespan.[7]

Indonesian infant feeding policy does not build on these subtle observations because it takes its lead from shared global public health policy documents that come from United Nations agencies. Indonesian policy makers are also unlikely to build on the Islamic approach to shared breastfeeding, including the customs around milk siblingship. Islamic Shariah law recognizes three alternative ways to establish relationships—through blood, affinity, and milk. Substances like breast milk serve to create special relations between mothers and infants, but they go beyond the mother-infant bond. There is no more intimate act than consuming milk from someone's breast. In the past, some Muslim societies used this intimacy to acknowledge the power of relatedness through milk siblingship. Through the act of breastfeeding another child or even an adult taking milk from a lactating woman's breast, strangers can be turned into relatives, enemies into allies, marriageable relatives into ineligible ones.

The milk sibling relationship contrasts with the Thai case where the woman who breastfeeds another woman's child has no formal permanent relation to the mother or the child, but simply sets a good habit for the child out of loving-kindness.

Implications for Public Health Practice

I have chosen a few exotic examples of cultural differences—stories of people unlikely to reside in North America—to remind us how breastfeeding is embedded in women's lives and communities in unique ways. They provide glimpses into different cultural worlds. The cultural details may not all be use-ful to policy makers in an instrumental sense. Rather, ethnographies describe the everydayness of breastfeeding in its normal cultural context, rather than as a problem to be solved. They are reminders that breastfeeding has a life of its own. It is not culturally constructed by individual mothers and communities, but is part of a set of practices with distinct local histories.

Anthropology, feminism, and public health need each other, and they could work better together. What can we take from a feminist social science approach to cultural differences that might be useful for transforming the way public health institutions and practitioners approach breastfeeding and infant feeding? Considerations of how we use culture, research practices, and policy making are places to start the conversation.

Culture

Ethnographies remind us that local cultural logics operate to guide breastfeeding. Anthropologists are useful for describing these cultural logics and developing middle-ground models that capture regional patterns. Public health policy works with and through cultural differences, many of which are less relevant to infant feeding than poverty, racism, and gender inequality. When working in interdisciplinary teams, the following suggestions might be useful:

- Find the balance between fetishizing cultural differences and ignoring them. Think of culture not as a variable but as deeply embedded systems of meaning.
- Reconfigure culture as a resource that women use to empower themselves, not as a constraint on women or on breastfeeding.
- Explore well-developed customs and traditions that create social relations and alliances between people through breastfeeding.
- Develop clinical cultural competency around skills such as sensitivity, empathy, and language, not stereotypes about categories of people.
- Understand how the culture of biomedicine shapes the discourse and culture of public health and breastfeeding advocacy groups.

Research Practices

Ideally, research on breastfeeding should be conducted in interdisciplinary teams. This means that the methods of psychology, ethnography, and geography, among others, may be combined with those of epidemiology and health surveys.

- Put most emphasis on examining the activity of breastfeeding, rather than on its determinants and consequences.
- Refine and broaden the definition of evidence, so that women's stories about their breastfeeding experiences can be treated as evidence, not anecdote.
- Attend more carefully to language and metaphor and how these shape discourses surrounding breastfeeding and infant feeding.
- Take leads from the questions people ask each other. (For example, in Canada, a First Nations colleague suggested asking something like, "Excuse me, who are your people?" after establishing a relationship where researchers explained who they were.)

- Asking how your mother fed you and how your grandmother fed your mother and you might be more important than asking about your ethnic or cultural identity.

Policy Making

In some localities, breastfeeding is an unproblematic aspect of human existence; in others, it is highly valued and highly charged symbolically, imbued with values beyond nutrition; in still others it is a risky process that needs careful management or is an act that evokes disgust and irrational prudery. How, then, could there be one policy for all mothers? Health professionals all want to improve infant health through improved infant feeding practices. Biomedicine is not the villain in the work of breastfeeding promotion, although health practices and out-of-date information may be obstacles. Thus,

- Avoid messages such as "breast is best," or "the one best way"; these slogans have little impact on mothers simply trying to nurture their children, not attain perfection.
- Assume that policy makers may respond to personal experience and stories as readily as statistics in setting priorities.
- Focus more attention on how breastfeeding solves problems for women rather than causes problems for women.
- Reinsert breastfeeding in global health agendas in many different places, including reproductive health, where it is strangely absent.
- Ensure that when cultural information is provided to policy makers, it is not presented as wrong information that must be corrected, or as raw material for developing training courses providing technical skills in cultural competency.

Conclusions

Within diverse stories and styles seen in ethnographic work, we search for language to begin to broaden the debates on cultural differences in infant feeding practices. We learn that women breastfeed in highly local life worlds in very specific niches. These local regimens occupy the middle ground between the uniqueness of every mother-infant pair and the uniformity of cultural traditions, all framed within biocultural universals. Ethnographic work provides the local contexts that fill the conceptual gap between individuals and populations.

Biomedical approaches to public health can inform global health and nutrition policy. Is there room for a more politicized feminist public health that can replicate past victories like immunization and sanitation in the field of gender-sensitive infant feeding policy? Is there room for other voices in these policy discussions, voices more attuned to mothers, meals, emotions, and pleasure?

Ethnographic cases show how local regimens fit breastfeeding and child nurture into other activities. Women and infants do not live in isolation; infants are born into preexisting families, households, and communities. They do not just live in communities with other mothers and babies. All mothers have to solve the problem of how to integrate their productive and reproductive lives in an organic whole of lived experience. Ethnographies show how breastfeeding is embedded in these local complexes, each with their distinct gender ideologies, religious beliefs and practices, and systems of household production and consumption. These brief examples remind us of the futility of many short-term interventions designed to tweak or improve infant feeding practices in isolation, without also addressing underlying conditions such as poverty or global marketing of commercial baby foods. Each cultural pattern touches a truth about the human condition and reflects back to our shared primate and human heritage. They remind us that there are infinite ways to think about and practice breastfeeding.

Notes

1. Van Esterik and Elliot, "Infant Feeding Style"; Kitzinger, *Ourselves as Mothers*; Quandt, "Patterns of Variation," 448; Riordan and Auerbach, *Breastfeeding and Human Lactation*, 42–43.
2. Nathoo and Ostry, *One Best Way*, 10. See also Wolf, this volume.
3. Code, *Ecological Thinking*.
4. Riordan and Auerbach, *Breastfeeding and Human Lactation*, 32.
5. Ryan, Bissell, and Alexander, "Moral Work."
6. See Howard-Grabman et al., "'Dialogue of Knowledge' Approach"; Payne, "Japanese Culture and Breastfeeding."
7. Bateson and Mead, *Balinese Character*, 107, 124. See also Sullivan, "Of External Habits and Maternal Attitudes," 240.

The Dangers of Baring the Breast

Structural Violence and Formula-Feeding among Low-Income Women

Athena is a twenty-six-year-old single mother who lives alone with her five children. After a high-risk pregnancy and premature delivery, she fully breast-fed her newborn, Clifford, for four months while attending a community college full time and caring for her four other children. She did this absent a partner or family support while relying on the supplemental nutrition program Women, Infants, and Children (WIC), public transportation, and day care. After four months, she added solid foods to Clifford's diet. At seven and a half months, she switched Clifford over to formula and discontinued breastfeeding. She said of formula, "Yeah, I don't have a problem with it."[1]

If Athena had shown up in a national database on infant feeding as a set of numbers and demographics, she would have fallen into several groups at high risk for not initiating or sustaining breastfeeding. Despite having partially breastfed her other children, she had four strikes against her in trying to breast-feed her newborn: she was low-income, African American, had no actively involved partner, and had a premature infant in the Neonatal Intensive Care Unit (NICU). Rather than view Athena as a set of numbers and risk factors, we look in detail at her story, her own voice. The focus on the gritty biographical details of a single low-income mother serves multiple objectives. First, it gives voice to those whose suffering is often ignored. Second, it is only through these details we can trace the links between structurally distal events of the social ecology, such as unequal drug laws and the disappearance of fathers from poor communities, and more structurally proximal events, such as the breakdown of families and the decision to feed formula. Third, this approach underscores the constant tension between individual choice and lack of opportunity to exercise it. Using the Social-Ecological Model in conjunction with the concept of structural violence, we will highlight how, despite her commitment to breastfeed, Athena's efforts were thwarted rather than supported by the very institutions that she depended on and the community in which she lived. We hope to show that the choice to use formula under these conditions, despite the documented risks, is a rational choice made among a plethora of risks over which she has minimal control.

Structural Violence

Structural violence originated in the work of sociologist Johan Galtung, founder of peace and conflict studies.[2] Structural violence refers to the indirect violence perpetrated on the poor through the higher order structures of the social ecology that leave the poor materially disadvantaged and at great risk for harm. By decreasing the number of available options for action, denying access to resources, and inflicting emotional and physical suffering on individual people, structural violence limits agency and negates the idea of choice. A number of anthropologists working with poor and relatively powerless communities throughout the world have used this framework to better understand the rapid global spread of HIV among poor women; drug addiction and its community consequences in East Harlem; and excess infant mortality in Brazil and Syracuse, New York.[3] Structural violence coming as it does through the structures of society has no identifiable agent, which makes it difficult to think in terms of preventive interventions. Nevertheless, understanding the problem of infant feeding in terms of violence originating at multiple levels beyond the individual gets us away from the "educating the mother" interventions so often used. Shifting the focus can stimulate interventions designed at multiple levels to change policies, institutions, and cultural attitudes.

Athena's Story

Athena was highly motivated to breastfeed, but beyond her individual motivation she also had to develop strategies to manage multiple risks in her environment. Over the past ten years we conducted dozens of interviews with poor women about the challenges and successes in maintaining their health and the health of their children. Athena's interview is remarkable for her indefatigable persistence in trying to breastfeed her youngest child. In a sixty-minute home interview, surrounded by her children, Athena described the social context in which she made decisions about infant feeding:

> I have epilepsy and I averaged about thirty-six seizures in the seven
> months that I was pregnant with [my fifth child, Clifford]. It just so

happened that the day that I went into labor with him, I actually had a seizure while getting my blood drawn at a regular prenatal visit. So he was, like, induced. . . . two days later I woke up and like, "hey, you got a baby." So it was kind of, whoa . . .

I had went through a lot when I was pregnant with him, like, his dad got incarcerated . . . my stress level was up, you know, and I was suffering from depression, majorly. So I really wanted to give him the extra that I wasn't giving him when I was pregnant because of the fact that I was so depressed. I was [using] . . . painkillers here and there trying to put me to sleep to get over the depression, and you know, even a little alcohol use and a little marijuana use when I was pregnant with him. I'm sure that he could feel my pain in my womb. So my whole desire to want to breastfeed came from me saying, "Okay, my life is not so horrible. He does not deserve this. I want to make sure that he has the same attention and the same love as the rest of my children."

After I came home [alone], because he was in the NICU . . . being that I had children at home, of course, I had to come back and forth, you know, take care of everything and then go back up to the hospital.

To have to see him laying in a feeding . . . just with all the tubes on his face and through his belly button, his mouth, and having to push the milk through the tube. That was the most horrible experience I ever experienced in my life. And I think that that was the main reason why I tried so hard to stay with the breastfeeding with him.

I was definitely going to keep with the formula being that he was already in the NICU getting the formula, but [my obstetrician] said, "You know, as long as you are lactating, then you can breastfeed." I didn't know that. I figured that if you didn't start breastfeeding from day one, you know, the baby would completely reject the milk or he wouldn't take it. . . . But she told me that that wouldn't be an issue. Being that he was in the NICU, I couldn't feed him as often as I would like, so my [obstetrician] told me, "Well, why don't you just buy a breast pump and store the milk." That was something that I also did not know you could do. I really didn't. I never used a breast pump until Clifford . . . I never even knew that was even a possibility.

Athena introduced solid foods into Clifford's diet at four months. She discontinued breastfeeding and introduced formula at seven and a half months, noting, "If my schedule wasn't as busy as it is, I'd probably still be breastfeeding [him] at one [year]." She continued: "I believe when you're breastfeeding, it can be draining. . . . For some reason, I find it harder to keep up with a newborn than it is with an eight-year-old. I mean that is just the one point in your life that you're actually on *their* time. There is no training them; there is no getting them on a schedule. Those first couple months there is nothing you can do."

She spoke about the use of formula: "I just don't believe that, like, when I combine breast milk and formula, it would be—I would breastfeed my child at one eating and at the next eating I might give him some formula. Yeah, I don't have a problem with it. You just have to go according to what the baby desires. If the baby is comfortable with breast and formula and it's helping you to get the sleep that you need when the baby first comes, then by all means, you work it out."

At another point Athena noted, "but, it was his [Clifford's] decision. He just completely stopped with the breast milk, and I could see that he was getting fuller and sleeping longer with the [formula]. So it was getting him full. And I needed to sleep."

Athena also described the stress of lactation management while going to school and using public transportation. Breast milk leaked through her blouse while she was in public, which she found embarrassing. She felt uncomfortable pumping in public bathrooms when she was engorged. She spoke at length about the harassment she encountered traveling to and from school on city buses:

> I actually breastfed my son when he was crying out of control, and I actually breastfed him on the bus—and you do not know how many people will stare at you and call you so many obscene names, and like, "oh, that is so disgusting. Put your breast away." They were just sitting behind me gossiping, "Oh my goodness, that is so disgusting. Do you know what she's doing? She has the blanket over—do you know what she's doing under there? She's breastfeeding the baby!" I once got off two stops early and walked down because I got tired of hearing them, "whisper, whisper."

Acceptable Risks in the Social Ecology

We are amazed that Athena was able to breastfeed at all. What new insights can Athena's story offer us? We already know that low-income women in the United States are significantly less likely to breastfeed their infants than are middle- and upper-income mothers, despite the documented risks of formula-feeding. Across studies and across ethnicities, most low-income mothers know "breast is best." So why do so many women choose to feed their infants formula, even when they are breastfeeding? The framework of structural violence illuminates the multiple daily risks low-income women face across the spectrum of the Social-Ecological Model.

Our goal here is to examine the cultural logic and social constraints that construct formula-feeding as an acceptable risk for low-income mothers. This is an important goal in breastfeeding research because it addresses three identified gaps in the research. First, while there is ample research on the barriers and facilitators to breastfeeding, what remains underexamined and unexplained is why so many women—especially low-income women—prefer feeding with formula or have no qualms about mixed feeding. Second, the public health emphasis on education as a way to change health behaviors has had only modest impacts on breastfeeding rates over the past thirty years. Education alone cannot change infant feeding practices. What many feminist researchers identify as missing in this work is a sufficient understanding of the complex social contexts in which infant feeding is enacted.[4] In addition, some public health researchers have critiqued as inadequate the simple, linear models typically used to capture social and cultural context.[5] Our approach, we believe, captures the complex trade-offs mothers need to make in raising their children with limited resources. Third, public health research unduly stresses the role of individual agency in making healthy choices, wrongly assuming that an agentive, independently acting woman is the sole determinant of infant feeding. She is not. In some situations, women's agency is actually punished.[6] Understanding agency as contingent on context prevents us from romanticizing poor mothers as heroines or casting them as passive victims, both of which oversimplify context and action. Using the framework of structural violence allows us to trace the pathways between the upper levels of the Social-Ecological Model and the lives of individual mothers and gives us a way to address the three gaps in the extant literature described above.

Neighborhood as a Site of Structural Violence

Many of the low-income mothers enrolled in our studies live within the Crescent, a geographic swath of the city extending from the northeast quadrant to the southwest. The Crescent is characterized by concentrated poverty, a high proportion of lead-contaminated housing, a single chain supermarket, and not enough government subsidized housing to meet demand. Mothers are confronted with increased risks of lead poisoning, food insecurity, and homelessness while trying to meet the most fundamental needs of their young families: shelter and food. The increased risk for harm is the result of structural violence, which operates, for example, through flawed housing policies that concentrate the poor in certain neighborhoods. Mothers have limited power to change policies and institutional practices. What agency they have is realized in their daily negotiation of this territory using strategies that minimize harm to themselves and their children. They change homes often, use WIC services, sign up for food stamps, and access food pantries.

The Crescent is also characterized by direct violence. It contains only one-third of the city's population but is the site for 80 percent of its murders. Drug-related arrests are frequent. Demographically, men between the ages of twenty-one and forty-five are missing from the census in Crescent neighborhoods.[7] Most of these missing men are incarcerated. Others are dead. Many mothers are thus at high risk for parenting alone without the support of fathers, grandfathers, brothers, or uncles.

When breastfeeding women experience a sense of vulnerability, the feelings of vulnerability go beyond the physical baring of the breast. In the words of one mother, "You let down your guard." In other interviews we heard fathers talk about protecting their women while they breastfed, including preventing interruptions, undue exposures, and young males that "leer." Athena had no one protecting or supporting her, contributing to her physical tiredness and her sense of vulnerability.

The absence of males in the community also places mothers and their children at risk for direct violence. The relationship between household and community violence and sustained breastfeeding remains underexplored; unfortunately, it is rare for breastfeeding promotion programs to screen women for domestic violence. It is not unreasonable to speculate, however, that fear of battering may inhibit a woman from breastfeeding.

Institutions as a Site of Structural Violence: Ignoring Suffering

The links between Athena's experiences and higher order social structures are described repeatedly in her story and include structural violence stemming from policies, institutions, and culture. The most immediately apparent instances of structural violence came from institutions. Despite multiple contacts with health care providers and the court system, no one recognized that Athena's many burdens put her at an increased risk for depression, and, by her estimate, dramatically increased the number of seizures she had during her last pregnancy.[8] She was unscreened, undiagnosed, and untreated for depression. Had her depression been diagnosed in a timely manner, a second barrier would have been finding a mental health provider that accepts Medicaid insurance. A significant number of pregnant, low-income women are depressed and untreated.[9] This form of structural violence is embedded in institutions that do not screen and do not refer; it also impacts at the policy level, where women at significant risk for depression are not provided with adequate coverage. Athena was untreated and ended up self-medicating her depressive symptoms with alcohol and street drugs, which is not unusual. Her suffering was ignored by the institutions established to support her.

Ignoring human suffering and silencing the voices of the sufferers is a hallmark of structural violence. Since there is no easily identifiable agent of this violence, no one within these structured interactions is responsive to the women who pass through the institutions, are processed according to policies, and whose treatment is rationalized by a cynical cultural view. It is not clear the extent to which Athena's providers even discussed breastfeeding with her prenatally or if they viewed her as single black mother with other children and assumed that she would not be able to manage breastfeeding. Once her obstetrician mentions that she can actually breastfeed, even with her child in the NICU, she works with the nursing staff to breastfeed. Her actions of self-advocacy in this and other situations demonstrate how she was able to overcome the barriers created by the structural violence in her world.

Policies as a Site of Structural Violence

Two of Athena's "baby-daddies" were incarcerated at the time of this interview, leaving Athena alone with the care of five children. The mass incarceration of black males is another form of structural violence, the result of specific drug laws and penalties. Incarceration of black males from low-income neighborhoods has had adverse effects on black communities in the United States.[10] The United States essentially warehouses black men in prison out of proportion to their numbers in the general population. For black women, the risk of single parenting is high, and lack of household support in the form of hands-on care of children and financial contributions from the father can impede a mother's ability to breastfeed. Such a situation makes formula-feeding attractive. WIC programs supply free supplemental formula, and with bottle-feeding the care and feeding of the infant can more easily be shared with older children. Athena offers that she would have breastfed Clifford longer had her schedule not been so busy—busy with her four older children, busy with her full-time college studies, and busy getting back and forth to college using an inadequate, time-consuming public transportation system.

Despite the fact that Clifford was her fifth baby, breast pumps were new to her. She had not been offered the support of a free breast pump from either the hospital or WIC, despite having an infant in the NICU, demonstrating another form of structural violence—institutional policies that neglect the needs of poor women trying to breastfeed. Having access to a breast pump makes lactation management easier for many women, especially by letting them feed their infants in public using a bottle with breast milk. Cultural norms that see breastfeeding as disgusting subject mothers to disparaging remarks and daily humiliations. This assault on a mother's dignity can be a powerful deterrent for all U.S. mothers; for poor mothers, it is another risk to manage. So even though Athena suggested that she received more education about breastfeeding when she was pregnant with Clifford than with her earlier infants, her lack of knowledge about pumps and their availability contributed to her vulnerability.

Not touched on in Athena's interview, but apparent in other conversations we had with low-income mothers, is the tension between the lack of adequate low-income housing in Rochester and the release of fathers from incarceration. Reintegration of men back into households and communities after their release from prison is difficult. It is difficult for men to find employment. It is difficult for newly reunited couples to manage their relationship. It is difficult for the couple to find housing large enough to accommodate the now expanded family. These exigencies result in frequent moves from place to place, from shared housing with friends to shared housing with extended family. Yet shared housing is often crowded and fraught with interpersonal tensions. Under these conditions breastfeeding at home is more akin to breastfeeding in public. The hypermobility that results also puts women at risk for disruptions in their social networks as they move from neighborhood to neighborhood. One low-income woman told us that on her street a block party was held that excluded those renting homes. Many women also lost their supportive relationships with service providers when they relocated to another part of the Crescent or outside the city limits.

Inadequate as Metaphor for Poor Women's Lives

Athena demonstrated considerable agency in negotiating multiple risks in her daily life wrought by structural violence. She managed to breastfeed her infant despite his premature birth, her own poor health, care of four older children, reliance on public transportation in getting to school, and incarceration of her children's respective fathers. Her agency was constrained, however, by a lack of intervention for her depression, by an aggravation of her epilepsy during pregnancy resulting in premature birth of her son, by lack of access to a breast pump, and by public harassment while breastfeeding. Even though she gave birth in a hospital, her son was in the NICU, and she accessed WIC, no one told her about pumping as a way to manage lactation nor offered her an available free pump. Two of the men she had children with were swept into the prison system.

We can only speculate on the material impact of reduced financial assets and lack of logistical support in raising five children alone. Our hypothesis is that after managing these daily risks, the risk of formula-feeding seemed insignificant by comparison. The use of structural violence as a model shows how risks are created that are beyond the control of an individual mother, and even Athena, this most strategic manager of risks, needed to resort to formula, despite her dedication to breastfeeding. Structural violence, considered in conjunction with the Social-Ecological Model, provides an alternative to simple linear models of health behavior.

The word most low-income women use to describe their breast milk— "inadequate"—is a metaphor for their lives as poor women.[11] They have inadequate protections against dangers in their environment, dangers that originate in spheres beyond their control. In such a context the risks or dangers of formula-feeding are not obvious or as urgent: "The question of *inadequacy* has dual significance for social life. On the one hand we can ask if the lives of low-income women are inadequate in terms of material items we as US citizens deem minimal for negotiating daily life, such as housing, safe neighborhoods, transportation, health care, training, and employment. On the other hand we can ask if low-income women feel inadequate in fulfilling the multiple social roles that are demanded of them as workers, mothers, partners, and family members."[12] The ethnographic literature reveals a staggering burden of inadequate safety—a description of lives so riddled with direct violence and structural violence that low-income women's complaints of inadequate breast milk might be a physical reaction to the context in which they feed their infants. Furthermore, the data strongly suggest that breastfeeding (and its attendant benefits) is a class-based privilege, and the public health focus on ethnic differences has masked the larger influence of social class as a determinant of infant feeding practices in the United States. No matter what a particular group's cultural beliefs are about infant feeding—breast is best or comfort with formula-feeding—below a certain level of income the structural violence is so constraining that beliefs about the benefits of breastfeeding cannot be put into practice. Agency is thwarted. Low-income mothers struggle and suffer with inadequate income, housing, food, safety, health care, transportation, and dignity. Even for the mother wanting to breastfeed, formula-feeding becomes the logical choice, because the day-to-day risks found in the lives of low-income groups far outweigh the risks of formula-feeding.

Notes

This work was supported by PHS Grant #RO1-HD055191, Community Partnership for Breastfeeding Promotion and Support, and a grant from the Susan B. Anthony Institute at the University of Rochester.

1. Athena's story was collected as part of a larger study described in Holmes et al., "Barrier to Exclusive Breastfeeding." We thank Dr. Holmes for permission to use Athena's interview in this chapter. Nancy Chin and Ann Dozier have worked with low-income mothers in a variety of settings and on a variety of public health issues. We thank Anna Solomonik for help in formatting the manuscript.
2. Galtung, "Violence, Peace, and Peace Research."
3. Farmer, "Chapter One: Women, Poverty, and AIDS"; Bourgois, *In Search of Respect*; Lane, *Why Are Our Babies Dying?*
4. Law, "The Politics of Breastfeeding."
5. Glass and McAtee, "Behavioral Science." Also see Green, "Public Health." Glass and McAtee draw a distinction between "risk regulators" and "risk factors." For example, they argue that the search for proximal risk factors such as sedentary behaviors and low-nutrient, calorie-dense diets to explain obesity at the individual level neglects the broader social environment from which risky behaviors arise. They use risk regulators to identify the more distal, contextual factors that contribute to population-level obesity.
6. Ortner, "Gender Hegemonies."
7. Klofas, "Community Structure."
8. The court system in Rochester has since established a system for depression screening and referral. Uptake was immediate and robust among women.
9. Brown and Moran, "Single Mothers."
10. Roberts, "Social and Moral Cost."
11. Chin and Solomonik, "INADEQUATE."
12. Ibid., 42.

Racism, Race, and Disparities in Breastfeeding

Discussions of racism and race are uncomfortable for most Americans who idealize equality of all peoples, yet individual and institutional racial discrimination abound. It has been called the elephant in the room, in part due to collective social guilt surrounding historical injustices that now can be openly discussed, and in part to a collective desire to feel that we have moved beyond the social and structural embeddedness of racism. Racism is evident in the framing of issues surrounding breastfeeding disparities, manifesting as the continuing overreliance on race as the defining identity categorization. Although racism and racial categorizing have been widely debated and discussed throughout the social sciences and humanities, with a few notable exceptions the health science disciplines have not participated in these dialogues.[1] Although many complex and dynamic influences have created these differences, the overreliance on empirical research approaches and epistemologies, along with the long-standing hierarchical power structure of the health sciences, have led to and perpetuate the lack of attention given to understanding the effects of racism in the health science breastfeeding literature.

The focus of this chapter is how these socially embedded realities have affected and continue to affect public health endeavors to support and promote breastfeeding. Conceptual assumptions framing this discussion are drawn from feminist treatments of power and gender inequity within social institutions, including the theory of intersectionality and Social-Ecological Model, all of which are related to the primacy of social justice.[2]

Racism: The Elephant in the Room

Racism, an inherent value and power structure based on racial social stratification, has deep historical roots that permeate all aspects of American society—one might say it is a defining feature of American society. Despite many well-intentioned efforts, we as a society have yet to move beyond the resultant embedded them/us power dynamics. Within a breastfeeding context racism is gendered, making it a feminist issue and adding dimensions of complexity.[3] We know certain populations, defined simplistically using racial categorizations, have lower breastfeeding rates, but what is far less obvious is why.

Most breastfeeding researchers do not explicitly reference racism. They refer to cultural differences and/or cross-cultural misunderstandings, defining culture using generic racial categories (so-called African American culture, Latina culture). Some suggest that "race-associated differences in health outcomes are in fact due to the effects of racism."[4] The first step in understanding the effects of racism is to define how it manifests. Camara P. Jones, an epidemiologist and a physician, developed a theoretical framework that articulates three levels of racism (institutional, personally mediated, and internalized) based on multilayered levels of influence similar to levels within the Social-Ecological Model. Using her framework, I explore historical and contemporary perspectives in the following sections.

Racism: The Ground upon which Breastfeeding Disparities Grow

Each of the three levels of racism has many manifestations within the context of breastfeeding disparities, too many to adequately describe. Jones states that *institutionalized racism* is the most fundamental level that must be addressed before the other two levels, largely because it reflects the basic assumptions upon which the other forms of racism grow. Language usage provides a clear example of this type of racism. The language we use to describe a circumstance reflects our underlying assumptions about the world.[5] The words used in the health science literature (vulnerable, inequity, disparity, less fortunate) have inferred embedded racism with an inherent them/us distinction, which distances and privileges the researcher. The terminology contributes to a situation where those in a privileged position do not recognize their contextual positionality.[6] For example, qualitative researchers interviewing nurses and physicians about racially based, unequal treatment found participants first denied that this phenomenon ever occurred. After being presented with a number of studies where racially differential treatment was obvious, most participants explained these occurrences by referring to patients' personal attributes or by making a global statement about inadequate access to care. Only one out of twenty-six participants acknowledged that racial bias occurs in health care delivery.[7] Institutionalized racism occurs without a designated perpetrator and is normative to the point of becoming invisible.[8]

Access to breastfeeding services provides another substantive example of institutionalized racism. In 1994 Michael D. Kogan and colleagues reported racially based differential breastfeeding advice was given prenatally by health care providers. Ten years later, Anne C. Beal, Karen Kuhlthau, and James M. Perrin reported that African American women were less likely to receiving breastfeeding advice and that they were more likely to receive bottle-feeding advice from physicians and Women, Infants, and Children (WIC) counselors than were their white counterparts.[9] One might call this racial profiling. Over this ten-year period, the evidence suggests that health care providers' attitudes and practices had not changed significantly.

Once in the hospital, differential treatment continues. In 2010, during an examination of how nursing staff cope with increased patient loads and inadequate staffing, researchers found nurses made decisions about whom to assist based on their perceptions of how much time assistance would take. The predominantly white nursing staff thought that women of color would require more of their time. As a result, nonwhite persons received less care. A similar finding was demonstrated by researchers surveying the hospital-based lactation services in a major metropolitan area. Researchers found an inverse correlation across hospitals between the number of women receiving public assistance and the number of professional lactation staff available to assist breastfeeding mothers. Their findings suggest that a disparity in access to hospital-based professional lactation services existed communitywide. By looking across studies, a pattern emerges that suggests, if not reflects, structural bias or blindness characteristic of institutionalized racism.[10]

Personally mediated racism (interpersonal discrimination) has a direct and consistent relationship with negative health outcomes.[11] Personally mediated racism (along with the other forms) has been analyzed by social science and humanities scholars focusing on the manifestations and power differentials inherent in breastfeeding mothers' lives.[12] Unlike public health research, most breastfeeding research (in the health sciences) has not addressed personally mediated racism. Far too often providers are unaware of scholarship outside of their practice-oriented domain. As the examples above demonstrate, it is difficult for practitioners to step outside their role as providers and to reflect on the assumptions that drive their practice, particularly when those assumptions are pervasively held. Perhaps researchers within a practice-oriented profession have a similar difficulty in exploring the assumptions driving their worldview.[13] Therefore, race-related issues raised by those outside the health science field are not heard. Established quantitative and epidemiological methodologies, grounded in reductionist empirical categorization, continue to dominate: "Despite such critiques, researchers continue to use the scientific discourses of the physical sciences to legitimate all forms of social research."[14]

Internalized racism is more difficult to study because it resides within individuals' psyches. It is a complex constellation of personal beliefs and psychological conditioning, making it difficult to study using quantitative methodologies.[15] Feminist and critical race theories have taken issue with the legitimacy of empirical research, suggesting these approaches are rooted in nineteenth-century white European cultural biases and privilege.

One form of internalized racism, historical trauma, has been debated and analyzed in the humanities and social science literature but is infrequently discussed in the mainstream health science literature. Yet it is repeatedly a concern of indigenous and other postcolonial people who speak and write about health inequities and for whom historical context is perceived as immediately present.[16] Internalized racism has been equated with the Stockholm syndrome associated with persons held captive, in which the traumatized individual internalizes the beliefs of her or his perpetrator.

Racism has been addressed in breastfeeding promotion and support programs in ways that are covert or implicit, and which have been aimed predominantly at personally mediated racism.[17] Breastfeeding intervention studies with racially based samples have focused on creating culturally relevant programs that aim to reduce discrimination through education of health care and public health providers. While education is essential, it is only minimally effective when it is the only method used to affect behavioral change. Many education programs aimed at broadening individuals' perspectives risk stereotyping, which reduces the possibility of meaningful mutual understandings, or cultural relativism, which may limit possibilities for health (breastfeeding) promotion by accepting any cultural practice as equally appropriate.[18]

Although cultural competency generally has not been framed explicitly in terms of reducing racism, racial discrimination remains an underlying reason for and assumption of these programs. Notions of cultural competence frequently lump race and culture together, perhaps to soften the underlying assumptions and stereotypes covertly made about participants' values, beliefs, and behaviors.[19] For example, some government and privately produced breastfeeding promotion materials contain inherent assumptions about the nature of personal values based on racial categorization. It is likely these messages will be viewed by targeted populations as racist.[20] U.S. public health agencies have been striving unsuccessfully to correct existing health and breastfeeding disparities for many years, but lack of attention paid to all manifestations of racism by the majority of breastfeeding researchers contributes significantly to insufficient progress in reducing disparities and improving health outcomes.

Racial Categorization: A Slippery Slope

"For over 100 years the public health system has routinely reported national health data by race."[21] Contrary to nineteenth- and early twentieth-century perceptions, race is now recognized as a social construct, not a biological determinant carrying inherent cognitive, moral, or social value. Racial categorization has been confused with culture in defining research variables and in explanatory narratives. Again, unclear and inconsistent definitions have perpetuated confusion. In 1999 the Institute of Medicine, in an attempt to avoid the defunct notions of biological determinism, advised abandoning the use of racial categories in favor of using "ethnicity" as the broad descriptor. Using the term "ethnic group" may further muddy these waters, replacing biological with cultural determinism. Recently, others have argued that using the more socially acceptable term ("ethnicity") does not change American views, as substituting terminology does not change the underlying biases. These issues have been debated in the public health literature without a clear resolution, resulting in both terms being used together (race/ethnicity), further obfuscating meaningful understandings.[22] The generalizing effects of stereotyping with a "false" biological or cultural categorization has created an environment of distrust in the relevancy and responsiveness of our health care systems.[23]

Racial Categorizations Oversimplify Breastfeeding Disparities

Using reductionist race-based metrics to determine breastfeeding disparities has led to oversimplification and to methodological confusion. Racial categories usually defined according to the U.S. census are major demographics collected in all national data sets that include breastfeeding variables. An extensive body of research focused on racial differences in breastfeeding patterns exists, resulting in widely recognized racially based *profiles* of who is most likely to breastfeed.[24] Referring to the "emergent myth that needs to be weeded before it roots," Anne Merewood cautions against stereotyping all minority women as having low breastfeeding rates.[25] As Donna J. Chapman and Rafael Pérez-Escamilla explain, collapsing and simplifying racial categories obfuscates important differences among the various Hispanic, Pacific Islanders, and African American populations. For example, African-born and Hispanic immigrants have higher breastfeeding rates than do native-born women categorized into the same racial group. This nuanced difference is lost when racial categories are the predominant demographic descriptors and immigration status is ignored.[26]

Other, potentially more meaningful, demographic variables (socioeconomic distinctions, geography, and marital status) remain hidden. In breastfeeding research, both descriptions of and determinations about socioeconomic status (SES) distinctions are underdeveloped. Two reasons have been suggested: meaningful measures of SES are difficult to create, because within national surveys definitions of socioeconomic groups and methods for collecting these data vary considerably; and SES has been viewed as a surrogate for social class.[27] Generally, Americans prefer to think of their society as classless, despite growing evidence to the contrary. It is another uncomfortable topic opposing American ideals.

We have inadequate knowledge about the ways poverty affects breastfeeding. We know more about the affluent breastfeeding mother than her low-income counterpart. Repeatedly, the well-established direct relationship between affluence and higher breastfeeding rates has been viewed simplistically, as a matter of education and racial categories. Although many researchers have reported differences in breastfeeding, others report that initiation rates between native-born white and African American women disappear when stratified by income. Still other researchers using aggregated national data have reported that "racial/ethnic differences in breastfeeding exist independent of other socio-demographic factors."[28] These discrepancies raise more questions than answers and provide many opportunities for further research. Viewing SES through compartmentalized categorically based epidemiology does not reflect the complexity of embedded power and privilege within socially situated behaviors.

Another relatively understudied demographic distinction is geography. Recently, Johnelle Sparks explored differences in infant feeding behaviors in urban and rural environments, finding different patterns for urban white and African American women from their rural counterparts.[29] Multiple factors seem to be influential: increased perceived racism, historical trauma, poverty, and immigration status. Decontextualizing identity categories and examining only one or two at a time is easier to measure, more convenient to study, and simplifies complexity. National and local governmental agencies, which have set the breastfeeding research agenda through programmatic and grant funding, drive and perpetuate the use of these methods.[30] Viewing women's breastfeeding behaviors through this lens leads to inaccurate generalizations, negating the inherent interplay of identity categories.

A Matter of Conceptual and Methodological Approaches

Throughout this chapter, I have made references to how both conceptual and methodological approaches have affected breastfeeding disparities research and framed our understandings. Here I briefly examine the paradigmatic assumptions upon which empirical (positivist and postpositivist) research and alternative paradigms are situated. My focus is on the nature of reality (ontology) and what we can know about it (epistemology).

Within the positivist and postpositivist paradigms, reality consists of an objective world that researchers "can describe (or quantify) more or less accurately and more or less objectively."[31] This notion has its roots in the Cartesian duality that separates object and subject into different and independent entities. Viewing the world from this perspective, social relationships and processes exist independent of human interpretation. Postpositivists assume that we can imperfectly understand these realities. Researchers working in these paradigms view race and racism as entities that exist independent of the meanings we make of them. Epidemiologic and quantitative methods, which predominate in the health sciences, are driven by these paradigms. Some qualitative research, particularly in the social sciences, is derived from these assumptions. In Western societies most education is framed within this perspective. Many professional and disciplinary fields (such as medicine and basic sciences) operate nearly exclusively from this perspective. We do not realize how these assumptions shape our understandings because of our familiarity with them.[32]

Following World War II an alternative worldview, which had been simmering below the threshold of most Western peoples' awareness for many years, became widely recognized. Led by European philosophers (Heidegger, Sartre, and Beauvoir), an interpretive paradigm emerged that rejects the notion that an objective reality exists independently from the context in which it occurs. In this framework all knowledge is situated within a social and geographical environment and within a temporal space. Race and racism occur only contextually and cannot be separated from those contexts. From this interpretive paradigm, breastfeeding disparities are viewed as multifaceted, unique to time, place, and circumstance, and knowable only by using methodologies that embrace complexity.

Intersectionality provides a framework which is congruent with these interpretive paradigms. As both a feminist theory and research methodology, intersectionality focuses on the multiple and contingent ways that identity categories (race, gender, class, geography, immigrant status, and sexual orientation) mutually influence one another.[33] Kimberlé Williams Crenshaw, a black feminist theorist, coined and popularized the term in 1989 when discussing why racism and gender cannot be separated into discrete categories or decontextualized.[34] Over the years, intersectionality has evolved into a useful research approach. Its assumptions include the ideas that different components of social life cannot be decontextualized and no one category of social position is more important than another; understanding the relation of these different components is not an additive process and the relational constructs of social inequality are intersectional; and a social justice perspective is implicit, so that within the theory is an activist intention to facilitate social change.[35] "Sorting through the layers and levels of oppressions and privileges and understanding them collectively without fracturing them as additive and separate components are crucial if we are to appreciate fully the shared and unique experiences of women as whole beings in their diverse roles and identities."[36] Examining breastfeeding disparities from this perspective would enable meaningful understandings about racism to emerge.

Although most studies using this methodology have been conducted in the social sciences and humanities, there are a few established public health research approaches that are consistent with this means of examination. Community participatory research methods and social marketing intervention strategies are good examples. The *Best Start* breastfeeding promotion programs have incorporated both of these strategies. Educational materials and intervention strategies are created with members of the community. The *Best Start* program has focused on developing an understanding of the particulars of specific communities, along with incorporating established marketing strategies, and is an approach that has successfully change breastfeeding behaviors in African American and low-income communities. It is a methodology that maintains the inherent complexity and diversity within a specific environment by incorporating mutual respect and voice.[37]

Other methodologies less frequently used in public health also could be helpful in developing a more nuanced understanding of the intersectionality of identity categories. A few possibilities are phenomenology, hermeneutics, feminist, and indigenous approaches. Health science–based breastfeeding researchers need to collaborate with our colleagues in social science and humanities, who work within these alternative paradigms, to design studies that encompass the complexity and nuance of breastfeeding women's lives.

Conclusions

Throughout this chapter I have raised concerns about the appropriateness of using only data gathered using quantitative methodologies to create interventions aimed at facilitating behavioral change. Of course, epidemiology and other quantitative methods provide necessary information to health care and public health providers. I am not suggesting that we abolish this approach; rather, we need to broaden our perspective. In the United States there is a resistance to acknowledging racism within the health care system, the same system that is tasked with supporting and promoting breastfeeding. Coupled with the continued emphasis on racially defining breastfeeding disparities, obfuscating other possible explanatory hypotheses, the contextual complexity of women's lives and their infant feeding behaviors is easily lost. Compartmentalizing and labeling mothers' identities according to outdated notions of racial differences does injustice to mothers and to the fundamental need for meaningful research into the effects of racism on breastfeeding practices and support. It is on this particular point that meaningful discussions of breastfeeding disparities need to begin.

Notes

1. Smedley, Stith, and Nelson's *Unequal Treatment* is the most notable exception.
2. Lounsbury and Mitchell, "Introduction"; Hausman, "Feminist Politics"; Grzywacz et al., "Serving Racial"; Jones, "Moral Problem."
3. Intersecting identity categories are the focus of the theory of intersectionality. Hankivsky et al., "Exploring the Promises." For a further discussion, see Smedley et al., *Unequal Treatment*.
4. Jones, "Levels of Racism," 1212.
5. Pascale, *Cartographies,* 160–163; Van Esterik, "Contemporary Trends," 258–259.
6. Positionality refers to how the researcher or individual is situated within a specific and particular context. Researchers need to acknowledge their power, previous experiences, and values to the reader. Pascale, *Cartographies,* 20–22, 154; Tomaselli, Dyll, and Francis, "Self and Other," 352.
7. Clark-Hitt et al., "Doctors' and Nurses' Explanations."
8. Jones, "Levels of Racism," 1213; Nuru-Jeter et al., "It's the Skin."
9. Beal, Kuhlthau, and Perrin, "Breastfeeding Advice"; Kogan et al., "Racial Disparities."
10. Beal, Kuhlthau, and Perrin, "Breastfeeding Advice"; Cricco-Lizza, "Black Non-Hispanic"; Dodgson and Struthers, "Indigenous Women's Voices"; Hurley et al., "Variation in Breastfeeding"; see also Dodgson et al., "Evaluation of Supportive"; Jones, "Invited Commentary"; Spitzer, "In Visible Bodies."
11. Williams and Sternthal, "Understanding Racial-Ethnic Disparities," S20.
12. Van Esterik, "Contemporary Trends"; Wolf, "What Feminists"; Hausman, "Feminist Politics."
13. Krieger, "Does Racism Harm"; Pascale, *Cartographies,* 25.
14. Pascale, *Cartographies,* 14, 20–21.

15. Green and Darity, "Under the Skin"; Jones, "Moral Problem."

16. Smith, *Decolonizing Methodologies*; Dodgson and Struthers, "Indigenous Women's Voices."

17. Modifying policy, regulations, and legislation are ways that public health providers and others have addressed the issue of institutional racism throughout the twentieth century with mixed success. Only recently have breastfeeding advocates focused on these types of interventions, and the effectiveness of their efforts has not been systematically evaluated. Koh et al., "Translating Research"; Minkler, "Linking Science."

18. Minkler, "Linking Science"; Betancourt et al., "Defining Cultural Competence."

19. Rubio and Williams, "Social Dimension," 10–13; Boulware et al., "Race and Trust," 362–364.

20. Boulware et al., "Race and Trust"; Cricco-Lizza, "Black Non-Hispanic."

21. Williams and Sternthal, "Understanding Racial-Ethnic Disparities," S20.

22. For a more extensive discussion, see Smedley et al., *Unequal Treatment*; Bhopal, "Glossary of Terms"; LaVeist, *Minority Populations*.

23. Limbert and Bullock, "'Playing the Fool'"; Oppenheimer, "Paradigm Lost."

24. The highest breastfeeding rates have been associated with white affluent and well-educated women, and the lowest rates with unmarried, low-income African American women who participate in WIC. See Scanlon et al., "Racial and Ethnic Differences." The interplay between race and education are in Chin et al., "Race, Education."

25. Merewood, "Race, Ethnicity," 1472.

26. Chapman and Pérez-Escamilla, "U.S. National Breastfeeding," 147.

27. Braveman et al., "Measuring Socioeconomic Status."

28. Williams and Sternthal, "Understanding Racial-Ethnic Disparities," S19; Lee et al., "Racial/Ethnic"; Grummer-Strawn et al., "Racial and Socioeconomic," 337.

29. Sparks, "Rural-Urban Differences."

30. Rubio and Williams, "Social Dimension," 1.

31. Pascale, *Cartographies*, 47.

32. Ibid. In Asian societies the postpositivist worldview does not predominate; rather, Confucian and Taoist ontology prevail. For more information, see Nisbett, *Geography of Thought*.

33. Hulko, "Time and Context," 46–47.

34. Crenshaw, "Demarginalizing the Intersection."

35. Hankivsky et al., "Exploring the Promises," 2.

36. Samuels and Ross-Sheriff, "Identity, Oppression," 8.

37. Dankwa-Mullan et al., "Moving Toward"; Ryser, "Breastfeeding Attitudes."

Part III

Medical Institutions and Health Education

Pediatrics, Obstetrics, and Shrinking Maternal Authority

When physicians do not allow mothers to breastfeed immediately after giving birth, when hospitals house newborns in nurseries apart from their mothers, and when nurses feed breastfed newborns formula without their mothers' explicit permission, it becomes obvious that the medicalization of birth and infant feeding impede breastfeeding. What is less apparent is how the historical development of the two medical specialties that interact most with mothers and their babies, pediatrics and obstetrics, has shaped attitudes toward breastfeeding. Since the late nineteenth century, mothers have sought infant feeding advice from pediatricians and obstetricians. Ironically, women began doing this in earnest just as the breastfeeding expertise of these specialists waned.

The first generation of American pediatricians and obstetricians shared a difficult reality: no job security. Although today everyone acknowledges that pediatrics and obstetrics are vital specialties, nineteenth- and early twentieth-century Americans dismissed both fields. When seeking a physician for a child, parents judged doctors' competence by their ability to heal adults. Treating only children seemed de facto evidence of incompetence. Medical professionals and laypeople alike consequently scorned pediatricians as "baby doctors." Obstetricians faced similar attitudes. Most general practitioners attended births as an occasional service for patients and thus tended to view obstetrics as a trivial sideline. Mothers had a similar view. As obstetrician Joseph DeLee lamented in 1903, he had difficulty attracting patients because women believed that childbirth was an event requiring little more specialized medical attention and treatment than breathing.[1]

This disdain for pediatrics and obstetrics would shape attitudes toward breastfeeding. As pediatricians and obstetricians attempted to attract patients, breastfeeding became an inadvertent victim of their efforts. Historians of pediatrics have recognized this phenomenon because change in infant feeding practices prompted public acceptance of pediatrics.[2] When historians of birth practices have studied maternal authority, however, they have understandably focused on the birthing chamber and ignored obstetricians' connection to the decrease in breastfeeding rates.[3] This chapter links the history of both pediatrics and obstetrics to mothers' move from breastfeeding to feeding with formula.

Nineteenth-Century Pediatrics

Medical schools discouraged interest in children's diseases in the nineteenth century. When Isaac Abt, for example, wanted to study pediatrics after graduating from Chicago Medical College in 1891, professors told him his interest would harm his medical practice, marginalizing him among colleagues and parents. In contrast, Europeans had long recognized the unique medical needs of children, and so Abt traveled to Europe to study pediatrics. When he returned to Chicago in 1894 to set up a practice, however, he found his mentors had been right. Mothers would not bring their children to him.[4] Not until pediatricians helped mitigate the nation's high infant mortality rate, a public health problem they often termed "the feeding question," did they enjoy significant respect and clientele.

The feeding question was deceptively simple. If a baby had no access to human milk, what food could the child safely consume? This was a new problem for medicine. Before the late nineteenth century, infant feeding was the mother's domain, and mothers breastfed for as long as their babies needed their milk. In the rare instance that breastfeeding was not possible, families hired a wet nurse or, particularly when a mother died in childbirth, relied on a sympathetic lactating neighbor to feed the baby. If a wet nurse was unaffordable or a neighbor unavailable, the baby died. While death for want of human milk was acknowledged as tragic, no one deemed it a misfortune that medicine could remedy.

This fatalism toward infant death ended in the last quarter of the nineteenth century. As the public became aware of the link between health and the establishment of water and sewer systems, municipalities sought ways to measure the success of this expensive infrastructure. Reasoning that babies were uniquely sensitive to changes in the environment, health officials began using the infant mortality rate to assess the effectiveness of public works projects.[5]

This benefited American babies, 13 percent of whom died before their first birthday in 1900. Infant mortality statistics demonstrated what pediatricians had long suspected: half of all babies who died were dying of diarrhea. The discovery prompted a change in thinking. Perhaps babies did not have a "natural weakness and sensibility" predisposing them to death. If diarrhea was their primary killer, maybe something was wrong with their food.[6]

Changing Infant Feeding Practices

Pediatricians were at the forefront of the movement to lower infant mortality, and initially they concentrated their efforts on convincing mothers to reject cow's milk and breastfeed. The headline of one public health poster distributed nationwide summarized pediatricians' assessment of the problem: "To Lessen Baby Deaths Let Us Have More Mother-Fed Babies." The poster depicted a long tube attached on one end to a cow's udder and placed at the other end in a baby's mouth. Between the udder and the baby, the tube snaked through an unkempt dairy barn, a railroad platform laden with cans of milk baking in the sun, and, immediately before the tube reaches the baby's mouth, an uncapped milk bottle covered with flies. Before pasteurization and refrigeration, the consequences of infants consuming cow's milk were dire. Fifteen artificially fed babies died for every one breastfed baby.[7]

Feeding cow's milk to babies in lieu of human milk was a relatively new practice. In the eighteenth century, mothers breastfed for at least two years, weaning only after a baby's "second summer." Not until then did mothers consider children hardy enough to tolerate adult food without human milk as a fallback, and mothers were especially careful never to wean in hot weather, when food spoiled easily and infant deaths rose precipitously.[8]

By the end of the nineteenth century, however, the habit of breastfeeding for at least two years had largely ended. Instead, mothers commonly weaned their babies at or before three months of age, and many women supplemented their breast milk with cow's milk before then. These practices were so common that in 1912 the *Journal of the American Medical Association* complained that breastfeeding rates had been declining since the mid-nineteenth century, and "now it is largely a question as to whether the mother will nurse her baby at all."[9]

The decline in breastfeeding prompted a public health crisis. In the absence of regulations governing the dairy industry, cow's milk was often spoiled and adulterated. As one doctor admonished at a 1910 meeting of the American Association for the Study and Prevention of Infant Mortality, "Nature gave infants as their birthright mother's milk . . . without a chance for contamination, without 100 miles intervening for the milk man to bring it."[10]

The reasons for mothers' new reliance on cow's milk sometimes varied by class—wealthy mothers hired servants to care for their children, precluding breastfeeding, and immigrant mothers who worked outside the home instructed older children to feed their tiny siblings cow's milk. The most frequent explanation given by women for artificial feeding, however, crossed class lines. Many insisted that their bodies were not producing enough milk, a problem that appeared with the introduction of infant feeding schedules.

Feeding Schedules and Insufficient Milk

Women embraced feeding schedules as the U.S. industrialized and scheduling became vital to factories and railroads. Rural inhabitants, who had never lived by the mechanical clock and who until 1920 were the majority of Americans, found it exceedingly difficult to structure their day around minutes and hours rather than natural events such as the sunrise. To ensure that babies adapted to this cultural development from birth, infant care manuals began to use industrial metaphors to encourage mothers to care for infants by the clock: "First, we must teach regularity, the cultivation of accurate habits in the baby; make a machine of the little one. Teach it to employ its various functions at fixed and convenient times."[11] Women consequently learned to breastfeed every four hours (although never at night), lest their babies not adjust to the industrializing world. These scheduled feedings were the likely cause of women's complaints of inadequate milk, for lactation is governed by the adage "supply equals demand"—the less a baby sucks on her mother's breasts, the less milk is produced.

Few physicians, however, recognized that change in human behavior prompted insufficient milk. They theorized instead that lactation failure had a physiological basis. A few physicians theorized that as children spent more time in school, girls' brains competed with their maturing reproductive organs, portending difficult births and lactation failure. Still other physicians argued that "overcivilization"—in other words, urbanization—forced women to live "unnatural lives," and their bodies were thus unable to perform natural functions like lactation.[12]

Pediatricians Garner Respect

These alarming hypotheses provided long-maligned "baby doctors" an essential task. With women increasingly, and apparently inescapably, unable to breastfeed, pediatricians became the specialists assigned the task of perfecting a replacement for human milk. Almost overnight, infant feeding became a serious medical problem only pediatricians could address.

The word "formula," as it applies to infant feeding, originated in this era. In the 1890s, Harvard pediatrician Thomas Rotch employed mathematical formulas to instruct chemists how to alter the percentages of fat, protein, and milk sugar in cow's milk according to the needs of a particular baby. "Formulas" contained variables that included (but were not limited to) the baby's weight, general appearance, expended energy, physical ailments, and the smell, color, and texture of the baby's stools. Rotch believed that "even slight changes" in percentages—minute fractions of 1 percent—given a change in any variable were "of real value in the management of the digestion . . . of the infant." A significant portion of pediatric training now entailed the intricacies of formula writing. Medical students complained that pediatrics was becoming "terrifyingly like treatises on mathematics or higher astronomy."[13]

Nothing captured the attention of the original members of the American Pediatric Society like the challenge of keeping artificially fed infants alive. In addition to their attempts to "humanize" cow's milk, pediatricians inspected dairy farms, lobbied municipal and state governments to pass pure milk laws, and distributed free pasteurized milk in urban neighborhoods.[14]

Newspapers joined pediatricians in championing milk reform. In 1892, "Scarcely Any Pure Milk" and "Stop the Bogus Milk Traffic" were two of dozens of headlines in Chicago newspapers alone. By the mid-1920s, efforts to clean up the dairy industry had succeeded and the traditional problems associated with substituting cow's milk for human milk had dissipated. In cities like Chicago, due to pasteurization, refrigeration, and the bottling and sealing of milk, infant deaths from diarrhea decreased 84 percent.[15]

The public credited pediatricians for the lowered death rate. With clean cow's milk now widely available, the complex mathematical "formulas" associated with infant feeding became passé even as the medical monitoring of babies became the norm. In stark contrast to their forebears, mothers now considered pediatricians indispensable. Even breastfed babies required medical supervision since lactation appeared to be an unreliable body function.

Breastfeeding became the inadvertent victim of the successful fight to purify the nation's cow's milk. New mothers and younger pediatricians who had never seen babies die for want of human milk presumed pure food laws rendered breastfeeding unnecessary. Only older pediatricians knew better. One of them, noting gratefully in 1936 that his colleagues had abandoned complicated formulas in favor of simpler mixtures based on pasteurized cow's milk, wished in vain that mothers would revert to the "ultimate in simplicity—breast feeding."[16]

Yet with cow's milk now bottled, pasteurized, and refrigerated, generations of mothers came to depend on this venerated product. While cow's milk had once been the threat, now human milk was suspect. One typical doctor warned in 1934, "The fact that the fluid comes from the maternal mammary gland does not make it good. It may be nothing but water." Doctors hailed the cow as "the foster mother of the human race." Breastfeeding knowledge disappeared from the maternal and pediatric lexicon.[17] In relinquishing their infant feeding authority to pediatricians, women became dependent on medical professionals just as those professionals lost knowledge of lactation and the importance of human milk.

Nineteenth-Century Obstetrics

The history of American obstetrics followed a similar trajectory. Just as they initially scorned pediatrics, most physicians and laypeople considered obstetrics unnecessary. One professor of obstetrics noted with dismay in the 1920s that the word *obstetrics* came from a Latin word meaning "'to stand before' or, as a sneering colleague once observed, 'to stand around.'"[18]

Given the disdain, medical schools offered almost no obstetric training. Joseph DeLee, one of the few physicians in the late nineteenth century who devoted his practice to obstetrics, complained of encountering recent medical school graduates who had never even witnessed a birth. One of those graduates recalled that while attending his first birth as a licensed physician, he found a massive tumor blocking the birth canal. Convinced that the baby could not be born and the woman would die, he froze. After the baby arrived safely without his aid, he discovered that the "tumor" had been the baby.[19]

The poor training negatively impacted maternal health, and medical charities stepped in to fill the void. The Chicago Lying-In Dispensary, opened in 1895 by DeLee, kept their clientele's mortality rate at a low .14 percent despite patients who were the poorest women in the city. At .59 percent, the United States had a maternal mortality rate more than four times higher.[20] DeLee's dispensary served two purposes: to provide free home birth care to poor women and to train medical students. Students from around the country paid to apprentice there, and students always accompanied a dispensary doctor to a birth. Admiring European physicians termed DeLee's venture the best of its kind in the world.[21]

In 1910 the American Gynecological Society paid homage to free home birth dispensaries when they concluded that urban medical charities, not medical schools, had been instrumental in training future physicians in obstetrics. Not until the 1920s did the isolated efforts of medical charities become unnecessary as didactics and clinical experience in obstetrics become an integral part of medical school offerings.[22]

The Effect of the Twilight Sleep Movement

While dairy industry reform provided the catalyst for the acceptance and growth of pediatrics, the twilight sleep movement did the same for obstetrics. Twilight sleep, a form of obstetric anesthetic employing elaborate medical ritual, sparked the interest of wealthy American club women in 1914. These activists organized the Twilight Sleep Movement, urging women around the country "to take up the battle for painless childbirth. . . . fight for . . . your sex, the cradle of the human race." The effect of this well-publicized campaign was profound.[23]

With the demand for twilight sleep came a new status accorded obstetrics. Twilight sleep required such intricate protocol that the treatment conferred respect to the obstetrician as opposed to the midwife or general practitioner who had neither the training nor inclination to administer the complex drug combination. As one obstetrician pointed out in 1915, widespread public interest in twilight sleep at long last signaled "proper appreciation of scientific obstetrics."[24]

Hospital-Based Obstetric Residencies

The institution of hospital-based obstetric residencies beginning little more than a decade later ensured that the respect now accorded obstetrics would not be fleeting. As hospitals became the exclusive training ground of obstetricians, the growing number of obstetrician-attended, hospitalized births hastened the view that if women wanted the most up-to-date treatments, birth had to take place in the hospital.

Full implementation of hospital-based obstetric residencies occurred over ten years. In 1921, the American Medical Association (AMA) Council of Medical Education, in response to the alarming maternal mortality rate, appointed J. Whitridge Williams, professor and director of obstetrics at Johns Hopkins University, to head the AMA Committee on Graduate Training in Gynecology and Obstetrics. Williams's committee formulated two proposals that ultimately reshaped views of birth. First, the committee recommended fusing obstetrics and gynecology into a single department in the nation's teaching hospitals; second, they recommended establishing three-year, hospital-based residencies in obstetrics and gynecology to be completed after internships. To implement these goals, the American Gynecological Society, the American Association of Obstetricians and Gynecologists, and the AMA formed the American Board of Obstetrics and Gynecology (ABOG) in 1930.[25]

The ABOG almost immediately announced that only doctors who limited their practice to women could receive their certification. This move, effectively barring general practitioners from the birthing business, secured the livelihood of obstetricians. The subsequent growth in obstetric residencies was swift. By 1935, 48 hospitals offering 104 training slots had been approved for obstetric residencies. Ten years later, 255 hospitals offered 773 positions.[26] Growth in the number of hospital births paralleled the increase in obstetric residents. In 1920 physician-attended home birth was the norm. Twenty years later, only 35 percent of births were physician-attended home births; ten years after that only 7 percent were.[27] In eschewing home births, the practice and sensibility of obstetricians changed; they ceased sitting at women's besides for hours and so lost familiarity with the rhythms of labor and the needs of laboring women.

The insular world of hospital-based residencies further ensured that obstetricians would come to view laboring women as potentially difficult cases in need of treatment rather than mothers to be seen comfortably through a normal physiological process. As one resident explained, the caseload and associated tasks inherent in medical residencies were customarily so overwhelming that "every second you spend being compassionate means that much less time to sleep. So you become very efficient at not really listening to people—just getting the information you need, and shutting them off." This phenomenon proved especially problematic when treating laboring women, for whom comfort and reassurance were often the most important—and sometimes the only necessary—treatment.[28]

Unlike home birth, with its emphasis on asepsis and "watchful expectancy," hospital birth highlighted medical intervention. This new emphasis on pathology rather than physiology occurred just as the ability of general practitioners to influence birth practices ended. With the growth of hospital-based residencies, the practice of leaving most births to general practitioners or midwives and turning over only pregnancy-related complications to obstetricians ended in the United States even as it became the norm in Europe. With birth now in the hands of obstetricians, all births in the United States came to be defined as risky. By 1950 the need for a board-certified obstetrician was unquestioned. Midwives and general practitioners did not seem to have the skill set to handle the ever-present threat of an obstetric emergency.[29]

Conjoining obstetrics and gynecology reinforced the assumption that a common trait of birth was its pathological potential. By 1946, 73.2 percent of medical schools had combined departments of obstetrics and gynecology as recommended twenty-five years earlier by Williams's committee. This link between obstetrics and gynecology ensured that, like gynecology, obstetrics would become a surgical specialty. Gynecology became a medical specialty in the nineteenth century to repair birth injuries caused by prolonged labors due to rachitic pelvises.[30]

Obstetrics and gynecology becoming a single specialty further altered the sensibility of the obstetrician. Although obstetrics and gynecology seem a logical duo today, traditionally the two specialties had contradictory underlying foundations. Obstetrics demanded intimate knowledge of physiology, gynecology of pathology. Their union allowed the pathological focus of the gynecologist to trump the physiological focus of the obstetrician.[31]

The Impact on Breastfeeding

Similar to the first generation of pediatricians who regretted their inadvertent role in ensuring that pasteurized cow's milk would replace human milk, Joseph DeLee, who once famously termed birth a "pathological process," assured a lay audience shortly before his death in 1942 that 95 percent of pregnancies required "only good obstetric treatment." He defined good treatment as management of complications before they endanger mother or baby, aseptic practice, and the presence during labor of a skilled physician who did not attempt to "streamline" birth.[32]

Younger obstetricians trained via hospital-based residencies, however, had come to accept the "streamlining" as necessary. These routines included chemically inducing labor, heavily drugging laboring women, and separating mothers and newborns for much of their hospital stay, all practices antithetical to successful breastfeeding.

Just as they defined birth as potentially risky, the pathologically oriented obstetrician/gynecologist similarly linked risk to the breast. In treating mastitis and diagnosing breast cancer, the physicians specializing in women's medicine came to associate the breast primarily with disease rather than biological function. Largely ignorant of lactation physiology, in their view breastfeeding compounded breast pathology, causing engorgement, mastitis, and cracked and infected nipples. In light of these conditions, breastfeeding did not seem worth women's effort, particularly given the low infant death rate compared to decades earlier.

Rather than learn how to help mothers prevent any problems associated with lactation, the risk-oriented obstetrician/gynecologist advised new breastfeeding mothers having any difficulties to simply switch to formula. Although there was no orchestrated collusion, both obstetricians and pediatricians encouraged women to avoid what seemed to them the problematic activity of breastfeeding. In sharp contrast to just a few decades earlier, pediatricians and obstetricians now deemed formula a safe, reliable choice in comparison to troublesome human milk.

Pediatrics, a long-maligned specialty, found success only after pediatricians discovered lactation pathology. Obstetrics found similar success only after its underlying presumption became pathology rather than physiology. Thus the two medical specialties that mothers interface with most garnered respect by presuming that the female reproductive system is so precarious as to warrant steady surveillance and frequent medical intervention. This sensibility did not bode well for pediatricians and obstetricians becoming breastfeeding advocates.

While infant feeding was once strictly a mother's domain, over the course of the twentieth century mothers came to rely heavily on breastfeeding advice from pediatricians and obstetricians. Simultaneously and ironically, these same specialists lost the expertise they once had in that arena. As lactation became the least understood and appreciated reproductive function by the very physicians who should have understood it best and appreciated it most, lactation also became the most dispensable reproductive function. And formula became indispensable.

Notes

1. Abt, *Baby Doctor*; Ziegler, "Teaching of Obstetrics"; "Discussion of 'The Early Recognition of Impending Obstetric Accidents.'"
2. Apple, *Mothers and Medicine*; Halpern, *American Pediatrics*; Meckel, *Save the Babies*; Wolf, *Don't Kill Your Baby*.
3. Leavitt, *Brought to Bed*; Mitchinson, *Giving Birth*.
4. Abt, *Baby Doctor*.
5. Meckel, *Save the Babies*.
6. Wolf, *Don't Kill Your Baby*, 42–46; Booker, "Early History."
7. *Bulletin* (June 3, 1911); Davis, "Breast Feeding."
8. Salmon, "The Cultural Significance"; Cheney, "Seasonal Aspects."
9. "The Care of Infants: Historical Data."
10. Wolf, *Don't Kill Your Baby*, 42–73; Fisher, "Address."
11. Eaton, "A Few of the Things."
12. Levenstein, "'Best for Babies'"; Clarke, *Sex in Education*; Newell, "Effect of Over-civilization."
13. Rotch, "Value of Milk Laboratories"; Rotch, *Pediatrics*, 231; Brennemann, "Periods in the Life."
14. Miller, "To Stop the Slaughter"; Waserman, "Henry L. Coit."
15. *Chicago Daily News*, "Scarcely Any Pure Milk"; *Chicago Tribune*, "Stop the Bogus Milk Traffic"; Wolf, *Don't Kill Your Baby*, 70–73, 208–209.
16. Poncher, "Relation to Supplementary Feeding."
17. Tow, "Rationale of Breast Feeding"; Kegel, "Milk."
18. Ziegler, "How Can We Best Solve."
19. DeLee, "Motherhood"; Prentiss, "A Report."

20. Tucker and Benaron, "Maternal Mortality."
21. *Chicago Lying-In Hospital Dispensary Second Annual Report*, 5–6; Tucker and Benaron, "Maternal Mortality"; *Chicago Lying-In Hospital Dispensary First Annual Report*; "Report of the Board of Directors," *Chicago Lying-In Hospital and Dispensary Thirteenth Annual Report*.
22. Cragin et al., "Report of the Committee"; Engelmann, "Birth- and Death-Rate."
23. Rion, *Truth about Twilight Sleep*; Wolf, *Deliver Me from Pain*, 44–72.
24. Knipe, "Twilight Sleep."
25. Randall, *Developments in the Certification*; Starr, *Social Transformation*, 356–357.
26. Starr, *Social Transformation*; Stevens, *American Medicine*, 202; "Hospitals Approved for Residencies in Specialties"; "Approved Residencies and Fellowships."
27. "Hospital Grows in Popularity"; "Maternity Department Shows a Great Increase"; American College of Obstetricians and Gynecologists, "Trends in Out-of-Hospital Births."
28. Wagner, *Born in the USA*, 15–17; Davis-Floyd, *Birth as an American Rite of Passage*, 226.
29. Arney, *Power and the Profession of Obstetrics*, 51.
30. Stander, "Undergraduate and Graduate Instruction"; McGregor, *From Midwives to Medicine*, 6, 33, 55, 110.
31. Mitchinson, *Giving Birth in Canada*, 57–58.
32. DeLee, "Prophylactic Forceps"; DeLee, "Mother's Day Address."

New Professions and Old Practices

Lactation Consulting and the Medicalization of Breastfeeding

Professional breastfeeding knowledge in the United States today is embodied by the lactation consultant.[1] Lactation consulting emerged on the global scene in 1985 as a new and highly gendered health care profession specializing in the clinical management of breastfeeding. Twenty-five years later, at the 2010 International Lactation Consultant Association (ILCA) conference, the more than fifty booths in the exhibit hall were a clear indication of how much the profession had matured. On display were breast pumps of different levels of complexity, plastic nipple shields, silicone breast pads, creams, milk storage systems, bras, clothing, pillows, herbal teas, and supplements—all designed to assist parents in feeding their babies human milk under varying personal, medical, and structural conditions. The amount and variety of equipment, technologies, and accessories available to breastfeeding women, and to the health professionals who work with them, point to the growing business of breastfeeding. Though nowhere near the $8 billion global infant formula market, the market for breastfeeding-related products is growing.[2] Most of these items, whether based on scientific evidence or invented out of breastfeeding experiences, are marketed directly to mothers, but manufacturers understand the benefit of marketing to lactation consultants (LCs) as well, in the same way that infant formula manufacturers recognize the advantages of marketing to physicians.

The investigation of an almost exclusively female profession whose expert knowledge is built on a women's health issue deserves a feminist analysis, and this chapter applies a feminist perspective to examining the relation-ship between professionalized breastfeeding support (in the form of lactation consultants) and the medicalization of breastfeeding.[3] Feminist attention to the control and transfer of knowledge, and resulting social constructions, provides the basis for an interpretation of the emergence of lactation consulting, its place in the existing biomedical system, and its role in reestablishing woman-to-woman knowledge transfer. In particular, this chapter focuses on constructions of natural processes (like lactation), and on professionals whose expert knowledge addresses those processes. This chapter also modifies feminist critiques of the medicalization of women's reproductive health that expose issues of gender and power to analyze how LCs simultaneously empower women and contribute to the medicalization of breastfeeding.

The Emergence of Lactation Consulting

Shifts in infant feeding knowledge and power ownership can be traced in two waves. First was the initial transfer from mothers to (primarily male) physicians, well documented in the literature.[4] La Leche League (LLL) had some success restoring woman-to-woman breastfeeding knowledge among certain groups, but infant feeding remained primarily in the medical realm. The subsequent shift from physicians, as well as from mothers, to (primarily female) lactation consultants has been rarely explored to date. This second shift served to remove, at least slightly, the breastfeeding mother/infant dyad from the authoritative biomedical gaze of physicians. However, instead of returning control to mothers, breastfeeding fell under the gaze of a newly constructed breastfeeding expert, the International Board Certified Lactation Consultant (IBCLC).

The profession's emergence in 1985 and its development over the last twenty-five years illuminates the ways in which the profession has been shaped by the medicalization of infant feeding through active appropriation as well as resistance. On one hand, the actions of the leaders in the professionalization of lactation consulting created a space for the new health profession within the existing biomedical system. On the other hand, the existing medical structures influenced their decisions, constrained the process, and affected the outcomes of their actions.

While physicians have been significantly involved in infant feeding since the late nineteenth century, breastfeeding expertise has never been fully claimed by obstetrics or by pediatrics.[5] Although nurses within many specialties (prenatal, labor and delivery, postpartum, nursery, and pediatric) often provide breastfeeding support, many do not have the time to provide adequate support, nor do they have the appropriate training to do so.[6] In fact, studies have shown that obstetrician-gynecologists, pediatricians, nurses, and even midwives often have minimal formal breastfeeding training and knowledge.[7] The professional LC addresses this gap in care, focusing on the breastfeeding mother/infant dyad.

In the 1980s increasing attention to breastfeeding as a national and global public health issue created a welcoming environment for a profession that would specialize in breastfeeding management. But the emergence of the lactation consulting profession represents more than just good timing; it is the result of the "collective enthusiasm" and actions of a group of LLL leaders. The breastfeeding movement can be traced to the mid-1950s, when the founding of LLL reflected a "growing reaction against the widespread employment of physician-directed bottle-feeding."[8] Since then, the breastfeeding movement has evolved into a much larger, and more formalized, global social movement.[9] Among other things, it successfully organized resistance to formula manufacturers, who were using increasingly aggressive global marketing strategies for human milk substitutes. It was out of this movement that the professionalization of breastfeeding support was initiated. Professional resistance to the cultural shift toward formula-feeding as the infant feeding norm is part of a larger cultural and political struggle that continues in the United States and globally.

LLL's informal mother-to-mother emotional and informational support soon became more formal, requiring "special training" to become qualified as an official (and unpaid) LLL representative.[10] In 1979 two LLL leaders, Chele Marmet and Ellen Shell, developed the first professional LC training program in California and founded the Lactation Institute and Breastfeeding Clinic. By 1982 the LLL International (LLLI) board of directors recognized that many league leaders were interested in professionalizing their breastfeeding skills, so they established a lactation consultant program. League leaders JoAnne Scott and Linda Smith organized a panel of health profession experts in 1985 to develop competency standards for safe and effective lactation consultant practice. Since then, these standards have been measured with a certification exam administered by the International Board of Lactation Consultant Examiners (IBLCE), which certifies the IBCLC, the only internationally recognized standard for lactation consultation competence.[11]

The first examination to certify LCs was offered in 1985, formally establishing a new profession. That year, 73 percent of exam candidates were affiliated with LLLI, but by the next year, the number of LLLI-affiliated test takers had dropped to only 41 percent; instead, 50 percent were affiliated with a hospital or clinic.[12] Currently, very few LLL leaders sit for the exam, as the clinical requirements have become more stringent. In fact, today many IBCLCs hold additional licensure or certifications: in 2007 in the Americas, over 8,000 of approximately 11,000 IBCLCs, were registered nurses and over 700 were physicians, and in Australia 90 percent of IBCLCs were also midwives or maternal-child health nurses. Besides having diverse occupational backgrounds and experience, LCs work in a variety of settings, including hospitals, public clinics, physicians' practices, and private practice out of an office and/or doing home visits.[13] The diversity in background, experience, and workplace does not extend to gender, however, as the vast majority of LCs are women.

Some of the LLL leaders who organized the exam also established ILCA in 1985 as the professional association for IBCLCs. Its current membership of over 5,000 primarily includes IBCLCs, but is open to others who support and promote breastfeeding. ILCA's mission is to "advance the profession of lactation consulting worldwide through leadership, advocacy, professional development, and research," but many of the 21,000 IBCLCs practicing in eighty countries are not members.[14] This is partly due to the high membership fees, as well as the growth of (less expensive) local, regional, and national affiliate groups. ILCA hosts an annual conference and meeting (also cost-prohibitive for many LCs—registration fees for the full 2010 conference ranged from $600 to $1020) and publishes the quarterly *Journal of Human Lactation* (*JHL*), the first peer-reviewed journal focusing on breastfeeding. The institutionalization of LC organizations has contributed to the formalization of breastfeeding knowledge, leading to a more exclusionary profession.

The Medicalization of Breastfeeding and Lactation Consulting

Most broadly, medicalization is the sociocultural "process whereby more and more of everyday life has come under medical dominion, influence, and supervision."[15] In the process of medicalization, a shift occurs away from non-scientific types of knowledge based on experience, instinct, or traditional knowledge and toward the more heavily valued, and thus "authoritative," biomedical knowledge.[16] Feminists have often characterized medicine as a patriarchal institution. They claim that women have been the main targets of the expansion of medicine, and they see the female body as a site for increasing technological intervention and biomedical surveillance.[17] From menstruation to reproduction, infertility, pregnancy and prenatal care, childbirth, infant feeding, and menopause, no part of the female life cycle has been spared.[18] In most of these medicalization stories, the woman no longer progresses through her natural life cycle or relies on experience, social supports, or her own body to cope with these events. Instead, medical experts possess the valued knowledge to guide her through these life changes, and her role becomes that of patient, both as seen by others and in how she constructs and understands her own identity.

Medicalization not only impacts the subjectivities of women as patients, it affects women as health care professionals. The medicalization of childbirth has greatly impacted the profession of midwifery, which now requires bio-medical training. While academic training has raised midwives' status and enhanced their autonomy, it has also incorporated them into the biomedical health care system, where they often end up practicing a medicalized model of birth.[19] Unlike midwifery, the much newer profession of lactation consulting was *established* with the intention of being part of the biomedical system. Evaluating the degree to which lactation consulting engages in the practice of a medicalized model of breastfeeding requires consideration of what the med-icalization of breastfeeding means, how it happened, and what effects it has on mothers, babies, and the breastfeeding relationship. Lactation, as a physiolog-ical function, falls more naturally in the medical realm. Breastfeeding, influ-enced by culture, changing social values, and political-economic context, has a much more ambiguous place, and its medical nature is more difficult to characterize. LCs, by (the profession's) definition, deal with both human lactation and breastfeeding, and their knowledge base clearly includes both.

The medicalization of *breastfeeding* is rarely conceptualized as distinct from the process of the medicalization of *infant feeding*, and when it is, a descriptive definition of what is meant by the medicalization of breastfeeding is not provided.[20] Anthropologist Penny Van Esterik describes the medicaliza-tion of *infant* feeding as the "expropriation by health professionals of the power of mothers and other caretakers to determine the best feeding pattern of infants for maintaining maximum health."[21] The medicalization of infant feeding, then, involves infant nutrition regardless of method or substance, and it encompasses the regulation of feeding schedules and the prescribing of human milk substitutes among other things. The medicalization of *breast*feed-ing involves medical intervention related to the feeding of human milk and includes at least three main interrelated aspects that have developed over the last 120 years, and with which LCs are involved today: professional or expert management; technological developments and interventions; and increasing scientific and medical research into breastfeeding and human milk.

Of course, medical conditions associated with breastfeeding do exist, and health problems associated with lactation should not be trivialized. Clinical and medical knowledge, scientific evidence, interventions, and technologies help us understand human lactation and assist mothers in overcoming prob-lems. It is important, however, to understand the socially and culturally constructed nature of the medicalization process through which breastfeeding is traveling, and to move toward a more specific, consistent definition of what we mean when we use the phrase "medicalization of breastfeeding."

Professional or Expert Management

The increasing role of medical practitioners in the supervision and monitoring of infant feeding contributed to the medicalization of breastfeeding. Through the medicalization process, breastfeeding has come to be "perceived as a mechanistic process, liable to breakdown but which could also be medically controlled" by health professionals who apply a medical model in providing care.[22] Having created a space for themselves in the health care system, LCs have had to adopt certain established biomedical norms to be accepted as legitimate health professionals. Indeed, the term "lactation management . . . was chosen in order to attract the attention of the largely male body of physicians whose lack of understanding and interest in breastfeeding has in the past half century only been surpassed by their power over it." The definition of "management" has to do with control, and thus using "management" in the context of breastfeeding support locates control with the health professional rather than with the mother.[23]

LCs, by virtue of their expert knowledge, take on an authoritative role. According to Palmer and Kemp, "ILCA . . . has tried to raise the profile of breastfeeding by . . . professionalizing support of the mother. The very existence of a 'professional' supporter motivates the expectation from clients for the mystique of complex information."[24] The LC's authority to label conditions (though not to diagnose) has both positive and negative implications. On the positive side, conceptualizing breastfeeding challenges as medically defined problems allows blame to be diverted from the mother. However, the LC's expert role changes the understanding and experience of breastfeeding. When a breastfeeding mother interacts with an LC, she assumes a patient role— her identity is no longer just "breastfeeding mother," but also "medically monitored patient."

Although LCs work primarily within the biomedical health care system with individual clients and have a clinical-based training, their maternalist roots and mother-centered philosophy of care place them in a unique position to bridge medicine and public health. LCs do not fully accept the system's existing culture; instead, they take a more holistic and humanistic approach to providing care than physicians, and they attempt to keep their care focused on the mother's choice. LCs uphold the primary underlying goal of empowerment of women to initiate and maintain breastfeeding, although this goal can conflict with the patient role that the breastfeeding mother assumes.[25] The lactation consulting profession's location both inside and outside the biomedical structure has led to a sort of identity "crisis" within the profession, since the professional identity of LCs "combines (sometimes uneasily) medical science and maternalist wisdom, formal expertise and respect for women's embodied experience."[26]

Technological Developments and Interventions

The medicalization of childbirth is partly characterized by the use of technological interventions, and so is the medicalization of breastfeeding, albeit to a lesser degree. Breastfeeding is still relatively low tech, but new technologies are currently being developed. For example, ultrasound is now being used to investigate the pathology of the lactating breast and to better understand human milk production and supply, and a controversial home test for the detection of alcohol in milk appeared on the market several years ago. Highly sensitive scales with "digital readout and computerized integration to account for infant movement" are used in infant test weighing; these pre- and postfeed weights are used to measure milk production and determine the amount of milk ingested.[27] Societal and structural changes that have created barriers to breastfeeding for many Western mothers have also encouraged technological developments. Breast pumps, for example, are marketed to women as an opportunity to continue providing milk after new mothers return to work.

With the development of scales, pumps, nipple shields, breast milk tests, and storage systems, as well as specialists who often advise the use of such products to help overcome problems, breastfeeding has become an activity characterized by systematic intervention, and human milk has become a valuable, measurable substance.[28] Part of LC training deals with the "identification of breastfeeding devices and equipment, their appropriate use, and technical expertise to use them properly," and as the products on display at ILCA's exhibit hall demonstrate, LCs play a key role in the use and promotion of these items.[29] Yet LCs do not necessarily control breastfeeding through the use of technology; rather, breastfeeding technology, and growing social acceptance of these technologies, influence how LCs provide breastfeeding support.

Increasing Scientific Inquiry

By the 1970s scientific research on breastfeeding and human lactation began to catch up with the existing and abundant scientific literature on artificial feeding.[30] Increasing scientific evidence of the nutritional, immunological, and other health benefits of human milk may have had a positive effect on breastfeeding rates among certain populations, but some scholars maintain that breastfeeding's shift to the medical and scientific realm has contributed to the decline of breastfeeding (particularly its duration).[31] The construction of human milk as a product to be studied separates the milk from the breastfeeding relationship and allows it to be monitored, measured, and even commodified.[32] As existing evidence on the many health benefits of breastfeeding continues to accumulate, so does the biomedical discourse concerning breastfeeding support and public health messaging.

The increasing scientific evidence regarding breastfeeding impacts the practice of LCs. For lactation consulting, as in other health professions, evidence-based knowledge has become the gold standard, and controlled experimental research designs are most valued.[33] Indeed, much of *JHL*'s content is clinical, evidence-based research. As this type of knowledge increases, and LCs both utilize and contribute to it, the medicalized approach to and understanding of breastfeeding increases. The profession takes a primarily clinical and scientific approach to resolving breastfeeding issues. This is reflected in the current IBLCE exam blueprint, which contains thirteen disciplinary areas, seven of which focus on medical domains (anatomy, physiology and endocrinology, nutrition and biochemistry, immunology and infectious diseases, pathology, pharmacology and toxicology, and growth parameters and developmental milestones). Two additional categories are technology related (breastfeeding technology and equipment, techniques).[34]

Lactation Consulting and Public Health

As breastfeeding supporters, promoters, activists, lobbyists, clinicians, experts, researchers, and policy leaders, professional lactation consultants have an important role in meeting the public health goals of breastfeeding promotion, protection, and support. The relationship between lactation consulting and the medicalization of breastfeeding, and the profession's position between medicine and public health, have implications for public health approaches to breastfeeding that can be explored by examining public health breastfeeding goals, policies, and women's ability to meet these goals.

The setting in which an LC works has implications for practice as well as for her ability to contribute to public health goals. LCs who practice in the medicalized context of a hospital have a different experience and provide a different type of care than private practice LCs who do home visits and work outside of formal medical institutions.[35] Hospital culture is regulated in terms of time, process, and function, which constrain LC practice, and hospital policies can limit the LC's role as a breastfeeding supporter.[36] Breastfeeding care provided in the hospital setting may contribute to increasing rates of breast-feeding initiation, but it does little to impact duration or exclusivity, which has implications for *Healthy People 2020* target goals. Private practice LCs, who work in nonmedical settings and do home visits, must charge set or hourly fees and are thus often limited to serving women who can afford their services. Women who are least likely to breastfeed—and perhaps have the most to ben-efit from LC assistance—are more likely to be minority, low-income, young, and less educated, and they often cannot access or afford LC services once they leave the hospital after childbirth. Lactation consultant visits are seldom cov-ered by health insurance, and many women are uninsured or underinsured anyway. LCs who work in WIC clinics fill in this gap to a degree, but they compete with free infant formula supplied to mothers who do not breastfeed. Such conditions constrain the ability of LCs to contribute to the public health goal of reducing health disparities by increasing the proportion of mothers who breastfeed their babies. Even if every mother had access to an IBCLC, the differences in the type of support provided (including the level of medicalized care) result in variability in the quality and equity of care.

The medicalization of breastfeeding has not been confined to medical practice and practitioners. Breastfeeding promotion, support, and protection have become public health priorities at national and global levels, beginning in 1981 with a series of World Health Organization (WHO) and UNICEF-led global initiatives. Breastfeeding promotion efforts, such as the U.S. National Breastfeeding Awareness Campaign, rely on the "discourses of scientific medicine."[37] The increasing prevalence of HIV has stimulated a new set of global infant feeding guidelines to protect infants from transmission through breastfeeding. LCs play a role in these national and international campaigns and projects, demonstrated by ILCA's participation in the development of breastfeeding policies with WHO, UNICEF, and the U.S. national breastfeeding committee.[38]

Women have themselves contributed to the medicalization of breastfeed-ing. In trying to meet mothering standards suggested by public health messages as well as breastfeeding recommendations set forth by the medical community, middle-class mothers have constructed breastfeeding as a "body-management project" that necessitates seeking professional help and purchasing supplies in order to be successful. Some mothers seek professional assistance with breast-feeding challenges in response to a lack of experiential knowledge and social support networks, or participate in the commoditization of breastfeeding technologies by purchasing breast pumps, special bras, and other gadgets to cope with certain cultural norms and structural realities. Often, rather than relying on embodied knowledge or mobilizing social networks, women seek the expertise of an LC to ease insecurities about technique or milk production and *not* for medical reasons. This reliance on LCs for their expert knowledge regarding nonmedical issues reflects a societal inclination toward medicalized breastfeeding, in which many mothers "construct the lactating body as a carefully managed site, and breast-feeding as a project—a task to be researched, planned, implemented, and assessed, with reliance on expert knowledge, professional advice, and consumption."[39]

Linking the processes of medicalization (of breastfeeding) and professionalization (of lactation consulting) helps us to understand how lactation consulting has both resisted and appropriated the dominant biomedical discourse and how it has become a legitimate health profession in the eyes of medical professionals, public health practitioners, and breastfeeding mothers. When recognized, the tensions embodied in the profession can operate as a system of checks and balances. Even if LCs contribute to the medicalization of breast-feeding, often working in a medicalized context, their maternalist roots and woman-centered philosophy of care allow them to think about breastfeeding in a broader, even feminist way—as a woman's right, a valued role, and a cultural issue that challenges women. The goal of providing care that empowers women might conflict with an LC's role as a breastfeeding expert; but in the broader cultural context of medicalized childbirth and breastfeeding support, empowerment might be achieved more successfully by an LC than by other health professionals more deeply embedded in the biomedical system. As well, such professional tensions allow LCs to "use medicalization for genuine empowerment."[40]

Notes

1. In this chapter, I focus on the IBCLC as the highest credential available in lactation consulting and use LC and IBCLC interchangeably.
2. See Kaminis, "Growing Boost for Baby Formula," for market figure.
3. Though the growing profession is global in its design and reach (according to Gross's "Statistical Report," the 2010 certification exam was administered in fourteen languages across forty-six countries and territories), nearly half of all IBCLCs in the world practice in the United States. This chapter's focus is on the United States.
4. Apple, "To Be Used"; Hausman, *Mother's Milk*; Meckel, *Save the Babies*; Starr, *Social Transformation*; Wolf, *Don't Kill Your Baby*; Wright, "Babyhood."
5. See Wolf, this volume.
6. Auerbach, "Role of the Nurse"; Coreil et al., "Health Professionals"; Meckel, *Save the Babies*; Mulford, "Swimming Upstream"; Wolf, *Don't Kill Your Baby*.
7. Anderson and Geden, "Nurses' Knowledge"; Cantrill, Creedy, and Cooke, "Australian Study"; Creedy, Cantrill, and Cooke, "Assessing Midwives"; Dykes,

Breastfeeding in Hospital; Freed et al., "Breast-feeding Education"; Hellings and Howe, "Assessment"; Marshall, Renfrew, and Godfrey, "Using Evidence"; Nakar et al., "Attitudes and Knowledge"; Patton et al., "Nurses' Attitudes."

8. Apple, *Mothers and Medicine*, 177.
9. Van Esterik, "Contemporary Trends."
10. La Leche League International, *The Womanly Art of Breastfeeding*, 390.
11. Bailey, "ILCA"; Marmet and Shell, "New Lactation Professional"; Countryman, Roibal, and Scott, "LLL Leader"; International Board of Lactation Consultant Examiners, "Facts and Figures."
12. Riordan and Auerbach, "Lactation Consultant."
13. Carroll and Reiger, "Fluid Experts"; International Board of Lactation Consultant Examiners, "Facts and Figures."
14. International Board of Lactation Consultant Examiners, "Number of IBCLCs"; International Lactation Consultant Association, "Mission and Vision."
15. Zola, *Socio-Medical Inquiries*, 295.
16. Jordan, *Birth in Four Cultures*, uses the term "authoritative knowledge" to describe socially legitimized knowledge systems that devalue systems and reflect power relationships.
17. Ehrenreich and English, *Witches, Midwives and Nurses;* Lock, "Situating Women."
18. Apple, "Medicalization of Infant Feeding"; Barker, "Ship upon a Stormy Sea"; Browner and Press, "Production of Authoritative Knowledge"; Davis-Floyd, *Birth as an American Rite*, "Mutual Accommodation"; Fraser, "Modern Bodies"; Furth and Shu-yueh, "Chinese Medicine"; Georges, "Fetal Ultrasound Imaging"; Handwerker, "Consequences of Modernity"; Katz-Rothman, *In Labor*; Lee, "Health and Sickness"; Lock, "Situating Women"; Lopez, "An Ethnography"; MacDonald, *At Work*; Martin, *Woman in the Body*; Morsy, "Deadly Reproduction"; Rapp, "Moral Pioneers"; Sievert, "Medicalization"; Van Esterik, *Beyond the Breast-Bottle Controversy*; Whitaker, *Measuring Mamma's Milk*; Whiteford and Gonzalez, "Stigma"; Zita, "Premenstrual Syndrome."
19. Benoit et al., "Designing Midwives"; Davis-Floyd, "Mutual Accommodation"; Katz-Rothman, *In Labor*; Triolo, "Fascist Unionization."
20. Exceptions include Green, "The Medicalization of Breastfeeding"; Bryder, "Breast-feeding and Health Professionals"; and Hausman, "Contamination and Contagion" and *Viral Mothers.*
21. Van Esterik, *Beyond the Breast-Bottle Controversy*, 112.
22. Bryder "Breastfeeding and Health Professionals," 192.
23. Green, "Medicalization of Breastfeeding"; Greiner, "Infant and Young," 7.
24. Palmer and Kemp, "Breastfeeding Promotion," 12.
25. Waggoner, "Emergence."
26. Carroll and Reiger, "Fluid Experts," 101.
27. Geddes, "Ultrasound Imaging"; Riordan, *Breastfeeding and Human Lactation*, 303.
28. Buckley, "Double-Edged Sword"; Sweet, "Breastfeeding a Preterm Infant"; Torres, "Pumps and Scales"; Van Esterik, "Expressing Ourselves."
29. International Board of Lactation Consultant Examiners, "IBLCE Exam Blueprint."
30. Mulford, "Swimming Upstream."
31. Apple, *Perfect Motherhood*; Avishai, "Managing"; Bryder, "Breastfeeding and Health Professionals"; Green, "Medicalization of Breastfeeding"; Palmer and Kemp, "Breastfeeding Promotion."
32. Dykes, *Breastfeeding in Hospital*; see Fentiman, this collection; Torres, "Pumps and Scales."

33. Wambach et al., "Clinical Lactation Practice."

34. From the International Board of Lactation Consultant Examiners, "IBLCE Exam Blueprint." The other four categories include ethical and legal issues, interpretation of research, public health, and one devoted to the social sciences (which includes psychology, sociology, and anthropology).

35. Literature does not exist empirically comparing the two, but Dykes, in *Breastfeeding in Hospital*, shows how hospital-based midwives experience provision of breastfeeding care. My own (unpublished to date) research, which includes interviews with LCs practicing in different contexts, shows differences in amount of time spent, history collected, patient demographics, etc.

36. Lauwers and Swisher, *Counseling*.

37. Giles, *Fresh Milk*; Hausman, *Mother's Milk*, 21; Van Hollen, *Birth on the Threshold*.

38. Bailey, "ILCA."

39. Avishai, "Managing," 143, 135.

40. Morgan, "Contested Bodies," 115.

Preparing Women to Breastfeed

Teaching Breastfeeding in Prenatal Classes in the United Kingdom

The seemingly paradoxical construct of breastfeeding as a "natural skill that needs teaching" has been examined in detail elsewhere and is evident by the plethora of books written by those who have been successful, giving advice to other mothers reflecting on their own experiences.[1] In these breastfeeding texts, breastfeeding is represented as the ideal way to feed one's baby, and women are encouraged toward making the "informed choice" to breastfeed.[2] But most women learn how to breastfeed from health care workers, many from teachers in prenatal classes. This chapter examines the teaching of breastfeeding to understand if something in the presentation of breastfeeding in prenatal classes contributes to high rates of early weaning.

The inclusion of prenatal teaching as one of the ten steps to successful breastfeeding demonstrates the importance of educating expectant mothers about lactation. As Riordan and others claim, most women decide on how they are going to feed their babies before and during pregnancy.[3] The instructor in prenatal classes becomes a support to the mother, correcting inaccurate information around breastfeeding and offering advice. Prenatal breastfeeding classes educate women about correct positioning and reaffirm that breastfeeding is a skill that needs to be learned, worked at, and supported by knowledgeable others if difficult. Most commonly, breastfeeding information given in prenatal classes is backed up with written information and access to postnatal support.[4]

There is a wealth of research suggesting that the teaching of breastfeeding has a positive impact on breastfeeding rates and women's reported experiences of it. Some research has found that prenatal breastfeeding education increased both initiation and duration of feeding. One study noted how thirty-one out of thirty-five women who had received prenatal breastfeeding support were still exclusively breastfeeding at the six-week mark, compared with ten out of thirty-five in the control group. Others found that those women who had attended such a class were 75 percent more likely to exclusively breastfeed their child. These latter studies note, however, that teaching had no effect on duration rates. Thus, the teaching of breastfeeding seems to have an important role in late pregnancy and early parenting, but its role in improving breast-feeding duration is as yet unclear.[5]

While the need for breastfeeding education is clear, the actual teaching of breastfeeding both in terms of subject matter and teaching style may benefit from further scrutiny. As the data in this chapter demonstrates, there appears to be a tension when discussing potential problems that may arise. The dilemma then becomes: How do we educate women prior to the birth of their babies around some of the realities of breastfeeding, offering them practical strategies to deal with difficulties, rather than only telling them to seek support and guidance? As studies have documented, some women are loathe to seek guidance, regarding health professionals' guidance as an intrusion, particularly in the early weeks of new motherhood.[6]

Support for breastfeeding from medical professionals is varied. Some studies have noted that midwives went against the official breastfeeding promotions, speaking of the need to "survive baby feeding."[7] Moves away from ideals set out by the Baby-Friendly Hospital Initiative were justified on the grounds of maternal care, so that the mother might rest and come to terms with the transition to motherhood. These justifications point to a lack of knowledge among health professionals regarding how to encourage breastfeeding. In the United Kingdom, for example, health professionals have gaps in specific knowledge around breastfeeding, often giving conflicting advice.[8] Louise M. Wallace, head of the Breastfeeding Best Start project in the UK, acknowledges that there are bureaucratic barriers in the support given to breastfeeding mothers.[9] Similarly, midwifery researchers Stephen Abbott, Mary J. Renfrew, and Alison McFadden argue that training and support to breastfeed are done informally by a few breastfeeding "champions." They argue that more support is needed.[10] The form that this support takes can vary. For example, one study found that in rural Australia, telephone-based support helped increase breast-feeding duration.[11] Another found there to be no difference in terms of duration between hands-off advice and physical demonstration.[12] These studies suggest that postnatal support to breastfeed may indeed be more useful than information given prenatally.

This chapter places its focus on the actual teaching of breastfeeding in prenatal classes. These are classes in which parents-to-be learn about and discuss issues around methods of infant feeding, labor, and types of birth. As such they offer a forum to study how advice is given and received by prospective parents. Prenatal classes are popular with first-time parents; in 2000, for example, 64 percent of first-time mothers in the United Kingdom attended such classes. The data for this chapter is a small-scale case study drawn from breastfeeding workshops run as part of prenatal *Parentcraft* classes in the United Kingdom.

The Teaching of Breastfeeding in Prenatal Classes

Much previous research into infant feeding has tended to focus on experiential interview accounts with new mothers, with little focus placed on teaching sessions. By concentrating on the *actual* workshops, the analysis offered here investigates how the teaching of breastfeeding is framed to expectant parents and considers the implications of this framing for public health promotion. In particular, I look at how the breastfeeding teacher, whose role it is to discuss the practice of breastfeeding, portrays the practice of breastfeeding as natural and valuable yet needing support and teaching, while at the same time reducing implied negative concerns raised by participants around the issue of discomfort. I discuss these findings further in relation to a broader consideration of the transmission of public health information concerning breastfeeding, and how such transmission is operationalized at the local interactional level.

In this sense, I consider prenatal classes a method of *empowering* women with the right to breastfeed and to give them a fully informed choice. However, this empowerment is not fully actualized if some women are not fully informed as to the realities of feeding and cease breastfeeding earlier than they had initially planned. Indeed, it cannot be offered as an informed choice if all of the information has not been presented. If at six weeks of age over half of all babies are not being breastfed because many women who initiated have stopped, we need to know if the way that difficulties are dealt with in breastfeeding classes contributes to early weaning.[13] Indeed, several discursive constructions of breastfeeding were apparent in the classes: that breastfeeding needed to be learned, supported, and worked at, and that issues of pain and discomfort were the result of physiological changes and poor positioning, rather than the actual act of breastfeeding itself.[14]

In the first excerpt, we can see an example of breastfeeding being put forward as a skill to be learned, but one that, with practice, will become routine and second nature. "BFT" here refers to the breastfeeding teacher, and Rob is one of the expectant fathers in the class.

> *BFT*: Any skill when you first learn to do something, how hard was it? Those first steps? And I think you have—that's why you've got to be kind to yourself and you've got to learn. You know when you see a small child trying to take their first steps they stumble first, don't they? But they pick themselves up and they have another go. And I think it's perhaps a bit like that with breastfeeding you've got to just think, "Okay, let's have another go," like you'd have another driving lesson. Cause I think the—there's good reason after the first one "I'm never doing that again. I'll just never be able to do this," cause I do remember thinking that my hands and feet and brain couldn't possibly do it, but how's driving for you now?
>
> *Rob*: It's second nature.
>
> *BFT*: It's like breathing, isn't it? It's like walking is for the toddler, and hopefully that's how breastfeeding will become.

The BFT constructs breastfeeding as a generic skill and emphasizes that learning any new skill is difficult in the early stages, the "first steps." The underlying view here is not to give up when things become difficult. The BFT goes on to explicitly deal with this view by using two analogies: learning to walk and learning to drive. She applies these analogies directly to breastfeeding, saying that "it's a bit like that," that you need to "just think, 'Okay, let's have another go,' like you'd have another driving lesson." This formulation is interesting. The BFT instructs the class members as to the kinds of thinking they should be engaged in, and she does this through voicing hypothetical thoughts like, "Okay, let's have another go." The analogy of a toddler taking its first steps contains the explicit message that if things do not go to plan, have another go. Walking obviously is a more natural skill than driving. We all learn to walk, we do not all learn to drive, and thus it demonstrates that natural skills need to be learned before they become part of our everyday conduct.

On the other hand, driving is a mechanical, learned, potentially gendered skill (which may be an attempt to appeal to the men in class) that becomes like "second nature," a learned skill that becomes natural. So here we have two analogies: walking (a natural skill that has to be learned and practiced) and driving (a learned skill that once learned can feel natural). Both of these analogies are useful here for the BFT. The driving analogy appears to be a popular one in breastfeeding discourse, as it enables the BFT to talk around the conflict between "natural" and "taught." When it comes to the issue of positioning, other analogies are used—for example, eating a sandwich to demonstrate how a baby's mouth positions itself correctly on the nipple.[15]

Constructing breastfeeding as a learned skill implies a responsibility for women to seek the appropriate support to carry on if it becomes difficult. The statement from the BFT that "you've got to just think" is set up as a generalized and normative rule that women should follow: if breastfeeding is difficult, have another go and try again. The BFT's formulation of this rule is constructed very much in personal, hedged terms, "I think it's perhaps a bit like that," rather than a definitive statement of fact.

Breastfeeding difficulties arose in the classes as concerns for many of the participants. The question to be managed is why, if breastfeeding is an unproblematic skill, are some participants reporting acquaintances who have claimed that it can be difficult? A key concern, then, that emerges from prenatal teaching is how issues around potential difficulties and problems are discussed in the sessions. This is a tricky issue for the BFT—how to deal with the "reality" of potential difficulties that some women may face without putting those attending classes off initiating breastfeeding. One way to accomplish both goals is to make clear that any difficulties will be transient before breastfeeding becomes established and to outline extensive support networks that the parents can access. Another way, as we see in the excerpt below, is to put issues around perceived discomfort down to poor positioning—something that can be fixed through teaching and practice.

The excerpt below demonstrates one of the rare occasions when the BFT deals specifically with concerns that have been raised about pain and breastfeeding. Issues around pain and discomfort were often brought up by the expectant parents when discussing what they had previously heard about breastfeeding.

> *BFT*: When breastfeeding hurts is when the baby is nipple feeding, when they've got the end of the nipple onto the hard palate so hopefully that helps you to understand a little bit . . . and the other thing is that you get in a hurry and you can imagine when your baby's crying and you just think, "Got to feed the baby. I've got to feed the baby." Now, if breastfeeding hurts, then the baby isn't on correctly. It will feel different and it, for some ladies when the milk actually comes down in the baby's mouth they get what's called a tingling and that's called the let-down. Now not all women feel the tingling, so don't worry if you don't feel the tingling, but lots of women do feel a tingling as the milk lets down. And it's just important you will learn these things and breastfeeding's a learned skill.

The BFT responds to a question about breastfeeding pain by putting any discomfort down to a technical fault—the nipple on the hard palate of the baby's mouth—and follows this with a demonstration using a series of photographs of a feed. Any pain is clearly associated with an error in technique, one that can be rectified by practice and experience, rather than with breastfeeding in general. She focuses on the "other feeling" of let-down, referred to as "tingling," rather than the initial issue of a painful latch, and finishes by reiterating breastfeeding as a skill. By putting any concerns with breastfeeding down to two options—bad positioning and physiological changes—the BFT avoids any criticisms of the act of breastfeeding itself.

The final excerpt is a further example in which pain is explicitly negated as being due to a problem in technique—in this case, a painful latch.

> *BFT*: Because if you don't latch your baby on correctly, that's when you're going to hurt yourself and the trouble is, mums, we just want to do this so much that we stop thinking about ourselves, and the other thing I want to say is that if it hurts, use your little finger and take the baby off, because if there's pain, that is your body saying to you, "The baby's not on quite right." Don't work through the pain. Will you all promise me you won't work through the pain?
>
> *Ann*: It should be a completely painless experience?
>
> *BFT*: It will feel different to anything else you have ever known, and some of you will have a tingly feeling, what they call the let-down. Okay. We've had the latching on and now we're doing the letting down.

Again, poor positioning is identified as cause of pain during a feed. Note that this is put as a matter of responsibility for the mother—"if you don't latch your baby, you're going to hurt yourself." Through this frame, painful or difficult breastfeeding is a matter of poor technique learned by the mother that can be corrected through practice and training. This excerpt demonstrates how problems are personalized to the mother.

However, the BFT is asked by one of the expectant mothers in the room ("Ann") if breastfeeding "should be a completely painless experience?" The BFT's response is technical. As with the previous excerpt, we see the notion of pain changed into something else. Note also the subsequent abrupt subject change in which it becomes clear that this particular line of questioning is shut down and the topic changed.

What these excerpts from the classes demonstrate are tensions evident in the teaching of breastfeeding. On the one hand, the obvious aim of the breastfeeding workshop is to encourage women to breastfeed and to instruct them in the mechanics of breastfeeding. On the other hand, potential tensions and difficulties in breastfeeding do not appear to be fully addressed. A common concern raised by participants in the classes is around the difficulty and discomfort of breastfeeding. The BFT has to manage a tension between teaching "realistic" breastfeeding when discussing potential problems that could arise without presenting the practice of breastfeeding in a negative light. While the author acknowledges that this is a small-scale study, the analysis is telling.

Public Health, Prenatal Classes, and the Teaching of Breastfeeding

As has been noted elsewhere, feminist arguments on rights discourse for all women being empowered to breastfeed do not always prove helpful to the rights of all women, and indeed may position some women negatively.[16] While my analytic focus in the study was very much on the micro-level of how breastfeeding discourses operate within prenatal classes, the implications from this work have relevance to broader concerns of women's rights, social constraints, and the medicalization of infant feeding.

Through the analysis of prenatal workshops we can see themes related to the teaching of breastfeeding. First, breastfeeding is presented as a choice, an informed choice, as well as a natural skill that needs to be taught, with benefits for both mother and child. Breastfeeding is also presented as a choice that needs support and perseverance to succeed. More than this, we see how the BFT negotiates the tricky matter of dealing with potential problems. In particular, there are tensions surrounding discussions of pain and discomfort in breastfeeding. The dilemma for the BFT is how to teach realistic breastfeeding without introducing potential negative ideas about breastfeeding itself. In part, all of these themes are effective strategies for encouraging breastfeeding, and certainly, as the evidence presented earlier demonstrates, such teaching is beneficial in encouraging the initiation of breastfeeding.

In these ways, the main role of prenatal breastfeeding education becomes tied to empowering women to initiate breastfeeding. However, a secondary and important challenge of prenatal classes must be to deal with potential problems so that mothers will adhere to breastfeeding and persevere if difficulties arise. From the analysis of classes here, it is apparent that breastfeeding is actively encouraged and discussed in terms of positive outcomes for mother and child. The focus on technical advice concerning positioning as an answer to all problems of pain or discomfort means that any potential negatives are to some extent glossed over. Instead of directly addressing evident pain and displeasure, there are references to taught nature, perseverance, and support being available if needed. It appears that there is a reluctance to discuss potential problems for fear of women being turned off from starting at all. The emphasis is thus on encouraging initiation, with concerns around obstacles to adherence left to the postnatal period. While such an emphasis might work in some cases, especially if there are levels of support in place to assist breastfeeding mothers in the early days, the large number of women who cease breastfeeding in the first few weeks suggests that the levels of support proffered differ or are not always taken up by mothers.

A more realistic version of breastfeeding may be appropriate. If problems do arise, they are not unexpected and may be more likely to be worked through. As studies have demonstrated, difficulties in the early days of breast-feeding can come as a shock to many women.[17] Thus, the challenge for teaching and preparing women to breastfeed is to find a way of introducing potential difficulties, but also to reinforce that usually these are not insurmountable.

A number of practical suggestions can be proposed for a public health perspective on the teaching of breastfeeding. The main suggestion from the analysis presented here is that the BFT should not shy away from teaching about potential difficulties. More direct attention to actual difficulties (for example, many women have pain with early breastfeeding even when their babies are latched properly) will help women to see that their problems are not mechanical deficits but simply aspects of the experience to be worked through. Only then can we claim that women have been empowered to feed their children and to make fully informed decisions about weaning. In addition, only then have we really armed women with knowledge that they can really use in their own experience.

Obviously "realistic" teaching can only do so much. More support needs to be available to new mothers, particularly in the sensitive period following birth. Advice from health professionals has been shown to differ greatly, along with the health professionals' own experiences of teaching and empowering women about breastfeeding, so more time and care need to be taken to discuss issues with new mothers and to listen to what they think is important. The medicalization of breastfeeding may have contributed to the focus on mechanisms of proper breastfeeding and the downplaying of potential problems as a way of offsetting challenges to the "breast is best" ideal. As new research on "biological nurturing" by Suzanne Colson attests, technical teaching with a focus on positioning is not necessarily the most helpful way for breastfeeding to succeed.[18] Breastfeeding is an experience, not simply a technical skill, and attention to maternal fears, apprehensions, and physical sensations should be at the forefront of the prenatal teaching of breastfeeding.

Additionally, prenatal classes could consider the use of peer education. This is put into practice in some places, but it would be useful if it were commonplace for expectant mothers to be able to discuss concerns in these classes with a new mother who has recently gone through the experience.[19] The BFTs might then be able to discuss breastfeeding in its social contexts, in relation to constraints that mothers might experience (like being in a pressured situation and needing to feed the baby) and thus treat expectant mothers' questions about pain and discomfort in more concrete terms.

There is a reason to discuss proper latch and the fact that breastfeeding should not be painful most of the time. But to ignore mothers' and others' questions about pain associated with breastfeeding is to neglect mothers' real experiences. It is possible that what is really necessary is to split the advocacy of breastfeeding—the use of prenatal classes as a context in which to convince women to breastfeed—from the teaching of breastfeeding. The need to portray breastfeeding as the preferable method of infant feeding leads supporters to downplay the reality of pain for some women, which means that the experience does not match the ideal rendered in the classes. The framing of breastfeeding as a mechanical skill that is accomplished through practice and support thus may lead, inadvertently, to early weaning for a significant number of women. It's time we paid attention to the unforeseen effects of mixing advocacy and practical skills in the prenatal classroom.

Notes

1. Bartlett, "Breastfeeding as Headwork"; Locke, "Natural versus Taught."
2. See Stanway, *Breast Is Best*; La Leche League International, *Womanly Art*.
3. See Riordan and Wambach, *Breastfeeding and Human Lactation*; Sheehan, Schmied, and Cooke, "Australian Women's Stories"; Sloan et al., "Breast Is Best?"
4. See Abbett, "Expressing."
5. Pugin et al., "Prenatal Breastfeeding Skills"; Duffy, Percival, and Kershaw, "Positive Effects"; Lu et al., "Provider Encouragement"; Lu et al., "Childbirth Education Classes."
6. See, for example, research by midwifery scholars Hoddinott and Pill, "Nobody Actually Tells You," for a discussion of women's early experiences of breastfeeding. Carter, in her text *Feminism, Breasts and Breast-Feeding*, notes how some women in the early stages postbirth do not want involvement from health professionals.
7. Furber and Thompson, "Breaking the Rules."
8. Dykes, "Education of Health Practitioners"; Montalto et al., "Incorrect Advice."
9. Wallace and Kosmala-Anderson, "Training Needs Survey."
10. Abbott, Renfrew, and McFadden, "'Informal' Learning."
11. Fallon et al., "Evaluation."
12. Wallace et al., "Breastfeeding Best Start."
13. This is a small-scale study based on four breastfeeding sessions (approximately ten hours of audio-recorded data). Each class was attended by approximately eight

couples. The data was analyzed using discourse analysis looking at the common constructions of breastfeeding in the classes.

14. For example, Kelleher, "Physical Challenges," talks about the experience of pain in early breastfeeding.
15. Wiessinger, "Breastfeeding Teaching Tool."
16. See Carter, *Feminism, Breasts and Breast-Feeding.*
17. Hoddinott and Pill, "Nobody Actually Tells You."
18. Colson, "Maternal Breastfeeding Positions."
19. See Riordan and Wambach, *Breastfeeding and Human Lactation,* 817–835.

Part IV

Roles and Realities

"Are We There Yet?"

Breastfeeding as a Gauge of Carework by Mothers

On my lifetime Social Security record, there are two gaps filled in with zeroes. They mark the years—three after the birth of each child—when I left the paid labor force to be a full-time mother. During these periods when my official record says I contributed nothing to the economy, I produced literally a ton of milk. I was not paying into our national pension scheme, but I was making a lifetime investment in two people's health and development, building human capital.

As far back as the 1930s, econometrician Simon Kuznets wrote that to calculate national income without including the value of care provided by housewives and other household members was to render the national account a less valid measurement of national productivity. In the 1980s New Zealand feminist economist Marilyn Waring criticized the United Nations' System of National Accounts (UNSNA) based on gross domestic product (GDP), because it omitted women's carework, subsistence farming, and the life-supporting properties of the natural environment. Policy makers are starting to get the message. In 2008 French President Sarkozy set up a commission led by three prominent economists (Joseph Stiglitz, Amartya Sen, and Jean-Paul Fitoussi) to explore better ways of tracking social and economic progress and well-being. One recommendation of the commission is to measure nonmarket activities such as unpaid carework.[1]

At various points in life, every person needs care from another person—a caregiver. Babies and young children require care for survival and for normal development. Some disabled people need assistance to manage the activities of daily living, and many of us will need care if we become frail, sick, or injured.

Traditionally women provide the majority of care, and caregiving is expected of women in many cultures.[2] Around the world, women, men, and children provide care to others both for pay and without pay.

Over the twentieth century, feminist writers paid increasing attention to caregiving, an important topic for feminist economists and for writers on gender and social policy. The word "carework" comprises unpaid family and community caregiving; caregiving jobs in the public, private, and nonprofit sectors; and domestic chores like cooking and cleaning, which count as carework when done for recipients who cannot care for themselves.[3]

Breastfeeding is an example of caregiving that puts into high relief the small social and economic value most people in the United States place on carework by mothers. In this chapter I examine how we might make breastfeeding more visible by bringing it into the conversation on carework.

Breastfeeding and Women's Economic Roles

Breastfeeding plays a part in women's seven roles identified by anthropologist Christine Oppong.[4] The focus for my discussion is on the three roles central to a woman's economic life: the maternal (parental), occupational, and domestic roles. These are economic because they involve the allocation of a woman's resources, time, and energy. The activities associated with these roles are the following:

Maternal role	Bearing (producing) and rearing children
Occupational role	Producing goods and/or providing services for pay
Domestic role	Unpaid production of goods and/or provision of services for household use

The concept of a social role has two aspects: activities and expectations. Thus, each role encompasses what a woman does and expects to do in that role, what others expect her to do, and the rewards and/or sanctions that motivate her behavior within the role. Gender beliefs may be expressed through role expectations—what is expected of a woman as opposed to what is expected of a man.

One strategy in women's quest for gender equality has been to draw a distinction between the reproductive activities of childbearing (done only by women) and child rearing (which anyone can do). Child rearing includes education—both practical and moral; supervision for health and safety; and daily care—feeding, bathing, dressing, transporting, amusing, soothing, and settling to sleep. Raising children is reproductive work insofar as it reproduces the human race, but, except in the case of breastfeeding, it is work that does not specifically require a maternal body.

Breastfeeding crosses the boundary between childbearing and child rearing. For months or years after birth, breastfeeding fulfills the feeding, soothing, and settling functions of child rearing, and it requires a maternal body to perform these functions (although not necessarily the biological mother's body). As long as mother and child must stay near each other to facilitate breastfeeding, it is only a short step to assume that the mother might as well take the major responsibility for child rearing, too.

For a variety of reasons, child care in the home is highly gendered. The traditional roles of women in many cultures reinforce child rearing as a gendered practice. Biology strengthens the assignment of baby care to mothers every time the act of suckling raises a mother's level of oxytocin, the "affiliation hormone."[5] Fathers in developed countries now do more child rearing than in the past, but not as much as women. Fifteen- to twenty-four-year-old American women put in about six times as many hours per week caring for children in their households as men of the same age; twenty-five- to thirty-four-year-old women do three times more than the men; and for thirty-five- to forty-four-year-olds, about twice as much.[6] Child care as employment is also gendered.[7]

Yet women with young children are increasingly taking on paid jobs. In 2008, 56.4 percent of U.S. mothers with children under one year old participated in the labor force. This is consistent with economist Susan Himmelweit's description of the changing roles of women in industrialized nations, where "successively the labour market participation rates of married women, then women with older children and finally those with pre-school children have risen." Role conflicts for working parents are a subject of research and media attention, and in 2003 the U.S. Congress unanimously named October National Work and Family Month. Senate Resolution 210 called "reducing the conflict between work and family life . . . a national priority."[8]

Although breast pumps and bottles make it feasible for lactating mothers and their babies to spend time apart, breastfeeding is still a source of work-life conflict for American mothers. Ninety-two of the 167 member states of the International Labor Organization (ILO) have national laws that provide nursing or pumping breaks for lactating employees. The United States lagged behind until 2010, when the Affordable Care Act (ACA) required employers to provide worksite accommodations and unpaid milk expression breaks for hourly workers. By a conservative estimate, this support will help 165,000 more U.S. mothers (less than 5 percent) to sustain breastfeeding through six months every year.[9]

In December 1997 the American Academy of Pediatrics first recommended that babies breastfeed exclusively for six months and continue breastfeeding at least until age one. The National Organization for Women (NOW) reacted strongly to this pronouncement, pointing out how ill-suited U.S. labor laws and workplace practices were to accommodate this level of breastfeeding. Noting this conflict of expectations between women's occupational and maternal roles, NOW called for better federal policies in support of breastfeeding.[10]

Like child rearing, milk making does not fit neatly within the boundaries of a single role classification. Considered as food, drink, and immune protection for a baby or young child, breastfeeding produces goods for use within the household. Considered as a source of comfort, a stress reducer and sleep inducer, breastfeeding provides a caregiving service. These attributes place it in the domestic role.

Lactation, the physiological milk-making process that makes breastfeeding possible, is a normal phase of reproduction that begins soon after conception. Breasts shift into high gear after birth and can sustain production for years as long as there is a continued demand for milk. Making and giving milk is the way any mother mammal keeps her baby alive. Thus, as the final stage in the bodily process of reproduction, lactation is a function of the parental role.

In cultures where wet nursing is a job option for women, breastfeeding is also an occupational role. Slaves fed their masters' babies in ancient Greece and Rome and the antebellum American South. Middle- and upper-class babies have been reared by wet nurses throughout history. Until the late nineteenth century, wet nursing offered the only reliable chance of survival for an orphaned baby.[11]

Lactation can open other doors. A porn actress or sex worker may be able to get better jobs or bonus pay if she is lactating. These are nonmaternal ways to profit from lactation, but there is no reason why a breastfeeding mother could not take on such activities in an occupational sense, either in between bouts of caring for her own child or after her child has weaned. Mothers working in a garment factory in the Philippines took turns staffing a crèche at the workplace, caring for each other's babies. In this occupational role they acted as wet nurses, breastfeeding if the baby's own mother was not free to take a break when her baby needed her.[12]

In a world with human milk banks and growing interest in the therapeutic properties of human milk, a lactating woman is the source of a foodstuff that can potentially be donated or sold. A Norwegian mother bought a new car by selling her milk to a local milk bank at twenty dollars a liter. At the same time, milk is a biochemical substance whose components can be studied or exploited, even patented. Milk is a convenient human tissue for assessing the chemical contamination of the environment. With the development of these uses for milk outside the household economy, lactating women have gained yet another economic role, as a community resource.[13]

Despite its potential to fit into so many of women's roles, breastfeeding has been mostly invisible in the Western world. It was not a focus of second-wave feminism. Breastfeeding rates fell well into the twentieth century, and manufactured formula became the default infant feeding option. Against a background of good public sanitation, relatively low rates of poverty, and access to pediatricians and antibiotics, artificially fed American babies seemed to be healthy enough. But gradually, starting in midcentury, the tide turned. Supported by lay self-help groups like Childbirth Education Association and La Leche League, and inspired by the life-saving value of human milk for babies in poor countries, American women picked up breastfeeding again, but increasing numbers were getting jobs, too.

Women who went to work while their children were infants entered a workplace that was designed for men or for women who could act like men. Lactation was the unseen function of a body part much better known for its power to attract men's sexual interest. If people thought about breastfeeding at all, it was considered a personal child rearing choice, not a public health measure, and certainly not a human right that should affect the structure of work or the relationship between work and family life.

Lactation was invisible in the late twentieth century, and so was the unpaid carework that people—mostly women—were doing to sustain their families all around the world. But unpaid carework was a topic that feminists did want to bring to the world's attention.

Carework Comes into View

Feminist economists and others are seriously examining the work that is involved in caring for others. Care within the family was long taken for granted, especially when people believed that women had a special aptitude for it or a duty to do it. A new term, "carework," signifies the recognition "that care is not simply a natural and uncomplicated response to those in need, but actually hard physical, mental, and emotional work, which is often unequally distributed through society. Because care tends to be economically devalued, many scholars who study carework emphasize the skill required for care, and the importance of valuing care." Careworkers are claiming notice both when the work is done for pay—usually for low pay and without much respect—and when it is unpaid.[14]

Canada has been a leader in giving attention to unpaid carework, starting with the published estimate by Statistics Canada in 1971 that the value of household work in Canada represented 41 percent of national GDP. Surveys and statistics are key tools for advocacy on unpaid work, and since 1996 the

Canadian census has included time-use questions about housework. In 1998 a tax credit for unpaid carework was added to Canada's federal budget.[15]

In 1993 the UNSNA was revised to measure two previously excluded categories of work: *undercounted work*, which includes the work of the informal sector, and *uncounted work*, primarily subsistence farming. Unpaid carework and domestic work were still excluded, but in 1995, at the UN's Fourth World Conference on Women, world leaders yielded to a twenty-year global grassroots campaign, agreeing that nations would measure unpaid work, employing time-use surveys that allow for the recording of simultaneous tasks, as when a parent cooks a meal while also supervising children. The survey results and the imputed value of the work would then be reflected in new satellite accounts, parallel to but not part of the UNSNA.[16]

Carework advocates point out that basing a budget only on the market economy gives an unbalanced view of all the work that is done and the needs of the workers who do it. Sociologist Mary Daly and economist Guy Standing wrote about carework as part of ILO's twenty-first-century focus on decent work: "There can be no 'decent work' agenda in any country of the world where the needs of those providing care to their fellow human beings are neither recognized nor protected. Care work is real work and . . . deserves to be fully integrated into the analysis of work."[17]

Carework differs from other work such as manufacturing because caregiving builds a relationship between the giver and receiver of care. This relationship is inherently asymmetrical, since the person in need of care often has little to offer to the person providing care. It is difficult to increase productivity in carework because adding more people to the caregiver's workload is likely to result in decreased quality, not economies of scale. Sociologist Paula England and economist Nancy Folbre describe caregiving as "long-term commitments or 'contracts' characterized by emotional connection, moral obligation, and intrinsic motivation." These qualities aptly describe parenting, including the breastfeeding relationship.[18]

Some writers assert that the right to give and receive care is equally important as the right to employment. Arthur Kleinman, Harvard Medical School professor, describing several years of caring for his wife with Alzheimer's disease, wrote, "Caregiving is . . . a moral practice that makes caregivers, and at times even the care-receivers, more present and thereby fully human."[19]

Breastfeeding as Extreme Caregiving

Typically, carework calls on the caregiver to provide physical services— bathing, dressing, feeding, and assisting with mobility. Breastfeeding provides protection, food, drink, and comfort by involving the lactating caregiver's body in ways that are both more intimate and more comprehensive than with other types of carework. The physical mouth-to-breast contact between care receiver and caregiver is highly personal, as is the temporal interlocking of mother's and child's rhythms of activity, relaxation, provisioning, and sleep. The physiological function of lactation draws on the caregiver's nutritional reserves, changes her hormone profile and her body shape, affects her fertility and her state of mind, and has an impact, predominantly positive, on her short-term and long-term physical health. These effects go far beyond the usual demands of a caregiving role, even one that involves a deep emotional relationship between caregiver and care recipient. The average exclusively breastfeeding caregiver requires support in the form of time and energy—time to tend the baby, plus about five hundred extra calories in her diet per day.[20] One way to describe the ILO's century-old concept of maternity protection is as an adjustment in a mother's workload that allows her this time and energy.

Breastfeeding differs from other caregiving roles in another important way. Unless the caregiver is a professional wet nurse, she doesn't get paid for her work, nor is her work perceived as having any monetary value. Although she is producing a foodstuff that can be measured, valued, even sold in the marketplace, it is economically invisible. Not even in the first six months, when an exclusively breastfeeding mother is her child's sole food source, does her milk show up in her nation's accounts of food production—unless she lives in Norway.

At the 1973 World Food Conference, Norway proposed "that human milk be included in the food production statistics and reported regularly as such." Two decades later, the National Nutrition Council of Norway began including human milk in their annual report on food production. Knowing that the average baby drinks about 800 grams of milk a day, researchers estimated that the 60,000 Norwegian babies born in 1992 drank 8.2 million kilograms of milk. Ninety-five percent of these babies initiated breastfeeding. Sixty percent were still breastfeeding at six months, and 10 percent at twelve months.

Human milk was "about 1.2 percent of the volume of cow's milk delivered into the Norwegian consumers market." This was considered a significant proportion. Valued at the price that Oslo's main hospital was charging for banked human milk at that time, about US$50 per liter, the milk produced by Norwegian mothers that year had a market value over $400 million.

The authors of the report wrote, "The inclusion of human milk in food production statistics in a country, even though the data may not be very accurate, is a way to make an invisible food visible. In the effort to promote breast-feeding, such data may be valuable, both to record the prevalence of breast-feeding and to bring this valuable food into the public eye."[21]

The blind spot that keeps other economists from noting the value of breastfeeding is especially ironic given the interest that some women have shown lately for exclusively pumping their milk and feeding it to their babies by bottle. Even pumped milk, although one can see, taste, and measure it, goes unnoticed as an economic output, as do the two or more hours per day (input) that an exclusively pumping mother must spend attached to her pump if she hopes to supply all of her baby's needs.[22]

Australian economist Julie Smith has studied the economics of human milk from several angles. Through a study of parents' time use, she tracked the time it takes to breastfeed. She also reckoned the excess costs of hospitalization for illnesses traceable to premature weaning. She estimated the output of human milk in Australia and calculated its value. As in Norway, Smith set the value of human milk at US$50 a liter. While the market price of commercially made milk for babies was considerably less, this valuation underscores the fact that commercial products are *not* equivalent to human milk, because they lack its health-protective features. By Smith's accounting, Australian women's milk production for 1992 would have been worth US$1.9 billion, a sum equal to 0.375 percent of GDP. If Australian women had matched the World Health Organization's recommended breastfeeding rate, the value of their milk would have equaled over 1 percent of GDP.[23]

Smith also noted that while human milk was invisible in the national accounts, commercial infant foods were not. The paradox in this situation is that if women were to breastfeed more—if they produced more food themselves and bought less commercial infant food—the GDP would fall. Smith called this "a ridiculous result."[24]

Economist Diane Elson has said of women's activities in general, "they are often not 'counted' in statistics, not 'accounted for' in representations of the economy and not 'taken into account' in policy making."[25] UN statisticians have asserted that the reason unwaged work and home food production were not included in the UNSNA is the practical difficulties they present for data collection.[26] Yet tools already developed in Norway and Australia could enable any nation that tracks its breastfeeding rates to estimate the amount of human milk produced and the carework involved in producing it. Whether or not mainstream economists' neglecting to account for women's milk production as contributing to the national economy is intentional, the outcome is that breastfeeding's value to families, communities, and nations is only marginally recognized. Since breastfeeding may conflict with women's performance in the workplace, some people conclude that its harm to women's advancement outweighs its benefits for all.

Conclusion: Strategies to Win Attention for Breastfeeding

Breastfeeding can happen anywhere, but chiefly it goes on in the places where babies and mothers spend most time together—out of the public eye, in the dark corners, at home, in bed. If we want people to think about breastfeeding when they make policy, we have to find ways to remind them about it.

In their report for President Sarkozy, Stiglitz, Sen, and Fitoussi discuss the need for a range of indicators to assess social progress and well-being, which could be as varied and as specific as female literacy rate, number of smokers in a population, and degree of overfishing in a fishery. An array of such indicators is called a "dashboard," where, as in a car, the different gauges keep track of a complex system while the car moves ahead. The rate of exclusive breastfeeding can be just such an indicator. It packs into one number a rich collection of information about food production, carework, and community, workplace, and health system support for mothers. The exclusive breastfeeding rate belongs on the dashboard for assessing human well-being.

To emphasize the value of breastfeeding and its place on this dashboard, breastfeeding supporters can estimate the amount and value of human milk that mothers produce in their region and publicize those figures to draw attention to the urgency of lowering barriers to breastfeeding. Ultimately, breastfeeding data show us more than the numbers of babies being optimally fed. They are an indication of the unseen carework that breastfeeding mothers are doing, day and night, awake and asleep, at home and away. Exploring the carework aspect of breastfeeding offers readers a critical way to describe the role of breastfeeding in the lives of women with infants and young children and to advocate for improvements in women's experience of mothering and in children's experience of receiving care.

Notes

1. Kuznets, "National Income," 4; Waring, *Counting for Nothing*; Stiglitz, Sen, and Fitoussi, "Report," 14.
2. Folbre, *Invisible Heart*, xiv.
3. Razavi, "Political and Social Economy," 3; Sloan Work and Family Research Network, "Glossary."
4. Oppong, "Synopsis," 12; see Smith, this volume, for an expanded discussion of Oppong's theory of women's roles.
5. Feldman et al., "Evidence," 965.
6. Sloan Work and Family Research Network, "Questions and Answers"; Krantz-Kent, "Measuring Time," 49. See also Rippeyoung and Noonan, this volume.

7. Fuller, Beck, and Unwin, "Gendered Nature," 300; Tünte, "Man's Work," 1.
8. U.S. Department of Labor, "Labor Force Participation"; Himmelweit, "Can We Afford," 11; Alliance for Work-Life Progress, "National Work."
9. International Labour Organization, *Maternity at Work*, 81; U.S. Breastfeeding Committee, "USBC"; Drago, Hayes, and Yi, "Better Health," 12.
10. American Academy of Pediatrics Work Group on Breastfeeding, "Breastfeeding and the Use"; Toledo and Erickson, "NOW."
11. Fildes, *Breasts, Bottles, and Babies*.
12. Giles, *Fresh Milk*, 171; Fernandez, pers. comm. with author, June 1998.
13. Karlsen and Pettersson, "Milk Record"; McClain, "Banked Donor"; International Lactation Consultant Association, "Position on Breastfeeding." See also Fentiman, this volume.
14. UN Research Institute for Social Development, "Political and Social"; Sloan Work and Family Research Network, "Glossary."
15. PEI Advisory Council, "Women and Unpaid Work."
16. Razavi, "Political and Social Economy," 4–5.
17. Daly and Standing, *Care Work*, 1.
18. England and Folbre, "Contracting," 62.
19. Razavi, "Political and Social Economy," 3; Kleinman, "Caregiving," 29.
20. Butte and King, "Energy Requirements," sec. 7.2.
21. Oshaug and Botten, "Human Milk," 482.
22. Casemore, "Exclusively Pumping."
23. Smith, "Mothers' Milk and Markets," 375–376.
24. Ibid., 375.
25. Elson, quoted in Budlender, "Critical Review," 1.
26. Razavi, "Political and Social Economy," 5.

Breastfeeding and the Gendering of Infant Care

Human reproduction is inherently gendered: women, not men, give birth, lactate, and breastfeed.[1] Domestic work and child care are also highly gendered activities, but not necessarily inherently so. Among two-parent families with children, wives perform about twice as much domestic labor and routine child care (such as feeding and dressing them) as their husbands.[2] Couples are particularly likely to take on gender-specialized roles during the transition to parenthood: women take on the majority of unpaid work in the home, and men spend more time in paid work. Research has clearly documented this pattern, but it has not fully accounted for the gender gap in domestic work.[3]

In this chapter, we argue that breastfeeding promotion and practice seem to exacerbate the already unequal division of child care between mothers and fathers. It is important that breastfeeding advocates and supporters are aware of this "dark side" of breastfeeding; otherwise, breastfeeding will fail to be a liberatory practice for women. Although the division of child care seems to be more egalitarian, on average, among couples who feed their infants formula, we do not think formula promotion and feeding is an adequate feminist solution to this social problem. Instead, we advocate a feminist alternative that addresses the problems of women's subordination more broadly in order to support all mothers with infant feeding.

The Dark Side of Breastfeeding and Father Involvement

Thus far, most research on breastfeeding focuses on the benefit of the practice and of human milk itself for infant and maternal health, the environment, sexual assault survival, and many other aspects detailed in this book. Far less research has examined the ways in which breastfeeding may constrain women. One exception is found in the work of sociobiologist Joan Huber, who argues that ancient patterns of human lactation (feeding infants for a few minutes every fifteen minutes) put women at a distinct social disadvantage. Historically, women breastfed their babies frequently and for long durations and so were necessarily excluded from public roles, such as engaging in battle with other human groups. Freed from the responsibilities of infant feeding, men were able to garner power and political leadership roles in society through their warring and relationships with other far-reaching tribes. Thus, Huber argues, the human need for lactation set a pattern of gender inequality that tied women to the care and nurturance of children and men to the social relations of power.[4]

However, she argues that these gender role differences are neither deterministic nor inevitable, particularly considering that lactation is less constraining in the modern era than it was in more primitive times. Today, mothers no longer need to be physically attached to their babies to nourish them, largely due to changes in technology that have led to safer bottle-feeding— through increased sanitation, breast pumps, and human milk substitutes (formula). Huber posits that these technologies are, at least in part, what led to the rise in women's leadership roles in politics and the military.[5] Thus, biology may not be destiny with respect to family and societal roles, but thus far the solution to the constraints of breastfeeding revolves around bottle-feeding.

Not only is there evidence from comparative-historical studies that breastfeeding has contributed to the gendering of public and private spheres, but there is qualitative and anecdotal evidence as well. Some argue that breastfeeding inevitably leads mothers to be considered the primary parent within the family, and fathers are considered to be a "helper" parent.[6]

In her highly controversial article in the *Atlantic Monthly*, for example, journalist Hanna Rosin discussed her resentment toward her husband when she had to wake in the middle of the night to feed her child. As she writes:

> About seven years ago, I met a woman from Montreal, the sister-in-law of a friend, who was young and healthy and normal in every way, except that she refused to breast-feed her children. She wasn't working at the time. She just felt that breast-feeding would set up an unequal dynamic in her marriage—one in which the mother, who was responsible for the very sustenance of the infant, would naturally become responsible for everything else as well. At the time, I had only one young child, so

I thought she was a kooky Canadian—and selfish and irresponsible. But of course now I know she was right. I recalled her with sisterly love a few months ago, at three in the morning, when I was propped up in bed for the second time that night with my new baby (note the *my*). My husband acknowledged the ripple in the nighttime peace with a grunt, and that's about it. And why should he do more? There's no use in both of us being a wreck in the morning. Nonetheless, it's hard not to seethe.[7]

Rosin is not alone in feeling that breastfeeding led to an uneven split of parenting duties between her and her husband. In their qualitative interviews of fifty-six fathers in the ante- and postnatal periods, nurse Pamela L. Jordan and nurse and lactation consultant Virginia R. Wall found that all the fathers recognized the benefits of breastfeeding prior to the births of their babies; however, after their babies were born they began to express concerns "about the lack of opportunity to develop a relationship with the child, feeling inadequate, and being separated from their mate by the baby."[8]

This sentiment has led those who choose to feed formula to their infants to justify their decisions not to do what is argued to be "best" for infants (breastfeeding) by suggesting that formula-feeding will encourage something else that is good for infants—involved fathers. Many qualitative accounts exist of couples who choose to feed formula in order for fathers to be more involved in bonding with their babies. For instance, in geographers Rachel Pain, Cathy Bailey, and Graham Mowl's pilot study of first-time parents in North East England, *all* of the women who fed their babies formula stated father involvement in child care as a reason for doing so. As one of their respondents, Lisa, reported, "I'm not guilty, I don't feel I should have breastfed. There's lots of closeness when you give a bottle and Sam knows me. He moves his head to my voice and I feel very close. But Tom, can have that too and that's lovely, like I said he's quite soft about it. We can share and that's really nice. We're very happy."[9] In sum, there is a sense from women who breastfeed and women who formula-feed that breastfeeding may lead mothers to take on a larger share of child care duties and may exclude fathers from important emotional bonding with their infant.

The Bright Side of Breastfeeding and Father Involvement

Although there are many stories and explanations for why breastfeeding may have a negative impact on father involvement in child care and father-infant bonding, others suggest that breastfeeding may have no impact on father involvement or even a positive impact. As anthropologist Vanessa Maher has pointed out, bottle-feeding is more fun than other parenting duties such as diaper changing or trying to soothe a colicky infant. Thus, by encouraging bottle-feeding, fathers are not challenged to do the more onerous infant care tasks. Maher writes, "It is interesting that in Western industrial countries, too, many women explain their decision to bottle-feed in terms, among other things, of their wish to share the parental role with others, in particular with the father of the child. They describe this form of child rearing as one step towards a more equitable division of labour. . . . They do not often expect the father to take on other aspects of the parenting role (cleaning and so forth) or to take over the housework to enable the mother to breast-feed. Bottle-feeding is often regarded as allowing a somewhat covert shift in the sexual division of labour, and as involving the father in parenting, by beginning with its most gratifying aspect."[10] Thus, Maher suggests that bottle-feeding does little to change the historical division of domestic work within families, wherein husbands perform the most enjoyable household tasks and wives are left with the grunt work.

Others also challenge the idea that breastfeeding necessarily plays a role in decreasing father involvement in infant care because fathers of breastfed infants take on more responsibility for child care when breastfeeding mothers are expending additional energy and time feeding the infant than they would if they were feeding formula.[11] Not only can fathers perform the majority of child care tasks, but Susan B. Draper argues that breastfeeding challenges traditional gender roles more so than formula-feeding by making fathers' roles essential in protecting the mother–nursing infant dyad. She writes:

> The work of breast-feeding is biologically and emotionally demanding for the mother. Optimally she requires the regular and active support of others who can bring her plenty of drinking water, make her nutritious and filling meals, provide quiet and uninterrupted nursing time by screening phone calls and watching older children, and take the infant away after night time feedings to ensure the most sleep for the mother. . . . While men cannot breast-feed, they can be supportive part-ners to breast-feeding mothers. Not being able to breast-feed does not take men off the hook in participating in childcare, especially infant care. On the contrary, it highlights the fact that they can do everything else required for childcare quite competently.[12]

This is echoed in Jordan and Wall's respondents' voices as well. Although the fathers felt left out of an important opportunity to bond with their babies, they often tried to make up for it in other ways. As one reported, "I change her diapers so much because it is the one thing that I can do that leads to her happiness. When she's hungry, I can't do anything about it."[13] Thus, these researchers argue that breastfeeding can have a positive impact on father involvement by providing fathers with an important child care responsibility that also supports the mother.

Our Analysis

Because of these stories in the academic literature and in the popular press detailing the ways in which breastfeeding may have negative or positive impacts on father involvement in infant care tasks, we wondered which stories held more truth for families in general in the United States. In order to examine this issue, we analyzed data from the Early Childhood Longitudinal Study—Birth Cohort survey. Our main goal was to assess whether fathers in households where babies are breastfed take on more or less responsibility for a variety of parenting tasks compared to fathers in households where babies are not breastfed.[14]

We estimated the difference in father involvement between these two types of fathers at two points in time, when the babies were nine and twenty-four months old. These two time points are the earliest available in the data set and are also theoretically important time points for our analysis. Exploring data at nine months allows us to capture "real time" differences in father involvement between fathers of infants currently being breastfed and fathers of infants currently being fed formula. At twenty-four months, most infants are eating regular food and are no longer fed human milk or its substitutes, so these data allow us to see whether or not the associations we find at nine months remain after breastfeeding ends.

Included in our measurement of father involvement in child care were every variable in the data set that asked fathers about their frequency of participation in their child's care. More specifically, we looked at father involvement in eleven distinct activities: dressing the child, preparing the child's food or bottle, feeding the child, changing diapers and toileting, washing and bathing the child, helping brush the child's teeth (when the child was two years old), putting the child to sleep, getting up in the middle of the night with the child, soothing the child, taking the child to the doctor, and staying home with an ill child.[15]

We found that, on average, fathers in households where infants are being breastfed do less *on every single activity* compared to fathers in households where infants are not being breastfed. Not surprisingly, the largest difference in father involvement exists for the two feeding-related tasks: preparing the

Table 11.1 Father involvement in child care tasks by type of infant feeding, ECLS-B, Wave One (infants are nine months old)

Child care tasks	Currently breastfeeding (%)				Not currently breastfeeding (%)			
	A few times a month or less often	A few times a week	Once a day	More than once a day	A few times a month or less often	A few times a week	Once a day	More than once a day
Dressing	23	40	24	13	19	36	27	19
Preparing food/bottle	24	28	26	22	10	16	22	52
Feeding	20	28	29	24	7	15	26	52
Changing diaper	16	21	25	38	13	16	20	52
Bathing	52	30	13	5	44	33	15	9
Putting to sleep	26	28	25	21	12	25	32	31
	Never/rarely	Sometimes	Often	Always	Never/rarely	Sometimes	Often	Always
Getting up in the night	42	32	17	9	25	34	26	14
Soothing	5	36	48	11	4	27	50	19
Taking to doctor	43	28	15	14	34	30	17	19
Staying home when sick	56	26	10	7	46	28	14	12

Note: The differences between the currently and not currently breastfeeding groups are statistically significantly different for all tasks at the $p < .01$ level based on a chi-square test.

child's food or bottle and feeding the child. About half of fathers of infants not currently breastfed perform the feeding-related tasks on a daily basis, whereas only one-quarter of fathers of breastfeeding infants do so. Large gaps in involvement exist for other nonfeeding-related tasks as well. For example, fathers of nonbreastfed infants are significantly more likely to change their child's diaper and put their child to sleep compared to fathers of breastfed infants. We then included the control variables and still found that the fathers of nonbreastfed infants are significantly more involved in every child care task, except dressing the child, compared to fathers of infants being breastfed.[16]

Finally, we performed the analysis using the data from the second survey, when the children were two years old to see if the effects carried on beyond infancy.[17] Findings showed no difference in the behaviors of fathers of infants never breastfed and the fathers of infants breastfed for less than six months.[18] Nonetheless, fathers of children breastfed for six months or longer remained less likely to (1) put their child to sleep and (2) soothe their child, even after controlling for the demographic and attitudinal variables.

Our findings demonstrate support for the anecdotal and qualitative evidence suggesting that breastfeeding is negatively associated with father involvement in child care, at least when the child is in infancy. The association between type of infant feeding and father involvement in child care does weaken as the child becomes older, but the association still exists for two bonding-related activities. We are confident that the association between type of infant feeding and father involvement in child care is not due to other differences between the two groups (i.e., demographic, cultural, or value differences), because we controlled for education, income, work status, and fathers' beliefs about whether they should be helping out more with child care.

Thinking about the Dark Side of Breastfeeding

Although there are a number of ways to think about our findings, two models emerge most readily. We term the first approach "the optimistic advocate" and the second approach "the formula-feeding feminist." We believe that both approaches are problematic and so offer a third approach, which we call "the feminist advocate." We believe this third approach is most likely to lead to women's liberation.

The optimistic advocate viewpoint highlights the fact that the negative association between breastfeeding and father involvement in child care is not long term in nature. In our analysis, we found very few differences in father involvement when the father's child was two years old. As Canadian sociologist Andrea Doucet uncovers in her qualitative analysis of stay-at-home-fathers, parenting is always fluid, and there are rarely divisions of domestic work that work out precisely fifty-fifty between parents at every moment in time.[19]

Although this picture of parenting seems perfectly reasonable, it does little for the Hannah Rosins of the world, seething in the middle of the night as they exhaustedly feed their months-old babies while watching their snoring husbands. The optimistic advocate ignores mothers' real frustrations with the extra child care breastfeeding creates for them (not the fathers), and, in doing so, does little to improve the practice and promotion of breastfeeding.

Additionally, by ignoring these real concerns, the optimistic advocate may lose credibility with women struggling with breastfeeding and its consequences for family life. Internet blogs on breastfeeding are flooded with complaints from breastfeeding women; often they are counseled to "just plod on." Denying problems associated with breastfeeding, like less father involvement in child care, may lead to the discrediting of the real benefits of breastfeeding, and the alienation of mothers who struggle with it. This is hardly the intended aim of the optimistic advocates.

An alternative interpretation of our findings could be made by the formula-feeding feminists. This group would point to the empirical association between breastfeeding and lower levels of father involvement in infant care. They would likely recommend, as French feminist philosopher Elisabeth Badinter does, that in order to create a more equal division of child care within couples, children should be formula-fed not breastfed.[20]

We do not see this approach as a viable or truly feminist option either, however. First, feminism has been primarily articulated as an ideology that aims to eliminate the oppression of women. Instructing mothers that formula-feeding is the *only* feeding method that will lead to equally shared parenting is not a feminist act. Importantly, as discussed throughout this book, many women experience breastfeeding as empowering. Breastfeeding allows women to take control of their bodies, away from abusive or controlling men, and has the power to affirm women's breasts as life giving rather than as simply sex objects for the male gaze.[21]

But even for the many women who do not take pleasure in breastfeeding, simply promoting formula as a feminist practice does not address the larger questions about who profits from women's choice not to breastfeed. Some argue that formula manufacturers profit from women seeing their bodies as faulty when women give up breastfeeding due to difficulties they experience.[22] Thus, bottle-feeding, at a societal level, can be seen as exploitative of women as well.

Most important, the reason why advocating formula is not a viable feminist alternative is because this does nothing to challenge the structures of male domination that allow fathers to do far less domestic labor than women. Even the less extreme, and likely more common, version of the formula-feeding feminist position that women should be free to choose between breastfeeding and formula fails to recognize the ways in which structural constraints in women's lives make this choice rarely free. As it stands, regardless of which infant feeding method individual women choose, that individual choice alone will not allow us to overcome cultural misogyny. Instead, feminist advocates need to be questioning broader cultural expectations of men to be less directly involved in child care than women, which helps them to maintain positions of privilege in society at large.

Evidence for this lowered expectation for men is that our results show that regardless of type of infant feeding, fathers are not equally involved in caring for their children. For example, although fathers of infants not being breastfed are about twice as likely to report engaging in child care tasks more than once a day compared to the fathers of breastfed infants, only about half of the former report changing a diaper more than once a day and just under half report bathing their infants a few times a month or less. Further, 42 percent of the breastfed babies' fathers and 25 percent of the nonbreastfed babies' dads *never* get up in the night when needed. Our results are based on self-reports by the fathers; had the researchers asked mothers to report how often their partner changed diapers or got up in the middle of the night, the findings might have painted fathers in an even less flattering light.

All in all, we argue that a feminist advocate approach is most useful for interpreting our findings and working toward gender equity, one espoused by scholars like Bernice Hausman and Penny Van Esterik.[23] Past foci of breast-feeding advocates on ensuring the legal right to breastfeed are important but limited because there are no laws that can require husbands to do more child care at home. Because our analysis simply demonstrates what *is*, not what *must* or *should* be, there is great room for social change.

A bridging of the aims of breastfeeding advocates and feminists is needed. This partnership should go beyond public health campaigns exhorting women to breastfeed and feminist calls for formula usage. Rather, public health campaigners need to apply greater attention to fathers' behaviors rather than reinforcing the idea that breastfeeding applies only to mothers. More inclusion of fathers has been advocated by some, but not taken up to a large extent in most breastfeeding campaigns.[24]

Although our findings show that there is a dark side to breastfeeding and the gendering of domestic labor, we nonetheless argue that formula-feeding is not the only answer to this problem of domestic inequity. Formula does resolve individual issues for many women (as it did for one of the authors of this paper who fed both of her sons store-brand formula), but as a feminist platform, promotion of formula fails to address larger structures of inequity that create and reinforce women's subordination. Mothers are some of the most highly scrutinized people in society, and shifting some of that scrutiny to fathers, employers, and a social structure that privileges men might address some feminist concerns that breastfeeding promotion unfairly places the responsibility for the health of society on mother's shoulders (and breasts) alone.[25]

Notes

1. Kunz and Hosken, "Male Lactation." Men have the capacity to produce breast milk, however whether the average man could provide much more than nonnutritive suckling is unknown.
2. Bianchi, Robinson, and Milkie, *Changing Rhythms*.
3. Ibid.
4. Huber, *Origins*.
5. Ibid. Economists Albanesi and Olivetti make a similar argument using econometrics in their paper "Gender Roles." They find that the introduction of formula explains approximately 10 percent of why women's labor force entry increased over the twentieth century.
6. Rippeyoung, "Feeding the State"; Rosin, "Case Against Breastfeeding"; Schmidt, "Gendering."
7. Rosin, "Case Against Breastfeeding," 3.
8. Jordan and Wall, "Breastfeeding and Fathers," 211.
9. Pain, Bailey, and Mowl, "Infant Feeding in North East England," 267.
10. Maher, "Breast-Feeding in Cross-Cultural Perspective," 8.
11. Baumslag and Michels, *Milk, Money, and Madness*; Belkin, "Equally Shared"; Draper, "Breast-Feeding"; Van Esterik, *Beyond the Breast-Bottle Controversy*.
12. Draper, "Breast-Feeding," 261.
13. Jordan and Wall, "Breastfeeding and Fathers," 211.
14. The ECLS-B is a sample of 10,688 infants born in 2001 in the United States. In order to take into account the complex sampling design of the data, they were appropriately weighted using the survey command in the statistical package Stata.
15. We first performed a chi-square test of association between type of infant feeding and father involvement in each of the eleven child care tasks using data from the nine-month interview. Our main independent variable indicates whether or not a father's child is breastfed, where we split the fathers into two groups: (1) fathers with an infant being breastfed at the time of the interview and (2) fathers with an infant not being currently breastfed.
16. To save space, the results are not shown here, but they are available from the authors upon request.
17. For this result, we carried out ordinal logistic regression models. Since the majority of infants were no longer breastfed, we grouped the fathers into three categories as our main independent variable, depending on whether their infant was never breastfed, breastfed less than six months (short duration), or breastfed six months or longer (long duration). We then also controlled for parents' level of education, parents' employment status, father's age, father's race, marital status (married or

cohabiting), number of children in the household, household income, and whether or not the father believed that he *should* do as much parenting as his partner.

18. To save space, the results are not shown here, but they are available from the authors upon request.

19. Doucet, *Do Men Mother?*

20. Badinter, *Le Conflit.*

21. Van Esterik, *Beyond the Breast-Bottle Controversy.*

22. Baumslag and Michels, *Milk, Money, and Madness*; Van Esterik, *Beyond the Breast-Bottle Controversy.*

23. Hausman, *Mother's Milk*; Van Esterik, *Beyond the Breast-Bottle Controversy.*

24. Greiner, "Father's Involvement."

25. Rippeyoung, "Feeding the State"; Carter, *Feminism.*

Working out Work

Race, Employment, and Public Policy

It is simple enough—breastfeeding is the biologic norm, and it is good for babies and mothers. On this point, most would agree. However, like many other relationships in women's lives, maintaining a breastfeeding relationship can be complicated. Many factors influence both initiation and duration of breastfeeding, including the employment of the breastfeeding mother.[1]

Women's employment is also influenced by many factors, including race, education, and economic conditions.[2] Seldom, however, have the factors that influence both employment and breastfeeding been addressed together in research studies, either in the health or public policy literature. In keeping with the Social-Ecological Model, this chapter first reviews the scientific evidence on how employment characteristics, race, and socio-economic status influence breastfeeding levels. In order to facilitate discussion and research, a conceptual framework for the relationship between these factors is presented below. We then discuss each set of factors and how they contribute to explaining breastfeeding rates, focusing on the ways in which they interact to re-create social inequities.[3] Second, we argue that women's emergence into the regular labor force over previous decades created social expectations for working mothers that fit uneasily with public policy, and we discuss recent actions at the state and federal levels to address this disconnect. We particularly highlight the ways in which breastfeeding policy simultaneously advantages some women while disadvantaging others, most often intersecting with socially constructed class and race identities.[4]

Race and Socioeconomic Status

Important racial disparities have been documented in breastfeeding rates, with black women being less likely to breastfeed than nonblack women, contributing to higher infant mortality in black infants.[5] In contrast, Hispanic women have been reported to be more likely than non-Hispanic to breastfeed, in spite of relative socioeconomic disadvantage.[6] Asian women have the highest breastfeeding initiation and continuation at three months of all racial and ethnic groups. Immigrant women also had higher breastfeeding initiation and duration rates than nonimmigrant women, suggesting that acculturation has a detrimental effect on breastfeeding outcomes.[7] Socioeconomic status (SES) is also acknowledged as a variable influencing breastfeeding, with higher income mothers breastfeeding longer, regardless of race.[8] While race and SES are acknowledged as important variables, it is clear that their relationship to breastfeeding and to each other is complex at best.[9] In particular, race and socioeconomic status influence the employment characteristics of childbearing and breastfeeding women.[10]

Employment Characteristics: Structural

Employment of the breastfeeding mother is known to influence breastfeeding initiation, duration, and exclusivity (breastfeeding only, or in combination with formula-feeding). Each of these breastfeeding outcomes is important to consider, as the health benefits of breastfeeding are dose-related, thus longer and more exclusive breastfeeding will potentially increase the benefits of breastfeeding to mother and infant. Interventions to promote and support breastfeeding would differ depending on which variable—initiation, duration, or exclusivity—is being addressed.

Research findings on the influence of employment on breastfeeding vary somewhat but suggest that returning to work outside the home decreases breastfeeding initiation, duration, and exclusivity. It appears that the more hours a woman works (work intensity), the greater the negative effect of employment on breastfeeding. The length of time a woman stays home prior to returning to outside employment also has an effect on breastfeeding duration. The most negative effect of employment on breastfeeding occurs during the first three months after birth.[11]

Women make breastfeeding decisions based on employment characteristics first, rather than making employment decisions based on their breastfeeding relationship.[12] More educated women, as well as women who were Asian or white were more likely to work full time, and more educated women returned to work sooner after birth, particularly if they worked full time.

Sociologist Barbara Reskin notes that occupational segregation occurs not only by sex, but also by ethnicity, resulting in women of color having jobs that pay less and have fewer benefits, fewer hours of work, and fewer opportunities for advancement.[13] Women who work in professional, managerial, salaried, or particularly fulfilling or autonomous occupations are more likely to breast-feed.[14] Mothers in small companies or those who work atypical hours are more likely to initiate breastfeeding, supporting the notion that women's breastfeeding decisions are based on having employment they believe will be compatible and supportive of breastfeeding.[15] Women of color are underrepresented in professional and managerial positions and overrepresented in hourly, low-wage jobs where they may not have access to or the ability to use a worksite lactation program, suggesting employment differentially affects women depending on socioeconomic status.[16] These findings highlight how racial and socioeconomic differences in employment patterns are important factors con-tributing to racial and socioeconomic disparities in breastfeeding.

Employment Characteristics: Psychosocial

Support for breastfeeding in the workplace can positively influence breast-feeding decisions, but it is rarely available. Women who do not anticipate that their employers or coworkers will be supportive of their dual role as mother and worker may opt not to even attempt to combine breastfeeding and employ-ment, or they may experience greater psychosocial stress and role conflict as they juggle these roles. This stress would be in addition to the challenges of negotiating hours, maternity leave, and access to the infant or the opportunity to express and store breast milk. While this stress may motivate the more empowered women to negotiate for a more supportive environment, women with less power may not be able to manage the conflicting demands and may give up exclusive breastfeeding or wean altogether.[17]

For working women, breastfeeding must often be integrated directly into a typical workday. Certain types of work environments or spaces make it more difficult to integrate breastfeeding or pumping. Women who work off-site, have no access to private rooms, spend a lot of time outside, travel frequently, or have limited time for breaks may find it more difficult to combine work and breastfeeding, and it is these types of jobs where marginalized, low-income women are most likely to work.[18] Women who do have a place to express milk oftentimes operate at the margins not only of the workday by taking numerous breaks, but also of the workplace. There is often a sense of banishment and shame perceived by women who pump at work because of their geographical removal.[19] In addition, lower income women may not be able to afford an electric pump and have to opt for manual pumps or hand expression, which take longer and make them less likely to continue.

Research has found reluctance by some employers to promote breastfeeding in the workplace, whereas others indicate they would be willing to take positive steps, such as setting up a private place for the expression of milk, with proper incentives. Those most likely to support breastfeeding in the workplace often already have had some personal experience with breastfeeding, either having breastfed or having a wife who had. Therefore, some sort of government intervention may be necessary to require employers to make workplace changes.[20] To create support for lactation at work, the Department of Health and Human Services has created the Business Case for Breastfeeding, an outreach program that provides information for employers and employees, as well as training sessions for professionals in government agencies or businesses.[21]

Becoming a mother is a developmental process that can be stressful. This stress is compounded by the struggle to balance work and family, which can be further exacerbated by socioeconomic status and racial discrimination, and by employment in a job with less control, autonomy, pay, and benefits, as demonstrated in figure 12.1. Breastfeeding women working in positions that do not provide maternity leave or workplace support for breastfeeding may find the strain too difficult to manage and choose to wean their babies.[22]

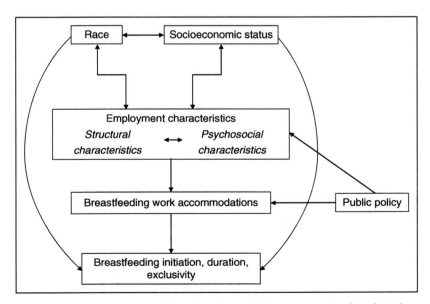

Figure 12.1 Interactive Explanation of Breastfeeding among Employed Mothers

Stress associated with breastfeeding at work cannot be traced just to individual decisions; its source is also socially constructed expectations about women, motherhood, and work. In the next section, we discuss how these expectations shape policy decisions related to breastfeeding at a structural level.

Social Constructions of Gender, Employment, and Breastfeeding

One of the major impediments to a consensus on breastfeeding policy is its social construction—in other words, how society understands, frames, and shapes our beliefs about it. Although medical research points to the health benefits of breastfeeding, any policy alternatives to encourage breastfeeding for working women must be linked to a socially apposite frame and proposed solution. Policy frames must fit with current social constructions of the policy targets, and the logic of the "problem" can then influence the types of solutions considered viable.[23] Comprehensive policy solutions in support of breastfeeding have been hindered by the difficulty that both feminists and breastfeeding advocates have fitting breastfeeding into the dominant strategies women's rights advocates and policy makers have used to advance women's equality: the individualistic economic and rights frameworks, and the rhetoric of choice. Breastfeeding policy is also disadvantaged because it is not clear how breastfeeding fits into the longstanding feminist debate over whether to emphasize women's similarities to or differences from men. The equality (similarity argument) advocates favor gender-neutral treatment under the law, thereby protecting women from discriminatory practices and preventing the emergence of "protective" rules that could render women second-class citizens. The difference argument acknowledges that men and women are biologically different, and therefore sex-specific benefits are required to address issues men do not experience.[24]

One overarching obstacle for promoting breastfeeding is how it fits uneasily with the dominance of economic and rights discourse in the United States.[25] Rights discourse often pits one right against another (for example, rights of the fetus versus rights of the mother). Constructing breastfeeding as an absolute right is complicated by the identification of groups of mothers who may be proscribed from passing along breast milk to their children, including women who are incarcerated, or who do not have full custody of their child.[26] Similarly, the dominance of economic rhetoric focuses on the breastfeeding only for its productive value. Women who want to breastfeed at work are encouraged to sell it to their employers as an economic benefit to the employer—for example, saving on time away for sick children.[27] Framing family policy through its economic benefits can help to build support for such policy, but it contributes to the perception that opportunities to breastfeed at work should be contingent on how beneficial it is to an employer's economic bottom line.[28]

Another obstacle to comprehensive policy solutions is the claim that breastfeeding is a woman's individual choice, akin to reproductive rhetoric. This framing has led us to view breastfeeding as a "lifestyle" choice that need not be accommodated by workplace or federal policy. This framing ignores the social consequences of infant feeding. As the Berkeley Media Studies Group notes, "Too often, the story on breastfeeding is narrowly framed around the mother and child."[29] By excluding the social realities that shape women's experiences, including structural factors discussed in the first section, "choice" rhetoric reinforces inequities by ignoring the constraints on breastfeeding decisions by relying on a masculine ideal worker that does not include children or family influences.[30] As legal scholar Joan Williams notes, "Allowing women the 'choice' to perform as ideal workers without the privileges that support male ideal workers is not equality."[31]

Historically, social policy in the United States defined mothers and workers separately, often assuming a traditional family structure. The ideal mother frame is also prominent in media coverage, focusing on the individual mother's choice to breastfeed, while masking the difficulties of balancing breastfeeding and work, such as unpaid maternity leaves and limited flexibility, because these policies are designed for the typical (masculine) worker.[32] This social construction therefore impedes their chances to succeed because policy has not adapted to mothers in the workplace.

Public policy solutions are often socially constructed in a way that favors some groups while marginalizing others.[33] The equality framework suggests solutions for women as typical workers, while the difference framework idealizes women as mothers, each precluding solutions specifically targeting working mothers. For example, the courts have struggled with the legacy of this debate on pregnancy cases.[34] The equality argument advocates gender-neutral treatment under the law, while the difference argument acknowledges biological differences, favoring sex-specific benefits to address issues men do not experience, such as pregnancy.[35] Lactation challenges the equality framework because it cannot be done by both sexes, so men and women cannot be treated equally. However, feminist organizations are invested in the equality frame, historically working to ensure discriminatory policy is not used to create an unequal playing field for women workers. For example, in one pregnancy discrimination case, several women's organizations filed amicus briefs against special treatment for the woman in favor of leaves of absence for all disabled workers, thereby supporting terming pregnancy a disability and asking that all disabled workers be treated the same, but also not arguing on behalf of the fired female worker.[36] Similarly, until the late 1990s the National Organization for Women had not been particularly vocal about promoting breastfeeding in the workplace and instead focused on supporting a parental leave policy that applied to both men and women.[37]

For many breastfeeding advocates and feminists who favor the position that "women are different from men," pumping at work is not equivalent to breastfeeding a child. They believe that the focus on pumping places focus on human milk as a product and on women as a vehicle, and away from breast-feeding as a relational process. Although survival is an important goal of breastfeeding, motherhood's nurturing role is undercut by simply conceptual-izing breastfeeding as the process by which a commodity is produced.[38] Activist organizations like La Leche League have historically tempered their support for breast pumps because it minimizes the emotional components of the mother-child relationship.[39] Although one of the most active breastfeeding groups, it was also not until the late 1980s that La Leche League took on workplace issues, focusing instead primarily on women who stayed home with their children. In sum, concern over undervaluing the nurturing aspect of breastfeeding has stifled support for workplace policies by those on the difference side, while those on the equality side have not promoted workplace policy because it undermines the case for complete equality by calling for accommodations for something only women require. The persistence of these frames has led to a lack of politically unified feminist activity on breastfeeding, the biggest example of which is the lack of mobilization by women's organiza-tions when formula companies suppressed pro-breastfeeding public service announcements in 2004.[40] Overcoming this divide will be necessary to create momentum in favor of employment policy to accommodate breastfeeding for all working women.

Current Breastfeeding Policy

In this section, we review current policies addressing breastfeeding, and the extent to which they address racial and socioeconomic inequities. Theories of intersectionality suggest that race, gender, and class identities can simultane-ously privilege certain characteristics, and when group status changes, old social constructions fit uneasily with new expectations.[41] We argue that women's growing presence in the regular labor force has created a similar disconnect between breastfeeding policy and social expectations of working mothers. Feminist theorist Patricia Hill Collins notes that "interlocking systems of race, class and gender" create and sustain a hierarchy that reproduces social domination.[42] Therefore, we also highlight the ways in which breastfeeding policy simultaneously advantages some women while disadvantaging others, most often intersecting with class and race identities.

Government policy can have a major impact on workplace polices that facilitate or hinder breastfeeding. At the federal level, the Patient Protection and Affordable Care Act requires that employers provide break time for employees, for up to one year, as well as a nonbathroom, shielded place for the employee to pump that must be free from intrusion. The legislation also authorizes funding for early childhood home visitation services to be directed to high-risk families including low-income households, which could help low-income women continue breastfeeding through counseling and assistance. Employers with fewer than fifty employees are exempt, if they believe it would cause undue hardship. Twenty-four states also have laws requiring workplaces to provide some level of support for breastfeeding employees, many similar to the new federal law. Some of these laws require unpaid break time and appropriate facilities (nonbathroom), while others use less restrictive language, such as "encouraging" or "allowing" employers to provide breaks or facilities. Regardless, many states exempt employers if it creates an unreasonable disruption, making enforcement difficult.[43]

However, for many low-income women these laws may not solve the problem. Federal law does not require that women continue to be paid while on the lactation break, no laws specify that women must also have additional breaks for typical reasons, and only a few of the state laws specify a place to store milk; one exception is Indiana, which requires paid breaks and access to a refrigerator to store milk. Federal law will require significant accommodation on the part of employees if they don't have readily accessible facilities.[44] It may also be that workplace pressures to conform and the temporary nature of breastfeeding may hinder workers from filing complaints, which may result in inequitable enforcement.

Additional breastfeeding legislation has been introduced in Congress. Congresswoman Carolyn Maloney (D-NY), the author of the first breastfeeding bill introduced in Congress in 1998, has introduced the Breastfeeding Promotion Act (BPA) each session since, which would provide tax credits for breastfeeding-friendly workplace facilities and prohibit employment discrimination by adding a provision to Title VII of the Civil Rights Act that includes lactation along with sex and pregnancy.[45] A new law would be important because thus far the courts have not been a favorable venue for successful breastfeeding workplace cases, which have based their claims on the pregnancy discrimination clause. The Civil Rights Act originally mandated women be treated the same as men in employment. The courts initially did not interpret denial of benefits to pregnant employees as sex discrimination, since they were asking for more than nonpregnant employees received (nonpregnant employees include both men and women). To rectify this problem, Congress passed the Pregnancy Discrimination Act (PDA) in 1972, which added pregnancy alongside sex as a protected category from discrimination and required that pregnant workers be treated the same as any other temporarily disabled worker needing accommodations for a medical condition. Pregnancy was reframed as a temporary disability, allowing it to fit well into existing disability law.

Unlike pregnancy, breastfeeding does not easily fit into the existing legal structure, as it cannot be easily framed as a disability. Plus many activists have objected to this term. Without a law prohibiting discrimination specifically for lactation, applying pregnancy law to breastfeeding cases has been difficult because breastfeeding is not a medical "necessity" for the worker. Congress noted the PDA applied only when "medically unable to work" and not for women who want to care for children at home because such care is not a medical need. A handful of cases have unsuccessfully tried to pursue breast-feeding as a medical necessity. In one ruling, the court excluded even the child's medical necessity—the child had a cleft palate, making it imperative for the mother to breastfeed, but the courts did not rule in her favor.[46] However, a recent IRS decision made breast pumps tax deductible because of their medical benefits.[47]

The federal government has attempted to promote breastfeeding among marginalized women, particularly through the Special Supplemental Nutrition Program for Women, Infants, and Children (WIC). The program reaches a significant number of women; in 2009 more than nine million low-income participants were enrolled to receive assistance. Today, mothers who breastfeed receive the most generous supplemental food packages through the program.[48] In 1998, recipients were allowed to purchase or rent breast pumps using federal funds.[49] However, women in WIC have a lower likelihood of breastfeeding compared to similar nonparticipants, a trend that has not decreased over the history of the program, in spite of promotional efforts.[50] Part of the problem faced by WIC administrators is balancing availability of infant formula for mothers who do not use breast milk exclusively without under-mining breastfeeding promotion, even though breastfeeding each infant enrolled in WIC would save money for WIC and Medicaid by cutting the cost of formula.[51]

There are other employment-related policies that may affect the decision to breastfeed. The federal government requires twelve weeks of unpaid maternity leave under the Family and Medical Leave Act (FMLA), which could allow new mothers to return to their jobs after breastfeeding at home with their children during that period, if they work for an organization with more than fifty employees. FMLA provisions are minimal compared to most western European countries, which at a minimum have paid maternity leave, in some countries for up to a year.[52] The assumption in the United States is that working mothers make the "choice" to stay home with their children and therefore should not be compensated.[53] Lack of paid leave restricts breastfeeding options if families cannot afford for mothers to take the full twelve weeks unpaid. This law also does not help women who do not want to take much time off but want to incorporate breastfeeding into their daily work schedule.[54]

Racial and socioeconomic disparities have been documented regarding how much leave time workers actually take. Those most likely to express needing more leave time include women with children, low-income workers, and African American workers; those with higher incomes and whites are more likely to actually have available leave time. Having children does not affect how likely one is to take time off, suggesting those with small children are not necessarily able to take advantage of FMLA.[55] Studies suggest managers may discourage leave-taking, even if the organization has policies in place to support it, and a supportive work environment is particularly important in predicting leave-taking.[56] Women who take maternity leave believe they are perceived as less reliable, committed, and competent afterward.[57] Thus, organizational norms and income needs may discourage some women from taking time off after giving birth, and the anticipated length of maternity leave can influence whether a women attempts to initiate breastfeeding or how long she nurses.

In the United States, there is also no comprehensive policy requiring employers to provide on-site child care or flexible work hours. Longer breastfeeding duration is associated with women able to feed their infants at work.[58] Child care policy in the United States is directed to low-income mothers through federal grants to states through the Child Care Development Fund, or through individual tax breaks, not typically through their employers. Although evaluating child care availability is difficult across states, estimates are that only 15 percent of eligible families are receiving assistance, with half of states having sizable waiting lists.[59] Accessing child care subsidies and accessible arrangements are also correlated with poverty and race.[60]

Although recent legislation has begun to address some barriers to breastfeeding for working mothers, the social construction of breastfeeding policy in many ways contributes to the persistence of social inequities, making it easier for some women to breastfeed than others. Most new mothers returning to work are often subject to unreasonable expectations about their roles as mothers and as workers, but these may be increasingly difficult to juggle as social support and resources decrease. The idea that women can choose to work, or are choosing whether to breastfeed in a vacuum, ignores social contingencies such as child care availability, a lack of paid leave, and the financial capability to take unpaid leave. Maternity leave and child care policies are typically aimed at middle- and upper-class families, which give them greater options concerning the decision to breastfeed.[61] Similarly, public policy rarely requires paid breaks or storage facilities for low-income women who do not have such access at work, and litigation in the states has not yet sided with women trying to balance work and breastfeeding. This situation suggests then that breastfeeding policy helps some women to fruitfully combine breastfeeding and work, but still excludes the less privileged.

Conclusion and Research Implications

Our discussion of breastfeeding and work points to a lack of substantial workplace accomodations for breastfeeding, although with recent progress at the state and federal levels. The theoretical model presented early in the chapter suggests that race, socioeconomic status, employment characteristics, and public policy interact to create a structure that exacerbates racial and economic inequalities in breastfeeding. As noted by Paige Hall Smith in this volume, advocacy can re-create social and gender inequities by making it easier for some women to breastfeed, but not others. Both public policy and employment characteristics may help some women to breastfeed, but often policy solutions and supportive workplaces assist those already privileged.

The link between the social construction of "the problem" at a theoretical level often influences how we think about "the solution." We have attempted to sketch out some of the complexity involved with defining "the problem" and in doing so hope future solutions will incorporate that complexity. While we can deduce that employed mothers of color may be disproportionately affected by employment in their infant feeding decisions, there is little research to support this assertion, suggesting a need for interdisciplinary approaches to the complex factors contributing to the problem. Additionally, the way we construct social norms to frame a problem often eliminates important potential solutions. Activists, policy makers, and academics must do more to intentionally consider the ways marginalized, less privileged women are either ignored or constructed as less deserving of the benefits public policy can bestow, so that all women who want to breastfeed have the opportunity to do so.

Notes

1. Thulier and Mercer, "Variables," 259.
2. U.S. Bureau of Labor Statistics, "Labor Force Characteristics," 30.
3. Johnston and Esposito, "Barriers and Facilitators," 9; Bentley, Dee, and Jensen, "Breastfeeding among Low-Income," 305S.
4. Lorber, *Paradoxes of Gender,* 1–10.
5. Forste, Weiss, and Lippincott, "Decision to Breastfeed," 291.
6. Phares et al., "Surveillance for Disparities," 11.
7. Singh, Kogan, and Dee, "Nativity/Immigrant Status," 540.
8. Grummer-Strawn et al., "Racial and Socioeconomic Disparities," 335.
9. Braveman et al., "Measuring Socioeconomic Status/Position," 449.
10. Browne, *Latinas and African-American Women,* 139.
11. Ibid., 139; Raisler, Alexander, and O'Campo, "Breastfeeding and Infant Illness," 25; Ryan, Zhou, and Arensberg, "Effect of Employment Status," 243.
12. Roe et al., "Is There Competition," 157.
13. Reskin, "Occupational Segregation," 183.
14. Heck et al., "Socioeconomic Status," 51; Guendelman et al., "Juggling Work," e28; Ortiz et al., "Duration of Milk Expression," 111.
15. Hawkins et al., "Maternal Employment," 242.
16. U.S. Bureau of Labor Statistics, "Labor Force Characteristics."
17. Ibid.; Guendelman, "Juggling Work," e28; Racine et al., "Individual Net-Benefit Maximization," 241; Gatrell, "Secrets and Lies," 393.
18. Boswell-Penc and Boyer, "Expressing Anxiety?," 551–567; Galtry, "'Sameness' and Suckling," 295–317.
19. Boswell-Penc and Boyer, "Expressing Anxiety?," 563.
20. Libbus and Bullock, "Breastfeeding and Employment," 247–251; Bridges, Frank, and Curtin, "Employer Attitudes," 215–219.
21. U.S. Breastfeeding Committee, "Business Case for Breastfeeding."
22. Racine et al., "Individual Net-Benefit Maximization," 241; Mercer, "Becoming a Mother," 226; Nelson, "Transition to Motherhood," 465; Schultz et al., "Social Context," 143; Perry-Jenkins, "Work in the Working Class," 453.
23. Stone, *Policy Paradox,* 164–187.
24. Vogel, "Debating Difference," 13.
25. Glendon, *Rights Talk,* 1–17.
26. Kedrowski and Lipscombe, *Breastfeeding Rights,* 117–125.
27. Best for Babes, "Breastfeeding on the Job"; Goodman, "Breastfeeding or Bust," 146.
28. Liechty and Anderson, "Flexible Workplace Policies," 310–315.
29. Dorfman and Gehlert, "Talking about Breastfeeding," 20.
30. Williams, "Reconstructive Feminism," 89–108; Greenberg, "Pregnancy Discrimination Act," 225–250.
31. Williams, "Reconstructive Feminism," 89–108.
32. Dorfman and Gehlert, "Talking about Breastfeeding," 13.
33. Schneider and Ingram, *Policy Design,* 102.
34. Lens, "Reading between the Lines," 40–45.
35. Vogel, "Debating Difference," 11–15.
36. Conway, Ahern, and Steuernagel, *Women and Public Policy,* 168.

37. Galtry, "Extending the 'Bright Line,'" 300–305.
38. Wing and Weselmann, "Transcending Traditional Notions," 257–263.
39. Hausman, *Mother's Milk*, 157.
40. Wolf, "What Feminism Can Do for Breastfeeding," 10–15.
41. Collins, "Moving beyond Gender," 261–284.
42. Collins, *Black Feminist Thought*, 1–50.
43. Vance, "Breastfeeding Legislation," 51–54; Weimer, "Summary of State Breastfeeding Laws."
44. Boswell-Penc and Boyer, "Expressing Anxiety?," 551–567.
45. Goodman, "Breastfeeding or Bust," 146–174; Christup, "Litigating," 263.
46. Ibid.
47. Stern, "Breast-Feeding Supplies Deductible."
48. U.S. Department of Agriculture, "WIC at a Glance."
49. Kedrowski and Lipscomb, *Breastfeeding Rights*, 66.
50. Fox, Hamilton, and Lin, "Effects of Food Assistance"; Jacknowitz, Novillo, and Tiehen, "Special Supplemental Nutrition," 285–289; Ryan and Zhou, "Lower Breastfeeding Rates Persist," 1138–1140; U.S. Department of Agriculture, "WIC at a Glance."
51. Jacknowitz, Novillo, and Tiehen, "Special Supplemental Nutrition," 285–289; Montgomery and Splett, "Economic Benefit," 379–385.
52. Jacobs and Gerson, *Time Divide*, 119–147.
53. Guerrina, "Equality, Difference and Motherhood," 33–40.
54. Greenberg, "Pregnancy Discrimination Act," 225–250; Hylton, "'Parental' Leaves," 275–293.
55. Gerstel and McGonagle, "Job Leaves," 528–532.
56. Fried, *Taking Time*, 39–43; Jacobs and Gerson, *Time Divide*, 100–117.
57. Liu and Buzzanell, "Negotiating Maternity Leave," 330–340.
58. Fein, Mandal, and Roe, "Success of Strategies," 559–562.
59. Vesely, "Child Care and Development Fund," 40–50.
60. Bainbridge, Meyers, and Waldfogel, "Child Care Policy Reform," 780–790; Radey and Brewster, "Influence of Race/Ethnicity," 285–290.
61. Durfee and Meyers, "Who Gets What from Government?," 736–742; Teghtsoonian, "Promises, Promises," 119–126.

The Impact of Workplace Practices on Breastfeeding Experiences and Disparities among Women

Since a majority of mothers of infants are in the labor force, work organizations play an important role in facilitating women's ability to breastfeed.[1] In most workplaces ideal worker notions assume male career patterns and treat women's reproductive activities as deviant.[2] Workplace "accommodations" of breastfeeding mothers are then based on deviations from a male standard.[3] Until passage of the 2010 Affordable Care Act, American law and policy did little to promote breastfeeding-friendly workplaces, thereby leaving it up to the workplace to decide whether it wanted to accommodate workers' reproductive activities, placing the burden on the employees to advocate for themselves or navigate breastfeeding-unfriendly environments.[4] As described by Jennifer Lucas and Deborah McCarter-Spaulding in this volume, differences in workplace flexibility and accommodation for pregnancy and breastfeeding have contributed to well-known racial, ethnic, and socioeconomic disparities in breastfeeding, whereby affluent white women are more likely to breastfeed and tend to do so longer than lower-income women and women of color.[5] The ways that organizations responded to public health's call for "more breastfeeding" before the 2010 law thus helped some women and not others. In effect, organizational strategies for accommodating breastfeeding workers affect the distribution of breastfeeding and disparities in breastfeeding rates.

The theory of gendered organizations argues that organizations themselves are gendered and typically assume an abstract male worker requiring no accommodations for reproduction or child rearing.[6] The implications of this ideal for workers who breastfeed are considerable. Breastfeeding mothers are a significant aberration from the expected behavior, which assumes a nonlactating male body.[7] Because the male body is the unstated norm for the ideal worker, and the law has required no accommodation for breastfeeding, employers, managers, and coworkers often resent having to allow time and space for expressing milk at work.[8] In addition, many managers and coworkers feel uncomfortable with lactating bodies in the workplace and make breastfeeding mothers feel unwelcome. This is partly because the "female body threatens the conventional (male) social order of things due to its metaphorical and material tendency to 'leak.'"[9] Without legal mandates, employers have had little incentive to accommodate the needs of workers who have deviated from the unstated male norm, and organizations have displayed, at best, ambivalence toward breastfeeding mothers.[10]

Many women report that they are unable to continue breastfeeding upon returning to work due to a lack of institutional support.[11] Organizational policy and support has an important influence on mothers' ability to breastfeed that is independent of her desire to nurse or her ability to produce a milk supply, and thus constrains any genuine vision of choice. There are also racial differences in working women's likelihood of breastfeeding that are related to organizational influences that undermine the ability of women of color to breastfeed, resulting in black mothers being much more likely to stop breast-feeding after they return to work than nonblack mothers.[12] White women are more likely to work in jobs where they have private space, scheduling flexibility, and storage facilities that accommodate breastfeeding, thus potentially contributing to known racial differences in breastfeeding.

Prior to 2010 there was no legal mandate for workplaces to accommodate breastfeeding. This situation stems from the legal doctrines governing equal employment opportunity that require gender-neutral, equal treatment of employees, even with respect to reproductive activities where women and men are clearly not the same, and has limited women's opportunities to combine breastfeeding with paid employment.[13] Under these doctrines, breastfeeding accommodations only address women and are therefore not mandated.[14] Breastfeeding is also something that not all women do, as substitutes (formula) are readily available and culturally accepted. As a result, there is a view of breastfeeding versus formula-feeding as just another consumer option rather than an issue of reproductive justice. In this regard, organizational and social policies that assume or require gender neutrality create reproductive injustice and contribute to reproductive inequalities among women.

The 1993 FMLA requires organizations with over fifty employees to provide twelve weeks of unpaid leave, but many women work for smaller organizations or simply cannot afford to take unpaid leave. The lack of paid maternity leave can make it difficult to establish breastfeeding before resuming employment and many women do not perceive that the choice to breastfeed is available because of lack of workplace accommodation. Women who return to paid employment soon after giving birth often experience role incompatibility when they try to continue breastfeeding and fulfill employment roles.[15]

Despite this ambivalence, some mothers successfully combine employment with breastfeeding, a practice workplaces can facilitate. For example, policy analyst Alison Jacknowitz studied the impact of workplace characteristics on mothers' ability to continue breastfeeding after returning to work. She found that the availability of employer-sponsored child care, being able to work some hours at home, and state laws encouraging breastfeeding in the workplace increased the likelihood that a mother would continue to breastfeed after returning to work.[16] At the same time, state laws permitting breastfeeding in public places and scheduling flexibility had no significant impact on a woman's decision to continue breastfeeding.[17]

Many workplaces accept the premise of the Business Case for Breastfeeding, which argues that offering employees private space to express milk and worksite lactation support leads to more satisfied, loyal employees and reduced turnover, thus reducing labor costs.[18] However, this philosophy applies primarily to the most privileged full-time workers because retaining employees, reducing parental absence for children's illnesses, and lowering health care insurance costs are most important to employers with experienced, benefit-eligible employees. Employers have little incentive to accommodate lower-skilled workers who are easily replaceable and often ineligible for benefits. Low-skilled, low-income women, who are disproportionately women of color, are more likely to work in jobs where they have no paid leave and little ability to afford to take unpaid leave, and also to hold jobs that offer no private space and insufficient control over their work time to express milk. Thus, equating the value of breastfeeding with its economic benefits is an organizational strategy that is applied primarily to high-wage workers with substantial control over their conditions of work; this strategy could therefore exacerbate existing racial, ethnic, and class disparities in breastfeeding. Yet little of the organizational material on breastfeeding-friendly workplaces has attended to these inequalities.

Intersections between Individual, Interpersonal, and Workplace Characteristics

We propose a conceptual model for understanding the individual, interpersonal, and structural factors that affect mothers' ability to combine breastfeeding with

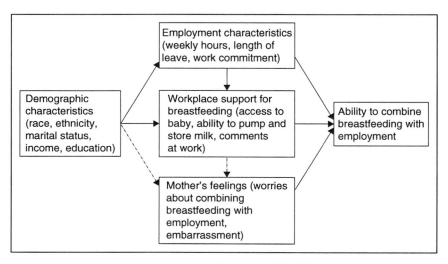

Figure 13.1   Conceptual Model

employment.[19] We then test this model using data from the Infant Feeding Practices Study. As indicated below, we group these influences into four categories: demographics, employment characteristics, workplace supports and/or obstacles, and mothers' feelings about combining breastfeeding and work.

Maternal age, race, ethnicity, marital status, household income, and education are all known to influence breastfeeding rates in the United States: white, married, high-income, highly educated, and older mothers are more likely to breastfeed than otherwise similar nonwhite, unmarried, low-income, less educated, and younger counterparts. Married mothers are typically more able to take unpaid leave because they tend to have partners with incomes. Because of racial stratification, non-Hispanic white women are also more likely to have the economic resources to take unpaid leave. Age, education, and household income are correlated with more resources and the ability to take unpaid leaves. Low-income women and women without stable partners are more likely to need their paychecks, preventing them from taking unpaid leave.

Demographic factors are also related to employment characteristics and work conditions that affect the supportiveness of the work environment. Businesses are more interested in retaining highly educated, highly paid workers and are more likely to accommodate their needs. Women who work in professional and managerial jobs are more likely to have private space and scheduling flexibility in their jobs. Low-skilled, low-wage employees are unlikely to have private space or scheduling flexibility and are more likely to be highly supervised, creating obstacles to combining breastfeeding with work. Lack of privacy can also lead mothers to feel embarrassed about breastfeeding and worried about already precarious job security.

Structural and interpersonal aspects of women's jobs can facilitate or hinder breastfeeding. Important structural influences are the length of maternity leave and the baby's age when the mother returns to work. Often, breastfeeding requires learning time, assistance from lactation consultants or other health professionals, as well as patience. Mothers who resume their jobs soon after giving birth have little opportunity to establish breastfeeding, feeling little incentive to start given the assumption that they will have to stop shortly. In contrast, women who take longer leaves have more opportunity to establish breastfeeding. Women who work fewer hours also find it easier to combine breastfeeding and paid work because they have more access to their babies.

Other structural factors include access to the baby during work hours and the ability to express and store milk at work. Mothers who have physical access to their babies, because they are able to take their babies to work, work from home, go to their babies during the workday, or have someone bring them the baby, can more easily combine breastfeeding with paid employment than those without access. Similarly, expressing and storing milk at work makes it possible to continue to breastfeed. Women who work in jobs where they have no private space or work on a tight or rigid schedule with high levels of supervision are less able to express milk at work and find it more difficult to continue breastfeeding at work. Difficulty expressing milk serves as an important structural obstacle to combining breastfeeding with employment.

There are also maternal characteristics that may affect breastfeeding at work. Women who are more committed to full-time paid work, those who find their jobs highly satisfying, and those who return to full-time or near full-time employment soon after giving birth may find it more difficult to prioritize breastfeeding, especially if they have had little time to establish breastfeeding. In addition, previous research has suggested that many women who return to paid employment soon after giving birth experience role incompatibility when they try to continue breastfeeding while fulfilling their employment roles.[20] This role incompatibility is a consequence of the ideal worker norm, discussed above, that is based on a male standard. This ideal worker notion, and some cultural taboos about breasts and breastfeeding, can discourage women from attempting to combine breastfeeding with employment in some work cultures. Mothers are sometimes concerned that their employment will interfere with breastfeeding, or that breastfeeding will negatively affect their job security. They may also feel embarrassed about breastfeeding when they are in the workplace because the physical aspects of breastfeeding deviate significantly from workplace norms that privilege the male body. Negative comments from coworkers or supervisors about breastfeeding or the presence of human milk in refrigerators provide significant interpersonal disincentives to women's efforts to combine breastfeeding with employment.

Testing the Conceptual Model

To test our conceptual model, we analyzed data from the Infant Feeding Practices Study II (IFPS), a longitudinal consumer-based study that followed mothers from the seventh month of pregnancy through the infant's first year of life.[21] The largest effect was that of marital status, whereby married mothers combined breastfeeding with employment for nearly seven weeks longer than unmarried mothers. Married women were also much more likely to have access to their infants during their work hours than unmarried women, and this access was the strongest predictor of continued breastfeeding. More educated mothers also breastfed longer after returning to work, with each additional level of education increasing duration by 4.22 weeks. It is possible that older and more educated mothers can afford longer maternity leaves and/or have more control over their conditions of work. More educated women were more likely to indicate that they had difficulties expressing and storing milk at work; however, they took longer leaves from paid work postpartum, giving them more time to establish breastfeeding, and they breastfed for a longer period after resuming employment. These findings provide support for our predictions that discretionary approaches to breastfeeding support primarily benefit women workers whose jobs might offer private space and scheduling flexibility.

In terms of employment characteristics, women who worked more hours tended to stop breastfeeding sooner, as did women who took longer leaves after giving birth. The first of these effects was expected: women who work more hours outside the home spend less time near their babies, increasing the burden of combining paid work with nursing. The second effect suggests that mothers of older infants may wait to return to work until they are ready to wean. In contrast, employed mothers of younger infants may view the early months as the critical period for breastfeeding.

We found that workplace support for combining breastfeeding with employment, and for access to babies during work hours, were the most important factors. A lack of access to their babies was a primary reason that many women stopped breastfeeding soon after resuming employment. We found that such access increased the length of time that mothers combined breastfeeding with paid work by more than twenty weeks. In addition to access, a combination of having a supportive child care provider, experiencing no negative comments or embarrassment about breastfeeding in the workplace, having a supportive employer, and having no difficulties expressing milk at work produced the most effective environment for mothers to continue breastfeeding after resuming employment. Being able to express and store milk at work increased the length of time that mothers combined breastfeeding with paid employment by nearly thirteen weeks. Interestingly, women who indicated that they had difficulties expressing or storing milk at work also combined breastfeeding and employment almost eight weeks longer than those who said they had no difficulties. We think this is because women who reported difficulties tried to express and store milk, in comparison to mothers who did not try.

Negative comments in the workplace were very uncommon and consequently had no tangible effect in our analyses. Mothers' own feelings about combining breastfeeding with paid work had small effects. Mothers who worried that breastfeeding would interfere with their job security tended to combine breastfeeding with employment for about nine weeks longer than those who did not. It is possible that mothers who were more committed to breastfeeding were also more likely to worry about its effects on their job security. However, as predicted, mothers embarrassed about breastfeeding at work tended to breastfeed six weeks less than those who were not.

We also identified the combinations of factors associated with breastfeed continuation.[22] This analysis suggests that the conditions necessary for continuing to breastfeed are the following: having a child care provider supportive of breastfeeding; receiving no negative comments from a supervisor about breastfeeding; having no worries or embarrassment about combining breastfeeding with employment; having an employer supportive of breastfeeding; and having no difficulties expressing milk at work. The women fortunate to have this combination of factors breastfed longer.[23]

Since we were also interested in examining how workplace structures differentially affect low-income women and women of color, we also compared white and nonwhite women and found that the causal conditions leading to breastfeeding cessation are similar for both. However, for nonwhite women, lacking access to their child and having difficulty expressing shorten the duration of breastfeeding after returning to work. When comparing women with a college degree to those without, we found that, in conjunction with a lack of organizational support, lower educational attainment is associated with stopping breastfeeding upon returning to work. Women with no college degree who did not have access to their child during the workday found it difficult to pump at work, and those without a supportive employer were more likely to stop breastfeeding soon after returning to work.

Conclusions

Our results suggest that maternal access to their babies and structural support for breastfeeding in the workplace are the most important factors affecting women's ability to continue to breastfeed after resuming employment. Our results also confirm that differences in breastfeeding rates by race, ethnicity, marital status, income, and education are associated with differences in the conditions of work.

Maternal access to babies is a critical issue and one that is often over-looked in policies and programs that focus only on milk expression. We found that women who had access to their babies during work hours, and women who worked fewer hours outside the home (thus having more access de facto), were more able to combine breastfeeding with employment over time. The importance of this access highlights the need for paid maternity leave, since that strategy, more than any other, increases the length of time postpartum that women have direct access to their babies. We also need more policies that facilitate access after return to work, such as on-site day care facilities and telecommuting. Social policy can play a significant role in improving employed mothers' access to their infants by offering employers incentives to offer on-site child care and telecommuting opportunities.

Another critical factor is women's ability to express and store milk at work, suggesting that more workplaces should offer a time and place for milk expression and storage. Historically, pump use has been more available to workers with private work spaces and scheduling autonomy, increasing breast-feeding disparities among employed women. Hopefully, the passage of the Affordable Care Act in 2010, which mandated workplaces to provide space and time for hourly workers to express milk, will support public health efforts to increase breastfeeding rates for all women, reducing breastfeeding disparities.

While we found few robust effects of race or ethnicity, white non-Hispanic mothers were substantially more likely to have access to their infants while at work than their nonwhite and Latina counterparts, and they breastfed six to seven weeks longer after resuming employment. Married women also tended to have more access to their infants than unmarried mothers. As a result, differences in availability of maternity leave and job characteristics, like work hours, access to the baby while working, and ability to pump and store milk, contribute to known disparities in breastfeeding. The most privileged workers are also more likely to have jobs that allow them the time, space, flexibility, and privacy to breastfeed or express and store milk at work. The primary way to equalize the playing field and improve public health outcomes for less privileged populations is to mandate paid maternity leave and encourage employers to increase access and opportunities for all women workers to express and store their milk.

Notes

1. Galtry, "Extending the 'Bright Line,'" 295–317; Gatrell, "Secrets and Lies," 393–404; Lindberg, "Trends in the Relationship," 191–202.
2. Acker, "Hierarchies, Jobs, Bodies," 139; Galtry, "Suckling and Silence in the USA," 1–24.
3. MacKinnon, *Feminism Unmodified*.
4. The Affordable Care Act requires employers to provide reasonable break time and a private, nonbathroom place for nursing mothers to express breast milk during the workday for one year after the child's birth. This provision only applies to hourly workers.
5. Blum, *At the Breast*, 103–109; Racine et al., "Individual Net-Benefit Maximization," 241–249.
6. Acker, "Hierarchies, Jobs, Bodies," 139; Bailyn, *Breaking the Mold*; Ely and Padavic, "Feminist Analysis," 1121–1143.
7. Gatrell, "Secrets and Lies," 393–404.
8. Ibid.
9. Ibid.
10. Galtry, "Extending the 'Bright Line,'" 295–317.
11. Ibid.; Gatrell, "Secrets and Lies," 393–404; Gillespie et al., "Recall of Age of Weaning," 4.
12. Blum, *At the Breast*, 103–109; Lindberg, "Women's Decisions," 239–251; Lindberg, "Trends in the Relationship," 191–202; Racine et al., "Individual Net-Benefit Maximization," 241–249.
13. Eichner, "Parenting and the Workplace," 14; Eisenstein, *The Female Body and the Law*; Galtry, "Extending the 'Bright Line,'" 295–317; Guthrie and Roth, "State, Courts, and Maternity Policies," 41–63; MacKinnon, *Feminism Unmodified*.
14. Eichner, "Parenting and the Workplace," 14; Galtry, "Suckling and Silence in the USA," 1–24; Galtry, "Extending the 'Bright Line,'" 295–317; Guthrie and Roth, "State, Courts, and Maternity Policies," 41–63; O'Brien "Other Voices," 1529–1552; Williams, "Equality's Riddle," 128–155.
15. Lindberg, "Trends in the Relationship," 191–202; Lindberg, "Women's Decisions about Breastfeeding and Maternal Employment," 239–251; Johnston and Swanson, "Cognitive Acrobatics," 447–459; Riad, "Under the Desk," 475–512.
16. Jacknowitz, "Role of Workplace Characteristics," 87–111. State laws regarding breastfeeding in the workplace varied among states, from acknowledging the importance of allowing workers to breastfeed at work to requiring employers to allow mothers to breastfeed at work and to make appropriate accommodations for them.
17. Ibid.
18. U.S. Department of Health and Human Services, "The Business Case for Breastfeeding."

19. Earp and Ennett, "Conceptual Models."
20. Lindberg, "Trends in the Relationship," 191–202; Lindberg, "Women's Decisions," 239–251; Johnston and Swanson, "Cognitive Acrobatics," 447–459; Riad, "Under the Desk," 475–512.
21. We used traditional statistical methods and Qualitative Comparative Analysis (QCA). The prenatal sample of IFPS includes 4,902 pregnant women age eighteen or over, among whom 1,807 continued with the study through their infants' first year. The response rate, calculated as

$$\frac{\text{number surveys completed}}{(\text{adjusted number mailed}) - (\text{number women disqualified})}$$

was 76.9 percent. Our analyses included the 752 women in the sample who resumed employment within one year after giving birth and who were breastfeeding at the time that they returned to work.

Relevant variables included the mother's age, race, ethnicity, marital status, household income, and education, the number of weeks that she breastfed, when she returned to paid employment after the birth, hours worked per week, whether or not the mother had access to her baby during the workday, could pump milk at work, had difficulties pumping or storing milk at work, had support for breastfeeding in the workplace, had concerns that work would interfere with breastfeeding, had concerns that breastfeeding might threaten her job security, felt embarrassed about breastfeeding among coworkers/supervisors, or heard negative comments about breastfeeding from coworkers or supervisors.

We ran statistical models to determine the effects of workplace support for breastfeeding and demographic characteristics on the duration of breastfeeding among these mothers. We also used fuzzy set Qualitative Comparative Analysis (fsQCA), a method that allowed us to examine combinations of conditions that led mothers to continue or cease breastfeeding after returning to work (Ragin, *Fuzzy-Set Social Science*, 56–59). QCA is a method based on Boolean algebra that examines numerous theoretical combinations of variables and identifies which actually lead to a specified outcome. Unlike regression models, which isolate the influence of single variables across a large number of cases and work with additive and linear assumptions, QCA assumes that multiple combinations of variables can independently lead to a given outcome. QCA is also intended to encourage in-depth understanding of specific cases in the data to inform decisions about coding and interpretation of results.
22. Using QCA method.
23. Mothers combined paid employment with breastfeeding for up to seventy-seven weeks, although over 50 percent stopped within twenty-three weeks of resuming employment and over 80 percent had stopped within a year.

Part V

Making and Marketing Mothers' Milk

Marketing Mothers' Milk

The Markets for Human Milk and Infant Formula

Today, breastfeeding, human milk, and its substitute, infant formula, are commodities. "Mother's milk" is marketed both literally and figuratively, as a good for sale, a normative behavior, and a cure for a variety of contemporary social and medical problems. Like previous exploitations of women's bodies, including their eggs and uteruses, the idea that human milk is a valuable good that can be given away, traded in a market, or subjected to scientific experimentation raises important ethical, moral, and policy questions. This chapter examines the emerging markets in human milk and the competing market in infant formula through a feminist lens. It asserts that women are autonomous decision makers, capable of making informed choices about the value of breastfeeding, human milk, and their own labor, in light of their individual needs as well as those of children and family. It advances the provocative argument that only by acknowledging that human milk has become a marketable commodity and offering women the chance to be paid for their milk in a regulated market can feminist aims be achieved.

This chapter reviews the markets in human milk and infant formula and considers how medicine and government have shaped the development of those markets. It asserts that recognizing human milk as a valuable commodity, for which women can be paid, promotes feminist ideals. The chapter concludes with a proposal for a regulated market that makes it possible for women to earn a fair wage for their productive labor in producing excess milk.

The Markets in Human Milk and Infant Formula

Markets respond to demand. This chapter contends that the market in human milk is growing because of a combination of demand drivers: increased advocacy by health care professionals and government for the human milk's benefits, coupled with the difficulty many mothers face in providing this commodity, due to cultural, economic, legal, medical, psychological, and workplace obstacles. The infant formula market exploits these obstacles by marketing that suggests that formula is nearly as good as "the real thing," human milk.

The demand for milk is constructed by both biological reality and subtle marketing signals.[1] Those who believe that breastfeeding is superior to bottle-feeding usually believe that human milk itself is a product that not only provides infants with important nutrition and immunities but also can function as a miraculous liquid in other circumstances. On "lactivist" blogs and mainstream news media, mothers and health educators tout human milk as a cure for conjunctivitis, rashes, and other childhood maladies. Human milk is used to treat burn victims, chemotherapy patients, and organ transplant recipients.[2] Some research indicates that milk might be used to treat cancer.[3] Prolacta Bioscience, a for-profit California company, takes donated milk and turns it into human milk fortifiers, which it sells to neonatal intensive care units.

At present, two sets of markets involve breastfeeding and human milk. The first are the formal and informal markets in human milk itself; the second concerns infant formula. The markets in human milk and infant formula both respond to the claim that "breast is best."[4] The human milk markets make their magic elixir available either as processed milk or as special fortifiers. The infant formula market promotes new products claimed to be identical to human milk, with nutritional enhancements that mimic human milk or organic variations offering a different type of "naturalness."[5]

Both markets confront the same demographic reality: a flat birthrate that predicts a stable demand for milk products for the foreseeable future. Physicians play a key role in increasing demand for human milk by asserting its superiority to formula, especially for premature and low birth weight infants.[6] Some physicians prescribe human milk to older children and adults.

For much of history the market for human milk focused on the services provided by wet nurses. In elite societies women who preferred not to breastfeed employed wet nurses.[7] In the United States, the use of slaves as "mammies" meant that many slave women could not care for their own children, a legacy that may contribute to some African American women's current discomfort with breastfeeding.[8]

Today, many nursing women donate or sell their extra milk to family, friends, or total strangers. These transactions are facilitated through websites as varied as craigslist and "lactivist" blogs.[9] The American Academy of Pediatrics and La Leche League counsel against informal milk exchanges, because of the risks that serious infectious diseases could be transmitted through unpasteurized human milk and that a liquid purported to be human milk is something else.[10] Nonetheless, many women are happy to offer their extra milk to others, and many mothers who cannot breastfeed proclaim the virtues of human milk.[11] Milk "sharing" also takes place directly, when women nurse other women's children for free or for pay.[12] One California employment agency provides wet nurses for new mothers, with weekly salaries of about $1,000.[13]

Supplementing these individual market arrangements, eleven not-for-profit milk banks in North America supply milk to hospitals and critically ill infants.[14] Milk banks were established early in the 1890s and expanded during the Great Depression, when mothers were paid for their milk.[15] After World War II, milk banks became less popular, but they rebounded in the 1970s as demand increased with the greater survival of premature infants.[16]

In the 1980s fears about HIV transmission through human milk led to a decline in milk banks' popularity.[17] Today, however, milk banks screen donors and donated milk for HIV, hepatitis, and other pathogens. Not-for-profit milk banks charge an average of $4.50 per ounce, a practice that can be quite expensive for full-term infants, who consume an average of thirty ounces of milk daily.[18] Recently some milk banks have faced shortages.[19]

In recognition of increasing demand, Prolacta was established near Los Angeles in 1999. Funded by venture capitalists, Prolacta has developed four nutritional fortifiers for premature infants as well as three "ready-to-feed" human milk products that can be given directly to these infants.[20] Nutritional fortifiers are highly concentrated versions of human milk sold in premeasured doses that can be added to donor milk or a mother's own milk to enhance the nutritional intake of premature infants.[21] Formula manufacturers previously made milk fortifiers from cow's milk; now Prolacta is attempting to demonstrate that its human milk fortifiers achieve better health outcomes.[22]

Prolacta has an ingenious system for obtaining donor milk. It operates a nationwide network of donation sites, which call themselves milk banks, and offer mothers a free breast pump and a convenient way to drop off their milk.[23] While the donors receive no compensation, the donation sites are paid for collecting the milk, which they ship to Prolacta's California processing plant.[24] Like not-for-profit milk banks, Prolacta appeals to women's desires to help other mothers.[25]

In addition, Prolacta has exploited Americans' desire to support African children with HIV. In an act that is either a stroke of marketing genius or an inspirational example of corporate charity, Prolacta has created a partnership

with the International Breast Milk Project to donate human milk to HIV positive infants. Prolacta processes milk donated by American mothers and ships
it to South Africa, where it is dispensed to infected infants.[26] Currently,
Prolacta ships 25 percent of all milk donated to the International Breast Milk
Project to Africa, and it processes the remaining 75 percent into human milk
fortifiers sold to American hospitals.[27] While not-for-profit milk banks sell
milk for about $4.50 per ounce, Prolacta sells its human milk fortifiers in
milliliter formulations, at prices equivalent to $184 per ounce.[28]

Infant formula is highly profitable, with sales of $4.9 billion in 2008.
Beginning with cow's milk, an inexpensive commodity, formula manufacturers add small amounts of other ingredients to simulate mother's milk. Retail
prices vastly exceed the actual cost of production and outpace inflation.[29]
Manufacturers develop "improved" formulations that appeal to parents
anxious to provide the best for their children.[30] These include "specialty"
formulas containing two fatty acids found in human milk, DHA and ARA.[31]
Organic formulas' sales are growing, even though they contain added sugar,
with potential long-term harmful effects.[32]

Three major firms compete for formula market share. Abbott Laboratories
and Mead Johnson are both pharmaceutical companies, while Nestlé is a global
food manufacturer.[33] All three companies promote consumer brand loyalty
through outreach to health care professionals, exclusive contracts with hospital
nurseries, direct-to-consumer (DTC) advertising, and strategic bidding in the
WIC program.[34]

Historically, Abbott and Mead Johnson marketed their products directly to
physicians through so-called "ethical marketing,"[35] in which drug representatives visited physicians with free samples and urged them to recommend
specific products to patients.[36] Formula manufacturers contributed heavily to
the American Academy of Pediatrics, paying about one-third of the costs of
building the Academy's headquarters in the 1980s, providing grants to the
Academy, underwriting pediatric conferences, and offering loans to medical
students and pediatricians.[37] In the 1980s, confronted with Nestlé's imminent
entry into the American infant formula market, Abbott and Mead Johnson
worked with the Academy to oppose DTC advertising, citing its negative
impact on breastfeeding.[38] In 1989 the Academy adopted a policy against
accepting contributions from formula manufacturers that engaged in DTC
advertising.[39] In 1993 Nestlé sued the Academy, Abbott, and Mead Johnson
under the Sherman Antitrust Act. Nestlé charged the defendants with conspir-
ing to block its entry into the American formula market, citing evidence of
the defendants' jointly developed opposition to DTC advertising. However, the

jury found for the defendants.[40] Formula manufacturers have been challenged in other antitrust actions, alleging price fixing and other collusion in both the WIC program and the Academy's "no DTC advertising" policy.[41]

Today all formula manufacturers use DTC advertising to reach parents.[42] Formula manufacturers also spend millions in covert advertising, providing free formula samples and discount coupons to pregnant women and new mothers at doctors' offices and via direct mail.[43] For years, manufacturers have supplied hospitals with free formula for nonbreastfed infants, as well as other institutional support, with the explicit quid pro quo that the hospital will distribute free formula to all infants upon discharge,[44] even though many studies demonstrate that these free samples discourage women from breastfeeding.[45]

The WIC program plays a key role in the infant formula market, affecting consumer demand and formula prices. WIC provides free supplemental formula to more than half of American infants.[46] Mothers participating in WIC consistently lag far behind non-WIC mothers in their rates of breastfeeding,[47] although it is not clear why this is. WIC participants are poor and frequently racial minorities who are less likely to breastfeed for other reasons; thus, the gap between WIC and non-WIC mothers could simply reflect the program's demographics.[48] However, structural aspects of WIC also discourage breastfeeding. These include the make-up of WIC "food packages," the public perception of their value, the system of WIC funding (a combination of federal grants, competitive bidding, and formula manufacturers' rebates, which tends to reduce support for breastfeeding), and the marketing advantages of WIC affiliation, which include preferential product placement at grocery stores.[49] In almost every state, the WIC-approved brand has the biggest market share. In *every* state, the prices of infant formula have outpaced inflation.[50]

Historically, the composition of WIC food packages created incentives not to breastfeed. Until the 1990s, breastfeeding women who participated in WIC were not given supplemental healthy food to support breastfeeding, even though WIC fully covered infant formula costs, thus making breastfeeding less attractive.[51] In 2007 WIC changed its package structure, responding to an Institute of Medicine report noting the substantial dollar value differences of the food packages given to breastfeeding and nonbreastfeeding mothers. Before the change, the annual value of the WIC subsidy was $1,380 for women who only used formula, $668 for mothers who breastfed exclusively, and $1,669 for mothers who breastfed but also used formula, making exclusive breastfeeding unlikely. Since women choose WIC food packages at the beginning of each month and formula is very expensive, rational women would choose the formula package if they thought there was any chance of using formula in the following month. Once formula is available it is more likely to be used.[52]

WIC spends less than 1 percent of its budget on outreach to encourage breastfeeding.[53] While many state WIC program personnel try to assist women with breastfeeding, some women have found that WIC staff members are ambivalent.[54] Often WIC programs fail to offer practical assistance with breastfeeding, such as providing nursing bras, breast pumps, or breastfeeding support classes,[55] even though such concrete support is essential if poor women are to continue breastfeeding after returning to work or school.[56]

The infant formula market demonstrates the ironic, if not surprising, situation in which major government agencies are at odds with each other. One arm of the government, the Department of Health and Human Services, spent millions on the National Breastfeeding Awareness Campaign, touting breastfeeding and human milk as absolutely necessary for infant and maternal health.[57] At the same time, another government agency, the Department of Agriculture, has developed the WIC program in a manner that actively discourages breastfeeding. Congress has generally failed to weigh in on breastfeeding policy, declining to adopt the Baby-Friendly Hospital Initiative, which would require hospitals to stop giving free formula and other gifts to new parents. However, in the 2010 Patient Protection and Affordable Care Act, Congress required that all employers of fifty or more workers provide a clean and private location "other than a bathroom" for nursing mothers to pump their milk, and to permit these women to take unpaid breaks to do so.[58]

The Commodification Debate

Over the last twenty-five years, an intense scholarly debate has raged over the commodification of anything connected with the human body. Proponents of free market economics assert that markets are desirable for almost all transactions,[59] while critics argue that commodification of anything connected with human personhood, particularly the female body, is inherently dangerous.[60]

However, a growing group of feminist scholars recognize that market exchanges may be valuable if they protect vulnerable populations.[61] Martha Ertman asserts that marginalized people may gain from markets, citing the market in sperm for artificial insemination, because it helps single women and gay and lesbian couples form intentional families that would be impossible through the adoption market.[62] Katharine Silbaugh rejects the notion that "talking about home labor as productive mean[s] commodifying it."[63] She notes that many commodification critics appear to object to a market approach *only* when it is *women* who are receiving money for their services;

this focus on purported harm to women may reflect "a romantic essentialism about femininity."[64]

Critical race scholars have also asserted that market principles should not be shunned simply because of previous market exploitation of vulnerable populations.[65] Writing about organ donation, Michele Goodwin suggests that playing "the race card" to preclude all private ordering will neither successfully prevent the exploitation of African American patients nor guarantee them access to desperately needed organs.[66] Indeed, she asserts that permitting organ and tissue donors to be paid for their gifts might actually enhance the supply of organs and tissues for the African American community.[67]

The essential question is not whether commodification of breastfeeding and human milk should occur, because it already does. Many groups promote human milk as a commodity—a product with economic value as well as scientific benefit. These include pediatricians who promote breastfeeding and human milk, the U.S. Department of Health and Human Services (in the National Breastfeeding Awareness Campaign), not-for-profit milk banks, agencies providing wet nurses, and for-profit companies like Prolacta. I propose that this commodification should be made explicit and permit market principles to illuminate the trade-offs involved in choosing to breastfeed, to sell, donate, or purchase human milk, or to buy infant formula.

Both not-for-profit milk banks and Prolacta depend upon women's generous desire to help other mothers by donating human milk. Not-for-profit milk banks' reliance on women's altruism makes sense because the banks barely break even. However, altruism cannot justify Prolacta's exploitation of the generosity of women who donate their milk expecting it to be given to starving infants in Africa, when instead most will be processed into human milk fortifiers and sold to hospitals at prices exceeding $180 per ounce. Women may feel betrayed if they learn that their milk was the raw ingredient for a biotech company's profits.

Despite the existing commodification of breastfeeding and human milk, the idea of treating either as commodities raises both eyebrows and moral reservations. I suggest that acknowledging and expanding the markets in human milk is so threatening because of how these markets sound in motherhood, raising concerns about the corruption or degradation of personhood.[68] There is a fear that allowing a market for a product will drive out noncommodified interactions in the same area, under a sort of "moral domino theory."[69] But I argue that permitting a market is actually consistent with feminism, whose core values include the recognition of each woman's independent perspective and the belief that women should make decisions based on their own values and aspirations, rather than the values mandated by external and hierarchical forces.

A Proposal for a Regulated Market in Human Milk

We must begin by acknowledging that milk production and donation *do* involve the use of human tissue and labor and offer both informed consent and reasonable compensation for what women are providing. I propose a regulated market that would exist alongside the current donative market, in which everyone benefits *except* the women providing their milk.[70]

A preliminary market model would work as follows. In order to transfer (either donate or sell) their breast milk, women would need to be *offered* a minimum of $2 per ounce. This would ensure that the woman could earn a minimum wage of $12 to $14 per hour, compared to the current federal minimum wage of $7.25.[71] Women would not be *required* to accept any compensation, but its availability would have several salutary effects. First, compensation might help not-for-profit milk banks enhance their milk supply, since some women might donate if they were compensated but would not do so if the only option was gratuitous donation. This scenario could result in nonprofit milk banks actually having more milk, helping them to meet rising demand.[72] Two dollars per ounce would lead to a relatively small increase over the $4.50 per ounce that not-for-profit milk banks currently charge hospitals and infants' families for their milk, and it might decrease demand for those infants whose need for human milk is not clearly established.

For women deciding whether to return to work or to take an extended unpaid parenting leave, the opportunity to earn extra money for a few hours of extra labor a day, without leaving home, might prove an attractive alternative. Other women might choose to donate to a not-for-profit milk bank rather than to a corporation like Prolacta once they learn that Prolacta is profiting enormously from their freely given milk. Still other women might decide to donate their milk either to Prolacta or to a not-for profit organization, concluding that the satisfaction of helping others is sufficient.

This market should be regulated by the government, to prevent the exploitation of women who provide their milk and protect infants from receiving potentially harmful milk. Prospective donors would be screened for diseases as well as for medications they could transmit through breast milk. Women would also be required to be examined by a physician or nurse practitioner to ensure their suitability as donors. This would safeguard the quality of the donor's milk *and* the health of the donating women, with the additional physical examination paid for indirectly by the purchaser.

Historically, it has been women, and poor women of color in particular, who have been excluded from positions of power and prestige in a market economy. Offering women who choose to produce and exchange their breast milk the opportunity to be compensated at fair market value for their services will only enhance their sense of agency and worth. By rejecting the false "dichotomy between the language of economic productivity and the language of [care]," the recognition of a market in human milk and a frank discussion of the costs and benefits of breastfeeding, human milk, and infant formula can enhance both women's agency and the public health by making human milk more widely available.[73]

Notes

This chapter is drawn from a longer exploration of the commodification of breastfeeding and human milk, "Marketing Mothers' Milk: The Commodification of Breastfeeding and the New Markets for Breast Milk and Infant Formula," *Nevada Law Journal* 10, no. 1 (2010): 29–81.

1. Tierney, "Message."
2. Brotman, "Natural Wonder"; Noor, "Breast Milk"; Slater, "Breast Milk Used"; Steingraber, "Benefits of Breast Milk"; Sundstrom, "Breast Milk Used in Cancer Fight"; and Whit, "Breast Milk Cures."
3. Labbok and Tully interview; see also Mulvihill, "Breast Milk."
4. Lepore, "Baby Food," 34.
5. An advertisement for Similac infant formula claims that it's "closer than ever to breast milk." PhDinParenting, "Sabotage," explains how mothers searching for breastfeeding advice on the Internet are directed to Similac's "Welcome Addition Club," which makes this claim for Similac.
6. See Child Trends Data Bank, "Birth and Fertility Rates"; Stobbe, "AP Impact"; Park, "Why the U.S. Gets a D." More than 12 percent of all births are premature. Some prematurity is due to inadequate prenatal care, while some reflects the increased number of multiple births due to artificial reproductive technology used largely by wealthier women. Institute of Medicine of the National Academies, "Preterm Birth," 1, 3.
7. Baumslag and Michels, *Milk, Money, and Madness*, 40–45.
8. Wolf, "Is Breast Really Best?," 621; Roberts, "Spiritual and Menial Housework," 56; compare Harris, "Finding Sojourner's Truth," 337.
9. Pearce, "Breast Friend"; Muñoz, "Mothers Who Share."
10. American Academy of Pediatrics Work Group on Breastfeeding, "Breastfeeding and the Use of Human Milk"; Arnold, "Becoming a Donor"; Henry, "Banking on Milk."
11. Lee-St. John, "Milk Maids."
12. Lloyd, "Modern-Day Wet Nursing."
13. Henry, "Banking on Milk."
14. Austin, "Sides Clash"; see the Human Milk Banking Association of North America website (http://www.hmbana.org). Each milk bank is governed by guidelines approved by the Centers for Disease Control and the Food and Drug Administration. Donated milk is processed in bulk and shipped to hospitals and individuals pursuant to a physician's prescription (Dunn and Evans interview).

15. Arnold, "Becoming a Donor"; Pollak, "Mother's Memory"; "Service Extended."
16. Porter, "Breast-Feeding"; Arnold, "Becoming a Donor."
17. Arnold, "Becoming a Donor." Maternal-fetal transmission of the HIV virus can occur during pregnancy, labor, and delivery and through human milk. The risk of transmission is reduced dramatically if the mother is treated with combination antiretroviral drug therapy during pregnancy (National Institutes of Health, "Recommendations for Use of Antiretroviral Drugs," 6–10, 26–28).
18. Dunn and Evans interview; Human Milk Banking Association of North America, http://www.hmbana.org.
19. Human Milk Banking Association of North America, "ALERT: Milk Donors."
20. Prolacta Bioscience, October 4, 2006, and May 23, 2007. Prolacta currently markets four infant fortifiers (see Prolacta Bioscience: Prolact + H2MF Human Milk Fortifier, as well as three "ready to feed" human milk products for premature infants. Prolacta Bioscience), "Standardized Human Milk Formulations."
21. Heird, "Progress," 500S.
22. Prolacta Bioscience, "Research and Development"; Sullivan, "Historically Controlled Cohort."
23. There are nineteen milk "banks" currently involved with Prolacta Bioscience. "Milk Bank Mothers"; Bernhard, "Human Milk." Mothers donating to a not-for-profit milk bank must pack their milk in dry ice, place it in a Styrofoam cooler, and ship it to one of these milk banks. Dunn and Evans interview.
24. Bernhard, "Human Milk."
25. Ibid.
26. International Breast Milk Project, "Donation Process."
27. Whit, "Should You Support"; International Breast Milk Project, "Donation Process."
28. MamaBear, "Thinking of Donating."
29. Burton, "Spilt Milk"; "Baby Food," 5.
30. "Baby Food," 2.
31. Ibid., 1.
32. Ibid.; Moskin, "All-Organic Formula"; Reyes, "Organic Baby Formula."
33. "Baby Food," 2; Jordan, "Nestlé Markets."
34. WIC is the U.S. Department of Agriculture's Special Supplemental Nutrition Program for Women, Infants, and Children.
35. U.S. Government Accountability Office, *Breastfeeding*, app. I27; Cutler and Wright, "U.S. Infant Formula," 41.
36. Cutler and Wright, "U.S. Infant Formula," 39–42, 46.
37. Burton, "Spilt Milk."
38. Ibid.
39. Epstein, "Women and Children Last," 25, 40–54.
40. Ibid., 48–49.
41. *FTC v. Abbott Laboratories*; Epstein, "Women and Children Last," 28–39; Siegel, "Formula for Disaster"; *Florida ex rel. Butterworth v. Abbott Laboratories, Inc.*; Burton, "Spilt Milk."
42. U.S. Government Accountability Office, *Breastfeeding*, app. I26.
43. Kent, "High Price of Infant Formula," 22; Cutler and Wright, "U.S. Infant Formula," 47.
44. Rosenberg et al., "Marketing Infant Formula," 290; Merewood and Philipp, "Becoming Baby-Friendly," 280–282.

45. U.S. Government Accountability Office, *Breastfeeding*, app. I9; Shealy et al., *The CDC Guide*, i.

46. WIC provides supplemental food packages, nutrition education, and health care and social services referrals. WIC applicants must be poor and at nutritional risk. Oliveira et al., *WIC and the Retail Price*, 6–8; McLaughlin et al., *Breastfeeding Intervention*, 1.

47. Ryan and Zhou, "Lower Breastfeeding Rates," 1136.

48. Ibid., 1144.

49. Oliveira et al., *WIC and the Retail Price*; Kent, "WIC's Promotion," 7.

50. Oliveira et al., *WIC and the Retail Price*, 59–60, 81–85; Oliveira, Frazao, and Smallwood, *Rising Infant Formula Costs*.

51. McLaughlin et al., *Breastfeeding Intervention*, 3; Labbok and Tully interview.

52. Revisions in the WIC food packages; see also Ryan and Zhou, "Lower Breastfeeding Rates," 1144–1145.

53. Arnold interview.

54. Bonuck, "Country of Origin," 321.

55. Arnold interview; Kukla, *Mass Hysteria*, 160–163.

56. Kukla, *Mass Hysteria*, 160; Kantor, "On the Job"; see Philipp et al., "Baby-Friendly," 680.

57. U.S. Department of Health and Human Services, "National Breastfeeding Campaign."

58. Flores-Paniagua, "Office Support"; see the Patient Protection and Affordable Health Care Act, s. 4207.

59. Landes and Posner, "Economics of the Baby Shortage," 323–324.

60. Sandel, "What Money Can't Buy," 122.

61. Ertman, "What's Wrong," 304.

62. Ibid., 303–317.

63. Silbaugh, "Commodification," 298.

64. Ibid., 299–301.

65. Goodwin, *Black Markets*, 193–203.

66. Goodwin, "The Body Market," 603–604, 626, 635; Goodwin, *Black Markets*, 198–204.

67. Fentiman, "Organ Donation," 1598; Oberman, "When the Truth Is Not Enough," 941; Goodwin, "The Body Market," 629.

68. Sandel, "What Money Can't Buy," 122; Radin, "Contested Commodities," 82–83.

69. Radin, "Contested Commodities," 83–84.

70. The uncompensated donation of human milk has striking parallels with the current system of organ and tissue donation, in which federal law prohibits the compensation of the organ and tissue donor, while physicians, hospitals, and organ and tissue suppliers are handsomely rewarded. See Fentiman, "Organ Donation," 1601; Goodwin, "The Body Market," 629; Oberman, "When the Truth Is Not Enough," 930.

71. When her child is a month old, a woman can pump three to four ounces in approximately half an hour. See, for example, Mohrbacher, "How Much Milk."

72. Mulvihill, "Breast Milk as Cancer Treatment?"; Institute of Medicine of the National Academies, *Preterm Birth*.

73. Silbaugh, "Commodification," 82.

Empowerment or Regulation?

Women's Perspectives on Expressing Milk

Recent research suggests that expressing breast milk may be an increasingly common practice during early infant feeding, yet relatively little is known about the reasons for this practice.[1] Moreover, there is little explicit analysis of early milk expression in the feminist infant feeding literature. That which does exist suggests contradictory theorization. It has been suggested that expressing represents a type of regulation, in that it imposes an external form of control upon breastfeeding. Thus, milk expression offers a way of managing future expectations about returning to work or normal life and activities while continuing to breastfeed. In addition, the use of breast pumps has been theorized as contributing to the commercialization, medicalization, and mechanization of breastfeeding and a focus on milk as a product rather than breastfeeding as a process.[2] On the other hand, expressing has the potential to be *empowering*, in that it allows for greater paternal involvement in infant feeding and increased freedom for women.[3] Our recent analysis of experiences of expressing milk with a group of first-time British mothers suggested that the women accounted for the practice of expressing in ways that, in feminist terms, could be seen as potentially both empowering and disempowering.[4]

In this chapter we analyze three case studies from our research and argue that, because of its potential to empower new mothers in contemporary Western contexts, the practice of expressing might sometimes be considered as a way to promote the continuation of lactation and breastfeeding by enabling women to navigate some of the perceived barriers to breastfeeding. However, this should not negate critical feminist engagement with factors that constrain breastfeeding.

Negotiating Early Infant Feeding: Expressing Stories

We present case studies of three women who have expressed milk extensively, based on data from audio diaries and interviews.[5]

Samantha's Story

Samantha was nineteen and lived with her grandmother, as did her new partner, who was not the father of her child. Samantha was living on an income of less than ten thousand pounds per year.[6]

Samantha initially reported that breastfeeding was "quite painful" and that she was "starting to feel really sore." By the third day she was exclusively pumping and feeding breast milk via a bottle. Samantha gave pain management as her primary reason for expressing milk. In a previous analysis we argued that expressing is a practice that can be deployed when experiencing difficulties to ensure the baby still receives human milk.[7] As Samantha put it, "I'm happy to do it like this for now, she's still getting all the nutrients that she needs from the breast milk . . . and it's a lot less painful expressing the milk than latching her on." This statement implies that, for Samantha, the practice of pumping to manage pain enabled her to fulfill her "moral duty" and position herself as a "good mother" who, as the sociologist Elizabeth Murphy argues, ensures that health outcomes are maximized for the baby.[8]

She also reported that "it feels like I'm restricted because . . . I don't feel comfortable feeding in front of people." She repeatedly said that expressing and using a bottle made it easier to feed if she went out, saying that she "would have preferred to have expressed it rather than breastfeed in public because I know there is quite a lot of stigma about it in some places."

Analysis of concerns about public breastfeeding in the feminist literature has been mainly associated with the sexualization of the breast in Western societies. The feminist sociologist Cindy Stearns links this anxiety to current constructions of the "good maternal body," which requires the careful management of breastfeeding in specific ways in front of others so that the nurturing rather than the sexual breast is evident.[9] Here Samantha avoids transgressing this precarious boundary by removing her breast from the act of breastfeeding.

Samantha mentioned that another advantage of pumping milk was that it enabled others to feed her baby, and that it gave her the freedom to do other things. She spoke about wanting to enroll in an educational course and implied that expressing would be a way of managing this activity. Expressing was therefore constructed as a way of having a break from the demands of motherhood and resuming other tasks and activities. Her rationale resonates with nursing scholars Janice Morse and Joan Bottorff's characterization of expressing as a practice that can open the "door to freedom."[10] However, feminists have also conceptualized these reasons for expressing as a form of regulation put upon breastfeeding in an attempt by women to return to a normal, generally productive life.[11] Within this context expressing offers opportunities to experience a degree of freedom while still aligning the self with "good mothering" and the "breast is best" imperative.

Samantha also spoke extensively about expressing facilitating the "bonding" of her partner and family members with her baby. This popular construction of "bonding" through feeding has been linked to cultural understandings of maternal instinct and love, which have their roots in scientific notions of attachment.[12] Though bonding theory suggests that it is the mother who is exclusively attached to her infant, the notion of "bonding" seems to have taken on a more general meaning following research focused on multiple bonds being beneficial for child development.[13] Samantha appeared to prioritize this meaning over the notion of developing an exclusive bond with her baby. It is also interesting that, despite concerns from breastfeeding scholars that expressing bypasses the relational aspects of breastfeeding, Samantha shows some ambivalence about this issue.[14] Although elsewhere she talked about feeding expressed milk as meaning an absence of "closeness and skin-to-skin contact," here it was the process of feeding that was associated with bonding rather than direct nurturing from the breast.

Samantha did not attain her goal of breastfeeding for three months or more. Later in the study she reported an inability to express milk and that she had resorted to feeding formula to her infant.

Hannah's Story

Hannah was in her mid-twenties and had been living with her partner for seven years. Both were employed in professional roles, and together they earned over forty thousand pounds per year.[15] Hannah had a Cesarean section at thirty-six weeks because her baby was in the breech position. Her baby was relatively small at 3,050 grams when born.[16]

By the end of the first week postpartum, Hannah was feeding her baby approximately half from the breast and half from bottles of pumped milk. She indicated that her baby had not always been latching on or sucking properly and thus was concerned that her son was not getting enough milk. Her anxiety was heightened because he had been born slightly early and was small. She stated several times that she was not confident that she was producing enough milk even when he was latching on: "I'm . . . not confident about the amount that he's actually getting . . . but I am expressing, and I'm managing to express, about three ounces, two or three times a day, so we are able to see what he is getting as well." An initial lack of confidence in the body's abilities to breastfeed, and concerns about producing enough milk, have been highlighted elsewhere as key reasons for giving up breastfeeding.[17] For Hannah, pumping milk gave her the confidence that her son was getting enough milk and may have been a strategy that enabled her to continue breastfeeding, which she was doing exclusively by the third week postpartum. In addition, by pumping milk Hannah was able to navigate potentially being positioned as a "bad mother" for either using formula or for failing to ensure the provision of adequate sustenance for her baby to gain weight.[18] For Hannah, as for women in other studies, pumping meant that her milk could be quantified and objectively measured.[19] Although measurement of milk can give women the confidence to continue breastfeeding, Fiona Dykes, professor of maternal and infant health, suggests that a techno-medical discourse of measurement can undermine women's confidence in their ability to understand and interpret their own bodies, and possibly negatively affect lactation.[20]

Hannah also spoke about pumping facilitating shared parenting as an early justification for adopting this practice: "I've also expressed with a pump today so that my husband can feed him . . . so we can both do it." Her explanation makes sense in the context of prominent discursive constructions of contemporary fathering, such as "being there" and "involved fatherhood."[21]

Yvonne's Story

Yvonne was in her mid-twenties at the time of the study. She had been living with her partner for ten years. She was educated to degree level and her partner to GCSE level.[22] Both were employed, Yvonne in a professional role, and the household income was over forty thousand pounds per year.[23]

Initially Yvonne reported she was getting on well with breastfeeding and that it had been easier than expected. A week after the birth she reported that she was exclusively breastfeeding, but a month later she was mainly pumping and feeding breast milk via a bottle. She said her baby was "constantly on the boobs, non-stop," and "I find the breast pump easier to use. . . . he's taking up to an hour and a half, two hours to have a proper feed. It is actually quicker to sterilize the equipment and express the milk." Such accounts of frustration at the inefficiencies of breastfeeding may relate to feminist scholar Alison Bartlett's argument that the breastfeeding body contradicts Western notions of a perfect female body that is under control. Breastfeeding, she argues, represents a challenge to the body, including being constantly available.[24]

Expressing milk is a practice that enables the retention of a sense of bodily control because it is seen as more efficient than breastfeeding.

Like Samantha and other women in our study, Yvonne spoke about pain from sore and cracked nipples and related problems latching her baby on as a key reason for expressing milk. In her diary, Yvonne indicated initially that she was trying to persevere with breastfeeding but that she was struggling to establish a feeding routine. However, when interviewed eight days later, she reported feeding mostly pumped milk. She made sense of this as "easier" for him, as "he's got to do less work," and said that because "he's having the bottle more than the breast now," he had developed a preference for it.

Infant Feeding Outcomes

We do not know the longer-term outcomes for the eight women who expressed extensively. Of the five who completed the study to six weeks postpartum, two had given up feeding at the breast, though one was still extensively expressing and combining with formula-feeding. One woman was exclusively breastfeeding, another was predominantly breastfeeding while giving some formula and expressing, and another was primarily expressing with some breastfeeding.

Implications for Public Health Promotion

For all three women discussed here, and several others in our research, expressing milk was a central practice enabling them to provide human milk to their babies. Given this, and the way in which pumping has to some extent been problematized in the literature, we offer some tentative thoughts on the role that expressing milk might play in public health initiatives to promote breastfeeding.

Expressing has often been discussed as an issue of particular relevance to women's return to work and to the provision of milk for preterm infants.[25] However, our participants' babies were born at or close to term and, as is the norm in the United Kingdom, none of the women had yet returned to work, nor did they anticipate returning in the near future.[26] Instead, they talked about expressing as supporting their breastfeeding in much more varied ways, which fits with recent large-scale surveys suggesting that the majority of women breastfeeding full-term infants express some milk in the first few weeks following birth.[27] Our data suggest that expressing can be useful to new mothers as a way of managing the demands of early breastfeeding, facilitating shared parenting, and negotiating public feeding. However, our data also highlight the importance of wider social and cultural factors. The perceived gains from expressing milk were often seen as such because they enabled the navigation of cultural pressures and contradictory demands, which can, paradoxically, make it difficult to combine breastfeeding with being a "good mother" and a "good partner."[28]

We began the chapter by noting the differing ways in which expressing has been portrayed—as an oppressive control on breastfeeding or as an empowering practice. Our data suggest that for some women expressing may be empowering *because* it gives them additional control over their bodies. As sociologist Linda Blum notes, "feminist discussions of motherhood . . . continually ponder how to retain the empowering or pleasurable aspects of motherhood without reinforcing the straitjacket of traditional gender arrangements and how to demand political and economic rights on a par with men's without denying the value of women's experiences."[29] Our data suggest that expressing offers women a way of managing this dilemma. Our participants valued breastfeeding and yet also valued control over breastfeeding—in particular, control over problematic aspects and the restrictions it placed on both their autonomy and on shared parenting.

However, we retain a degree of caution in advocating the unqualified promotion of milk expression as a practice that supports breastfeeding. First, concern has been raised that extensive expressing may interfere with breastfeeding when an artificial teat is used to deliver the milk, resulting in "nipple confusion" due to the different sucking technique required.[30] The World Health Organization (WHO) recommends cup feeding when milk is not taken directly from the breast. However, WHO suggests that although there is evidence for an association between use of artificial teats and early cessation of breastfeeding, the evidence for "nipple confusion" is not conclusive.[31] In fact, a positive association was found in a recent study between expressing milk and continuing breastfeeding for six months.[32] Moreover, it has been suggested that pumping, like suckling, can raise levels of the hormone prolactin, which then stimulates milk supply.[33] Until there is further research on the longer-term effects of extensive milk expression on breastfeeding, particularly where artificial teats are used, it seems wise to exercise caution about extensive use of expression as a replacement for feeding at the breast.

Second, suckling at the breast rather than at an artificial teat appears to be advantageous for development of both the jaw and oral musculature during infancy and may yield subsequent orthodontic benefits.[34] Third, promoting expression may also lose sight of the relational aspects of breastfeeding, particularly of the way in which breastfeeding offers women and their babies a means of embodied sensual engagement.[35] Although criticized by developmental psychologists, the notion of "skin-to-skin" contact in "bonding" originally proposed by pediatrician Marshall Klaus and others remains popular in lay discourse.[36] This suggests that the introduction of something nonbiological into the breastfeeding relationship (a breast pump and bottle) may have a certain meaning for some women which detracts from their experience of breastfeeding their child. It is important, though, not to overstate the value of the physical contact of breastfeeding for women's developing sense of their relationship with their child. Research has demonstrated that women who bottle-feed do not typically have poor-quality relationships with their babies and that some women experience the physicality of breastfeeding as unpleasant.[37]

As feminist scholar Donna Haraway suggests, we may need new ways of thinking about our relation to an increasingly technological world and might usefully question dualisms such as the natural or biological and the artificial or technological.[38] Thus, we might find ways of being able to conceive of embodied and relational experience that incorporates technology such as the breast pump but that is not constrained by unhelpful mechanistic metaphors and does not therefore privilege technical (in this case medical) expertise over women's agency and relational experience.[39] In a similar vein, Ashley Pinkston, in her master's thesis, suggests that our distaste for "mothering with machines" such as breast pumps, may be open to challenge by asking, "Does technology mediation change the very experience of human emotional bonding into something inhuman?"[40]

Perhaps one answer to Pinkston's question is that for the women concerned it depends on the meaning of the technology. As others have argued, in order to understand whether and how breastfeeding is in women's interests, we need to look at the particular circumstances of breastfeeding and their meaning for particular women, in particular contexts.[41] The same can be said for expressing milk. For many women, the practice may have the same emancipatory implications that early feminists attributed to formula-feeding: enabling women to assert their presence outside of the domestic sphere and to resist the notion that infant nutrition is their sole responsibility by virtue of gender. Other women may feel more concerned that "mothering with machines" means the loss of something important to their relationship with their infant and their body, or inappropriate collusion with the biomedicalization, commercialization, and surveillance of breastfeeding. We may indeed need to resist approaches to breastfeeding that have at times been driven by medical and economic interests and as such have undermined women's confidence in their bodies.[42] However, it may not be wise to attempt to achieve a more woman-centered approach to breastfeeding by promoting an alternative one-size-fits-all image of the technology-free breastfeeding mother that does not take account of women's varying circumstances or value their particular preferences. For *some* women, these circumstances and preferences may mean that pumping is an attractive option.

Fourth, although the practice of expressing can clearly be very useful to women in navigating cultural pressures in relation to being a "good mother," it does not necessarily help women to challenge these. For example, it is important that we continue to assert the right of women to breastfeed when and where it is appropriate for them and their infants, to resist unwarranted medicalized surveillance that undermines women's sense of confidence in their bodies, and to challenge objectified images of the sexual breast. While public health initiatives might raise women's awareness of the *possibility* of individual solutions (like expressing) to some of these sociocultural dilemmas, they could usefully prioritize solutions developed at the social and policy level. These might include legislation to protect the right to breastfeed in public and the right to paid maternity leave without risk of job loss. Similarly, although some of our participants found expressing a helpful strategy for managing pain, maternity services still need to be organized and resourced so that they provide adequate breastfeeding support.

A final point to make in relation to public health initiatives is the way in which our participants talked about expressing as a solution to a problem. Feminist breastfeeding advocacy focused around women's "right" to breastfeed, though politically useful, can perhaps distract attention from the significant difficulties some women experience breastfeeding. Our data show that for many women feeding their baby is a matter of balancing different demands, finding solutions. and struggling with choices in difficult circumstances. Raising awareness of possible difficulties with breastfeeding at the prenatal stage and the role that expressing might play in addressing some of these seems likely to be useful rather than counterproductive, so long as this does not negate solutions at the social and policy levels by suggesting that expressing is the only or best solution.

Notes

1. See Labiner-Wolfe et al., "Prevalence of Breast Milk Expression"; Win et al., "Breastfeeding Duration"; Binns et al., "Trends"; Clemons and Amir, "Experience of Expressing."
2. For example, Dykes, "'Supply' and 'Demand'"; Blum, "Mothers, Babies, and Breastfeeding"; Van Esterik, "Expressing Ourselves."
3. Dykes, *Breastfeeding in Hospital*; Morse and Bottorff, "Emotional Experience."
4. Johnson et al., "Expressing Yourself."
5. Participants were first-time mothers intending to breastfeed who had healthy, term or close to term, singleton births. Thirty-three women took part in a larger qualitative

longitudinal study. Eight reported expressing or pumping breast milk extensively, and the stories of three of these women are presented here. We analyzed the data from a feminist poststructuralist perspective. See Johnson et al., "Expressing Yourself," for further details.

6. Approximately US$15,000.
7. Johnson et al., "Expressing Yourself."
8. Murphy, "Risk, Responsibility, and Rhetoric."
9. Stearns, "Breastfeeding and the Good Maternal Body."
10. Morse and Bottorff, "Emotional Experience," 330.
11. Dykes, "'Supply' and 'Demand.'"
12. Wall, "Moral Constructions."
13. See Parker, *Torn in Two*, and Eyer, "Mother-Infant Bonding," for a critical discussion of bonding theory.
14. For example, Blum, "Mothers, Babies, and Breastfeeding."
15. Approximately US$60,000.
16. Six pounds and 11.5 ounces.
17. Dykes, "'Supply' and 'Demand'"; Dykes, *Breastfeeding in Hospital*.
18. Murphy, "Risk, Responsibility, and Rhetoric."
19. For example, Dykes, "Western Medicine and Marketing."
20. Ibid.
21. For discussion of this, see Barclay and Lupton, "Experience of New Fatherhood"; Earle, "Why Some Women."
22. General Certificate of Secondary Education: Qualifications taken at sixteen years of age, at the end of compulsory education. In the United Kingdom, GCSEs are not sufficient for university entry, which requires two more years of study.
23. Approximately US$60,000.
24. Bartlett, "Breastfeeding Bodies and Choice," 154.
25. For example, Blum, "Mothers, Babies, and Breastfeeding"; Rojjanasrirat, "Working Women's Breastfeeding Experiences"; Meier, "Special Care Nursery."
26. Current UK legislation provides women with job-protected maternity leave for twelve months, which is paid for six weeks at 90 percent of the mother's average pay, followed by thirty-three weeks on Statutory Maternity Pay.
27. Labiner-Wolfe et al., "Prevalence of Breast Milk Expression"; Win et al., "Breastfeeding Duration."
28. Of course, it is possible there were additional reasons that some women were more comfortable expressing than placing their infants at their breasts, which may have been difficult to disclose.
29. Blum, "Mothers, Babies, and Breastfeeding," 290.
30. See further discussion in Lawrence and Lawrence *Breastfeeding*, 277–278.
31. World Health Organization, *Evidence for the Ten Steps*, 74–78.
32. Win et al., "Breastfeeding Duration." Although the researchers provide no information about methods of milk delivery, significant use of artificial teats could be assumed.
33. Walker, "Breast Pumps."
34. See Genna and Sandora, "Breastfeeding"; Page, "Breastfeeding in Early Functional."
35. Blum, "Mothers, Babies, and Breastfeeding."
36. See Klaus et al., "Maternal Attachment." For critique, see Burman, *Deconstructing Developmental Psychology*; Eyer, *Mother Infant Bonding*.
37. See Else-Quest, Hyde, and Clark, "Breastfeeding, Bonding"; Kelleher, "Physical Challenges"; Schmied and Barclay, "Connection and Pleasure."

38. Haraway, *Simians, Cyborgs, and Women.*

39. Dykes, "'Supply' and 'Demand.'"

40. Pinkston, "Being Cyborg," 67.

41. Carter, *Feminism, Breasts, and Breast-Feeding*; Hausman, *Mother's Milk.*

42. For a discussion of some of the effects of commercial and medical interests on breastfeeding, see Renfrew, Woolridge, and McGill, *Enabling Women*, 8–11.

Part VI

Morality and Guilt

Feminist Breastfeeding Promotion and the Problem of Guilt

It is difficult to have a conversation about breastfeeding in any setting without raising the specter of guilt. From the point of view of the mother who does not breastfeed and says she resents being made to feel guilty about her feeding method, to that of the former head of the American Academy of Pediatrics, who urged that breastfeeding "should be a nurturing sort of experience; we should not use guilt," breastfeeding and breastfeeding promotion are clearly associated with the induction of guilt.[1] What is less clear is how breastfeeding promoters—particularly if they are feminist—ought to carry out their promotion in such a way that does not induce guilt in women. In this chapter, we provide an analysis of infant feeding–related guilt. Our analysis of the feelings that women describe about feeding formula suggests that the dominant emotion may be more accurately described as shame. Much more damaging than guilt, shame involves the failure to live up to an ideal and the understanding of oneself as a lesser creature. Thus, it is the induction of shame, not guilt, that feminist breastfeeding promoters must resist. We close by describing conceptual shifts that must take place in breastfeeding promotion to eliminate the shaming of women.

Breastfeeding Promotion and Guilt

Most breastfeeding promoters are already familiar with the challenge that guilt presents to their promotion efforts. From the anecdotal accounts of doctors reluctant to recommend breastfeeding to their patients to the large-scale attack on the National Breastfeeding Awareness Campaign (NBAC), the induction of maternal guilt is a commonly cited reason for moderating or even avoiding exhortations to breastfeed. This professed concern for women's feelings is often viewed with skepticism by breastfeeding promoters, many of whom implicitly assume or explicitly argue that the guilt argument is, at least in part, a self-interested rhetorical ploy on the part of those who stand to benefit from increased sales of infant formula.[2] Still, many promoters remain genuinely disturbed by the possibility that mothers may be experiencing their breast-feeding promotion efforts as emotional coercion with guilt as the (unintended) side effect. In either case, breastfeeding promotion—particularly if it is to be feminist—is faced with the challenge of finding a way to deal with guilt.

Some breastfeeding promoters have answered this challenge by relabeling guilt as a different emotion; rather than feeling guilt, some commentators insist, nonbreastfeeding mothers are really experiencing anger, regret, resent-ment, or the sense of being cheated by a medical system or society that fails to adequately educate or support breastfeeding mothers. Lactation consultant Dianne Wiessinger suggests, "Help a mother who says she feels guilty to ana-lyze her feelings, and you may uncover a very different emotion. Someone long ago handed these mothers the word 'guilt.' It is the wrong word." The 1999 La Leche League International (LLLI) Conference included an entire session dedicated to the question: Promoting Breastfeeding or Promoting Guilt? In her summary of that session written for LLLI's *New Beginnings* magazine, commentator Robin Slaw explains, "Regret is what you feel when the choices, and the consequences of your choices, are not explained to you." Breastfeed-ing counselor Lesley McBurney echoes this point: "Guilt should be reserved for something over which we have control."[3]

This relabeling strategy is persuasive, as it shifts focus to the contexts in which mothers' choices are made, but it fails to address the guilty feelings of those women who make informed and relatively unencumbered decisions about feeding their babies. Certainly, many women face cultural, economic, physical, and social constraints that make breastfeeding difficult. Still, not all mothers who feed formula are dupes, and not all reasons for opting for formula are related to these types of constraints. Further, there is evidence that mothers do, in fact, feel guilty for feeding formula. The popular resource babycenter.com lists "feeding your baby formula" as the first item in the piece "The Top 7 Mommy Guilt Trips—And How to Handle Them."[4] The babycenter.com message boards are teeming with posts from mothers who say they feel guilty for not breastfeeding. While many women are—or at the very least should be—angry about the lack of information and structural support available to them as new mothers attempting to breastfeed, their self-reported guilt cannot simply be explained away as something else.

Perhaps even more important, there is a widely held cultural assumption that mothers who feed formula feel guilty; feeding babies infant formula is something, it is clear, about which it makes common cultural sense to feel guilt.

In fact, this common-sense approach is another way in which some breastfeeding promoters tackle the guilt issue. From a public health standpoint, they suggest, guilt is a well-accepted and time-honored tool in the physician's bag of tricks. Pediatrician Nancy Wight notes, "As pediatricians we do not hesitate to make our patient's [sic] parents feel guilty about having their children wear bicycle helmets, using infant car seats and seat belts, obtaining immunizations and fencing in pools. We use guilt to help adult patients lose weight, exercise more, stop smoking, drinking alcohol, and taking drugs." What is it about breastfeeding, they ask, that makes guilt suddenly off limits? One answer is that feeding formula is not considered a risk in the same way as many of these other activities. Rather, Slaw argues, "breastfeeding is often treated as a choice that is above the normal standard of child care—like buying expensive educational toys or sending a child to an exclusive private boarding school." Breastfeeding is also, even in the best of circumstances, a time- and labor-intensive activity that can serve "to restrict women's autonomy," particularly in the way that our culture understands it. Further, when one considers the complicated matrix of material and ideological factors that have been identified by scholars and promoters as impediments to breastfeeding, the purposeful use of guilt as a tool of breastfeeding promotion becomes much more fraught.[5]

Ultimately, creating a context in which all mothers truly have the choice to breastfeed is an aim of many breastfeeding promoters. But the recognition that such a context does not exist for all or even most women works to complicate the notion of the guilt related to feeding formula. While breastfeeding promoters continue to emphasize the importance of education about breastfeeding's benefits—or formula's risks—the fact that mothers so often use the term "guilt" to describe their feelings in relation to feeding formula or breastfeeding cessation suggests that women have not only heard the message about its benefits but also think that not breastfeeding is a personal inaction that wrongs their infants. Though guilt has been defined in a number of ways by psychologists and moral philosophers, we characterize the feeling of guilt as a response to specific wrongdoings.[6] Feminist philosopher Jennifer Manion defines guilt similarly: "Usually, one's feeling of guilt concerns a rule or rule-like constraint that one has broken, the harm that has ensued, and the people affected by the harmful act." In the case of guilt inspired by infant feeding, the mother feels she has broken a rule-like prescription to breastfeed—the recommendations of her doctor, public health officials, or even "science" or "nature" more generally conceived—and that her failure to fulfill this prescription has harmed or will harm her child. Characterized in this way, guilt applies to things over which one has control. Or, as Manion puts it, "one feels guilty only when one recognizes one's responsibility for an action."[7]

The feeling of guilt, then, is commensurate with feeding formula when doing so is characterized as a woman's own personal choice and her own personal failure, but also when she is held primarily responsible for the health of her child. In a culture in which "we take mothers to be responsible for ensuring not just the health of their families, but the health of the next generation of citizens," there is the sense that mothers are, in fact, guilty as charged for failing to do everything possible to optimize the health of their children.[8] The sense of control provided by an enhanced understanding of the causes of disease, political scientist Joan Wolf points out, "means that poor health no longer has to do with luck or chance but is the personal responsibility of each individual"—or his mother—"to avoid."[9] The reality is that even the best mother cannot guarantee the health of her child, and even exclusively breastfed children get ill, sometimes critically. In addition, women don't always have absolute control over what doctors, public health officials, and breastfeeding promoters have insisted is the choice between feeding human milk or formula. This is something that breastfeeding promoters have recognized for decades: in 1981 Edward Baer reasoned that "the mother's choice is a function of her *opportunity* to breastfeed (material conditions that facilitate or interfere with breastfeeding) and her *motivation* to breastfeed (ideological conditions that reflect her attitudes, beliefs, and knowledge of breastfeeding and its alternatives)." This assertion is echoed by mothers and commentators who criticize what they perceive is a stifling cultural prescription to breastfeed in the absence of structural supports for doing so.[10]

Bernice Hausman makes a compelling point when she argues that it is easier to eschew breastfeeding promotion by citing a wish to avoid inducing guilt "in lieu of making substantive changes to the material circumstances of mothers' lives."[11] Certainly, the fear of inducing maternal guilt has become a trope that provides a politically effective way of appearing to care about mothers without actually having to do anything concrete to assist them; feminists and breastfeeding promoters alike must reject guilt as a rhetorical ploy in the way that she identifies. Yet, this view of maternal guilt leaves unanswered the legitimate concerns of feminists and breastfeeding promoters who worry about the toll that guilt takes on mothers. Of even greater concern, a more careful reading of self-described feelings of maternal guilt suggests that they may really be shame, an emotion that, for moral philosophers at least, is perceived to be more difficult and damaging than guilt.

Guilt, Shame, and the Total Mother

The term "guilt" fails to fully capture women's emotional experiences about infant feeding, particularly with respect to feeding formula. Political scientists Karen Kedrowski and Michael Lipscomb provide an instructive example in the opening of *Breastfeeding Rights in the United States*, which begins with a personal narrative of Kedrowski's own infant feeding experiences. When a string of illnesses and breastfeeding difficulties forced her to wean her first child early, she writes that she was "guilt-ridden," especially when he developed eczema and pneumonia. Her second breastfeeding attempt, with her daughter, proved more successful; however, she was chastised for breastfeeding her eighteen-month-old at her child care center. Kedrowski reports that the incident made her think, *"I am a perfectly bad mother.* I'm damned because I didn't breastfeed my son and I'm damned because I am breastfeeding my daughter."[12] Some further examples from online message boards, all typical of posts from mothers who have begun feeding their babies formula, are also instructive:

> I took my 6-month-old to the doctor today and she said he needs formula because he's not gaining enough weight; he should be at least 2 pounds heavier. *I kind of feel like a failure.* I've been breastfeeding him this whole time and things felt like they were right on track. I felt so guilty giving him the formula today I almost cried.[13]

> I've tried exhaustively—and unsuccessfully—to breastfeed my baby. It was always a struggle, even after I got professional help. During my pregnancy I was so excited about the idea of breastfeeding. *Now I feel like a failure*, especially because of all the information out there about breast milk being best. What should I do?[14]

> With the breeze that pregnancy and labor was I just assumed that I was on a winning streak and breastfeeding would be a breeze as well. I had read up and prepared myself or so I thought. It was so HARD! I feel so bad for only making it 5 days. *I feel like a failure as a woman.* I made my mother give her the first bottle because I was crying so hard I couldn't see or breath.[15]

All these examples indicate something other than just guilt. Kedrowski momentarily imagines that she is a bad mother, while the anonymous posters all say they feel like failures. In all cases, the mothers' emotions go beyond the feeling that a particular action, or lack thereof, has broken a rule and caused harm. Rather, they judge themselves as deficient: bad mothers, failures. Such negative global self-assessments suggest what philosophers Bartky, Deigh, and

Manion identify as shame, which according to Bartky "involves the distressed apprehension of oneself as a lesser creature" or is, in Manion's words, "a painful, sudden awareness of the self as less good than hoped for and expected." Guilt, then, is response to what one *does*, while shame is response to who one *is*. While Manion clarifies that "feeling guilty and feeling ashamed are not mutually exclusive," we want to focus on the shame that these mothers' experiences and comments suggest. They hold themselves up to a certain standard of motherhood and judge themselves as falling short, as failing. Joan Wolf provides a convincing portrait of this standard, arguing that our culture demands "total motherhood" as "a moral code in which mothers are exhorted to optimize every dimension of children's lives, beginning with the womb." This standard of total motherhood also casts children's needs in opposition to the needs of their mothers: "mothers have *wants* . . . but children have *needs*." The implication is that good mothers will endure any and all costs to ensure that their children's needs for "optimal" care are met. Joan Wolf's formulation of total motherhood is borne out in the following example: in her qualitative study of women's breastfeeding experiences, sociologist Christa Kelleher found that women described experiencing feelings of what they called guilt not only when they decided to discontinue breastfeeding, but also "when they acknowledged their own physical limitations or personal needs." In identifying their own needs, Kelleher's mothers failed to live up to the ideal of total motherhood; they used the word "guilt" to describe this failure, but the term "shame" is equally apt.[16]

Not breastfeeding or formula supplementation may also make mothers feel the shame of failing to achieve proper womanhood; one of the anonymous posters above specified, "I feel like a failure as a woman." As feminist scholar Pam Carter suggests, the link between breastfeeding and femininity that is assumed by many breastfeeding promoters means that nonbreastfeeding mothers are also less feminine, deficient not only as mothers but also as women. Kedrowski's account is again instructive. She explains that "the language of breastfeeding advocates, including phrases such as 'all women can breastfeed if they try hard enough' which was intended to be supportive, did nothing to assuage these feelings of guilt, and in fact compounded them."[17] The message that all women *can* breastfeed may be read by a new mother, already vulnerable to the demands of caring for a new infant, as meaning that any woman who cannot or does not is an incomplete woman and thus shameful.

Moral philosophers have often described guilt as useful in its ability to encourage moral behavior: "Guilt feelings, which focus primarily on the specific wrong act, encourage the guilt-ridden person to understand the nature of the harm done, to seek out the one who has been harmed and to attend to possible reparation." With a few exceptions, shame has been understood differently. Rather than provoking action, shame can often render the subject motionless. Manion also points out that many accounts suggest "that shame causes serious damage, especially in the form of self-doubt," and that it "might result in deference, withdrawal, and hopelessness about approximating one's moral ideal."[18] In addition, political theorist Jill Locke adds that shame can also blind the subject to the problematic social context that provokes her shame in the first place: "One of shame's most poisonous consequences is the way in which it overwhelms the subject so that she is unable to think beyond herself. Rather than focus on changing the world in ways that might lessen her shame, the shamed subject focuses on changing herself so that she might accommodate the demands of her milieu."[19] Locke's argument is especially salient with regard to the shame described above, the shame that results from identifying oneself as a deficient mother or woman, because it can prevent the subject from interrogating, criticizing, and even rejecting what she has been told it means to be a good mother or woman in the first place. Yet Manion suggests that shame, *when accompanied by a sense of self-concern*, can in fact "open up the possibility of genuinely healthy revision" of the standards by which one has been evaluating oneself.[20] By looking at just a few representative excerpts from responses to the Internet posts, Manion's meaning becomes clearer.

Do not feel guilty quitting breastfeeding. I persevered for 6 months with my first child. With my second, I quit after a month . . . only to realize that *it was my first child who missed out . . . on a happy mom! Because when mom is unhappy, everyone suffers.*[21]

You DO NOT love your child any less by not breastfeeding and if you're anything like me, *you will bond more with your baby when feeding him/her with a bottle because you will be able to enjoy each other's company without the worry and anxiety. Remember to take care of you and by doing so you can take care of your baby* and enjoy the beautiful experience of being a mother.[22]

The decision to switch was one of the hardest decisions I've ever had to make, but I will say that *any guilt I initially felt has been replaced with joy as I now treasure every moment with my new baby girl instead of living in fear of an upcoming feeding.* Congrats to all of you who have made a decision that is right for you and your baby. *Breastfeeding does not define a good mother!*[23]

In all of these examples, the posters use their own experiences of breastfeeding cessation to posit an alternative vision of what it means to be a good or ideal mother: a happy mother, a mother unimpeded from bonding with her baby because of pain or dread. Though the self-concern they exhibit is framed in terms of being a different sort of good mother, they nonetheless reject the ideal of total motherhood, incorporating their own needs into their revised motherhood ideals. It is this sort of revisioning with attention to self-concern that feminists and breastfeeding promoters must facilitate. As Joan Wolf points out, "risk calculations are evaluations of trade-offs or choices between imperfect options."[24] Infant feeding decisions are made in a cultural context, as argued above, but they must also be made with an eye to the needs and priorities of mothers.

Conclusion: Toward a Feminist Approach to Breastfeeding Promotion

Our analysis of infant-feeding-related shame suggests that mainstream breastfeeding promotion has colluded in the creation of a shame-inducing ideal of motherhood that inflexibly insists that the good mother is a breastfeeding mother, regardless of other social, cultural, economic, or even medical considerations. As Hausman has persuasively argued, the investment of breastfeeding promotion in a biomedical view has meant allowing medicine, not mothers, to define what it means to be a good mother. By so often privileging a medical model, breastfeeding promoters have focused on providing information to mothers to the exclusion of listening to mothers. Following the medical model, most breastfeeding promotion has prized the "natural" needs of infants over the needs of women, assuming that mothers are lacking in skills and instincts.[25] In the rare instances that the well-being of mothers is discussed, it is too often as a superficial carrot designed to incentivize breastfeeding— "Nursing your baby will help you lose weight!"—rather than fully considering the range of women's needs. Finally, in positing breastfeeding as a mother's choice, breastfeeding promotion has too often participated in the obfuscation of the structural factors that make breastfeeding difficult, placing the responsibility of infant health squarely on the shoulders of mothers, despite those structural factors.

If breastfeeding promotion is to take seriously the challenge of shame—as we argue it must if it is to be truly feminist—promoters need to commit to three significant conceptual shifts. First, breastfeeding promoters must place mothers at the center of our efforts rather than their infants. We should consider the interests, needs, and well-being of mothers as the objects of our promotion.

If one makes the reasonable (yet still somehow radical) assumption that the vast majority of mothers have the best interests of their children at heart, it becomes clear that in supporting mothers we are also attending to the needs of their infants. Further, by placing mothers at the center, we challenge the assumption of the total motherhood ideal that mothers' needs are irrelevant, creating a space in which they can define what good motherhood means *to them*. Second, as feminist breastfeeding promoters, we must take the lived experiences of mothers as seriously as we take evidence-based biomedical data. This shift necessitates working to create a flow of information that runs both ways, not just from medical providers and breastfeeding promoters *to* women, but *from* women as well. Only by listening to women can we discover what is important *to them*, what presents challenges *to them*, and what the breastfeeding experience is like *for them*. Doing so will allow us to acknowledge a full range of breastfeeding experiences, be they good, bad, or even ugly. Being honest about women's diverse experiences means that we will lessen the potential for shame among those mothers who do not have the idyllic experience that mainstream promotion holds up as the norm.

Finally, we need to approach our understanding of women's infant feeding choices aware of both the constraints that women face in developing their own infant feeding plans and the ways in which these constraints may recommend something other than exclusive breastfeeding. When we understand these constraints, we can work with individual mothers to develop strategies for dealing with them, as well as make the elimination of them a vital aspect of our promotion efforts. We must make it clear that micro-level shame is not appropriate for so-called individual choices, which actually have macro-level causes.

Notes

1. Dr. Carden Johnston, quoted in Orent, "Formula." We focus in this chapter on breastfeeding promotion, or planned social marketing in support of breastfeeding. In some cases, our conclusions regarding guilt and shame are also relevant to the practices of breastfeeding advocacy and support.
2. Hausman, *Viral Mothers*; Newman, *Breastfeeding and Guilt*; Slaw, "LLLI Conference"; Wight, "Guilt Issue"; Wolf, "What Feminists Can Do."
3. Wiessinger, "Watch Your Language!," 2; Slaw, "LLLI Conference"; McBurney, "Guilty Secrets."
4. Slaw, "LLLI Conference"; Lack, "Top 7."
5. Wight, "Guilt Issue"; see Hausman, *Viral Mothers*; Mojab, "Real Breastfeeding Issue"; Newman, *Breastfeeding and Guilt*; Slaw, "LLLI Conference"; Wiessinger, "Watch Your Language!"; Slaw, "LLLI Conference," 271; Blum, "Mothers, Babies, and Breastfeeding," 292.
6. Bartky, *Femininity and Domination*; Deigh, "Shame and Self-Esteem," 225.

7.   Manion, "Moral Relevance," 76.

8.   Kukla, "Ethics and Ideology," 158.

9.   Wolf, "Is Breast Really Best?," 613.

10. Baer, "Promoting Breastfeeding," 199. See also Rosin, "Case Against Breast-Feeding."

11. Hausman, *Viral Mothers*, 164.

12. Kedrowski and Lipscomb, *Breastfeeding Rights*, xi–xii, (emphasis added).

13. Ezramomma, "Breast or Bottle," (emphasis added; spelling and punctuation corrected).

14. Anonymous, "Question," August 24 (emphasis added).

15. Ruccadog, "Stopped Breastfeeding" (emphasis added).

16. Bartky, *Femininity and Domination*, 87; Manion, "Girls Blush," 21; Manion, "Moral Relevance," 76; Wolf, "Is Breast Really Best?," 615; Kelleher, "Physical Challenges," 2734.

17. Carter, *Feminism, Breasts and Breast-Feeding*; Kedrowski and Lipscomb, *Breastfeeding Rights*, xi.

18. Manion, "Moral Relevance," 78–82.

19. Locke, "Shame and the Future," 151.

20. Manion, "Girls Blush," 35.

21. Mac1444, "Question" (emphasis added; spelling corrected).

22. Anonymous, "Question," October 9 (emphasis added).

23. Klarose, "Question."

24. Wolf, "Is Breast Really Best?," 613. Wolf goes on to argue that "extensive research, moreover, indicates that babies are at risk for a variety of developmental and health disorders in homes where mothers are psychologically depressed or impoverished. For women who find the demands of breast-feeding overwhelming or who cannot reconcile breast-feeding with employment, bottle-feeding might constitute the less risky option" (614). See also Carter, *Feminism, Breasts and Breast-Feeding*.

25. Hausman, "Contamination and Contagion."

Breastfeeding in the Margins

Navigating through the Conflicts of Social and Moral Order

The moral tone implied in breastfeeding knowledge is rooted in power relations that also affect the identity of mothers. We present our arguments with examples of women living in poverty, since this is a population whose breastfeeding experiences are rarely addressed in the literature. Building from critical concepts developed by French thinkers Pierre Bourdieu and Michel Foucault, we examine closely how issues of power, morality, and identity are embedded in public health promotion of breastfeeding, and how that promotion might be changed to better address women's practices and needs.

Motherhood and Ritual

Medical anthropology demonstrates that the reproductive behaviors of women are heavily controlled through ritual. Reproductive rituals regulate and impose normative behaviors and often restrictive rules on women who are expected to follow them during pregnancy, birth, and the postnatal periods, constituting what French ethnographer Arnold Van Gennep called "rites of passage."[1] As a result, women around the world function under the scrutiny of family and community.

Women are expected to comply with specific rules relative to their social, bodily, emotional, nutritional, and spiritual behaviors during their biosocial transition to motherhood. In some cultures, for example, pregnant women are forbidden from attending funerals to avoid jeopardizing the health and survival of their unborn child.[2] In Vietnam, tradition dictates that mothers cover specific parts of their bodies to prevent illness in old age.[3] While the familial and community knowledge justifying these norms and rules varies according to cultural context, the aim to protect the mother and infant is fully transcultural. Such cultural knowledge, passed on from one generation to the next, serves to safeguard not only the mother and her child but also the reproduction and survival of a group.[4] This cultural pattern may also explain why, even in modern posttraditional societies, strangers commonly feel entitled to offer unsolicited advice to a new mother, to ask personal questions concerning her pregnancy, or even to touch her belly.

If mothers follow the prescribed traditional perinatal rules and rituals of their group, they gain what French sociologist Pierre Bourdieu refers to as symbolic capital. Symbolic capital is a form of power that comes with social position, affords prestige, and leads others from the same fields to pay attention to the agent who has such capital.[5] Indeed, such mothers will be considered "good mothers" by their group, since they are safeguarding themselves, their infants, and, correspondingly, the reproduction and survival of the family and community. Hence, by following culturally sanctioned infant feeding practices immediately after birth, a mother gains symbolic capital that imparts her with social stature and leads others from the same community to pay attention to and respect her. Conversely, mothers can lose symbolic capital if they fail to follow perinatal cultural norms. Rites of passage imply a moral dimension to motherhood and maternal practices.

Rites of passage are also known for the psychological protective and adaptive effect they have on women experiencing vulnerability because of their transition toward a new biosocial status and identity.[6] In the context of transition to a new identity, infant feeding decisions and experience—whether corresponding to or deviating from the local infant feeding habitus of their community—are not neutral for mothers, nor for their family or community.[7] In fact, when mothers choose to deviate from local cultural norms or the habitus of infant feeding, such a decision often has emotional implications for them in terms of their own identities as mothers, but also for other actors in their family and community. By adopting the traditional cultural rules regulating bodily and behavioral rituals, mothers contribute to the construction of their new maternal identity and gain symbolic capital. Through their actions they also confirm and reproduce the cultural identity of the family and community. For example, in our study examining breastfeeding attitudes and practices of mothers from Cape Town, South Africa, mothers of young infants reported that they adhered to traditional perinatal rituals, with more than half of the mothers using traditional infant herbal preparations despite clinical advice to the contrary.[8] Mothers did not disclose these practices to health care practitioners who were perceived to disapprove of these traditional practices.

The increasingly individualistic family structures in Western settings have meant a change in how families and communities dictate reproductive rituals. As family and community have become less publicly prominent as ritual forces, biomedicine and public health now serve these roles. This shift has provided health institutions access to private spaces. Institutions now dictate ways in which women should use their bodies in feeding their infants. These institutions have taken a leading role in the construction of infant feeding norms and behavioral rules for mothers, largely through the production of breastfeeding knowledge and discourse, but also through the promotion of breastfeeding as a health-enhancing practice central to public health goals.

Public health engagement in breastfeeding is motivated by its mandate to promote and protect the health of the vulnerable mother/infant dyad. However, we need to examine more closely the ways in which the authoritative and evidence-based knowledge that public health produces also infers, like rites of passage, a moral dimension of motherhood.

The Field of Health: Social and Moral Order of Public Health Discourse

Dual ontologies of breastfeeding exist in the public health literature: the medical model and the maternalist model. The medical model of breastfeeding, while recognizing the health benefits for women, primarily focuses on the nutritional and health benefits of breastfeeding for infants. Evidence-based studies that demonstrate infant benefits have influenced public health to prescribe breastfeeding as the optimal way to nourish infants.[9] Public health messaging tends to emphasize breast milk, not breastfeeding, and thus reduces the role of mothers to the provider of a substance that can also be provided through the technology of breast pumps.[10] This underlying ontology of the medical model has been criticized because it ignores the relational dimension of breastfeeding between mother and infant.[11] In this model, breast milk is presented as a source of optimum nutrients for infants, providing a "good start in life" by protecting infant health and enhancing brain development.[12] Not breastfeeding or delaying breastfeeding is thus associated with suboptimal health and mothers adopting a high-risk behavior that jeopardizes development.[13] The logic of this reductionist view ignores the relational and protective role played by mothers in the development of their babies. This discourse strongly suggests a moral obligation for mothers to breastfeed, an obligation to protect their babies according to rules that are supported by scientific knowledge and also by medical ethos that has replaced the authority of mothers and their families, their embodied knowledge, and their presumed capacity to care for their babies.

The maternalist model, on the other hand, builds on the embodied connection of breastfeeding between mother and infant as favoring "secure attachment" and enhancing the mother-infant bond.[14] While the bonding effect of breastfeeding is not supported by evidenced-based research, bonding theory prevails in much of health and breastfeeding discourse, as well as in popular knowledge. Bonding is a prominent justification of mothers' infant feeding choice.[15] For example, in our French-Canadian study, breastfeeding mothers considered their breastfeeding choice to be best because it fosters mother-child attachment. On the other hand, the majority of bottle-feeding mothers considered breastfed babies to be too attached to their mothers and not independent enough to face the hardships of life.[16] This persistent belief relating breast-feeding to secure attachment has also led to the idea that breastfeeding is a measure of successful and good mothering, contributing to the ontology of breastfeeding as a moral performance of mothering.

Both of these polarized ontologies of breastfeeding (the medical and maternal models) abound in public health literature and practice, thereby emphasizing and supporting the implied notions of good mothering and intensive motherhood.[17] We consider public health support for breastfeeding as a moral imperative of motherhood to be a serious problem for two reasons. First, ignoring the relational dimension of breastfeeding diminishes the contextual, technical, and individual constraints that women, particularly vulnerable women, face when they want to breastfeed. Framing the embodi-ment of breastfeeding within a largely biomedical view reduces breastfeeding to a biological, heavily moralized performance of mothers.[18] Hence, women who would like to breastfeed but are not successful at it may experience failure, guilt, or the fear of jeopardizing the physical and psychological health and development of their infants.[19] In our study of breastfeeding among French Canadians living in poverty, mothers' narratives often reference strong feelings of guilt about not being up to the task of breastfeeding. Such emotions also induced feelings of doubt in their abilities as mothers.[20]

Second, by constructing breastfeeding as a moral imperative of motherhood, public health succeeds in situating breastfeeding within the logic of the Western ethos of individualism. Such an embodied social practice cannot be reduced to the sole agency of mothers. Breastfeeding is a collective and biocultural endeavor. By adopting a moralizing discourse, public health blames mothers who abandon breastfeeding, making them feel responsible for the failure of their breastfeeding and, even worse, for failing to be good mothers. This perspective ignores the multitude of reasons women discontinue breastfeeding, many of which are related to societal constrictions and lack of support. The French Canadian mothers in our study who decided to feed with infant formula felt judged or stigmatized by nurses.[21] The rare mothers who participated in prenatal classes also felt the same judgmental climate and attitudes from health professionals and other mothers who intended to breastfeed.[22]

The abandonment of traditional perinatal rituals, combined with the more general moral vacuum of secular society and the strong belief in the value of individualism, creates fertile context for public health norms to function as moral imperatives during women's reproductive years. The shift of infant feeding from a traditional cultural practice to a public health imperative is noteworthy, especially since it involves the loss of embodied breastfeeding knowledge as well as the loss of traditional routes of support offered by family and community. Breastfeeding promotion efforts center on convincing mothers to breastfeed, but do not place emphasis on creating a cultural acceptance of breastfeeding. Hence, mothers may be expected to breastfeed because of public health messages or hospital practice, but they do not necessarily receive support, or even the moral stamp to do so, from their family and social environment or from their attending clinicians once they leave the hospital after birth. As we write this chapter, and despite the fact that breastfeeding is a public health priority in Quebec, a mother was recently forced to leave a children's store when she declined to stop breastfeeding. The mother, well aware of her rights, brought the case to the attention of the media; despite an apology, her story mobilized other breastfeeding mothers to stage a protest. One wonders: if this had been a low-income breastfeeding mother, would she have exercised her rights and engaged in such public action when she was already going against the habitus of her own group?

Conflicting messages concerning infant feeding often received from diverse fields are a strong indication that motherhood involves complex negotiations between medical ideas of risk, family expectations, demands relating to infant weight gain, rules regulating public spaces, and personal desires. Successful navigation through such complexities suggests that women are not passive recipients of discourse. It is more plausible to suggest that women employ power/knowledge at their disposal to guide their infant feeding decisions.[23] Such a response is a significant challenge when women have limited access to power and diverse forms of capital, as is the case of women living in poverty.

Mothers do not live in a perfect world, and their life contexts do not always provide congruency within the different fields they engage in. In countries where breastfeeding constitutes a relatively recent public health priority, ethnographic studies have shown that women negotiate their infant feeding choice with health professionals, as well as with key family and community members.[24] We thus need to rethink how public health knowledge about breastfeeding might guide actions in a way that recognizes both the embodied cultural knowledge of infant feeding in communities and the roles played by the actors with whom mothers engage in the different fields of their lives.

Navigating Fields to Construct Maternal Identity

The heavily moralized promotion of breastfeeding creates destructive tension between health care providers and mothers and, more important, misses the mark and opportunity of being truly supportive of breastfeeding practices. Public health linkage between breastfeeding and ideologies of intensive motherhood is shortsighted, since such a connection obscures the social and cultural complexities of breastfeeding and, moreover, conceals how infant feeding decisions and experiences contribute to mothers' identities within the different fields of their lives. By creating a heavily moralized breastfeeding discourse, public health asserts its power through knowledge directed at mothers. The implied morality becomes a mechanism of surveillance, used to control mothers' actions, creating difficult power relations between mothers and health providers. Mothers who deviate from these norms may feel alienated from other mothers and perceive themselves as failures, a detrimental self-perception of their maternal identity.[25] Mothers from the social margins are understandably vulnerable to such social scrutiny, even if they disagree with the "good mothering" discourse. Mothers' own formulation of maternal identity is highly dependent on the fields they engage in and the existing power dynamics within those fields. Thus, women living in the context of poverty experience the "good mothering ideology" differently from middle-class and wealthy women, as their access to symbolic capital is not as abundant as for those women and is often solely dependent on being perceived by others as a good mother.[26]

Despite power relationships between institutions and mothers, there is evidence indicating that women tend not to act as passive victims of dominant discourse. Instead, they participate in what Foucault referred to as resistance. Through resistance women create alternative discourses, whereby they construct new knowledge for their own use and thereby regain some power. Such processes allow mothers to reconfigure their identities through complex negotiations, and thus to include positive mothering concepts while maintaining preexisting identities and roles.[27] Some mothers in our South African work demonstrated their resistance to medical authority by deciding to breastfeed despite discouraging health care encounters. By practicing exclusive breastfeeding, these mothers used knowledge accessed from settings that were more empowering to them, places where safe breastfeeding for HIV-infected mothers was promoted, taught, and supported. Through resistance, mothers formulated a different discourse, one that addressed their own reality and therefore allowed forms of agency that helped them to reclaim some power within their social fields.

Through acts of resistance, mothers in our South African study deviated from cultural norms of mixed breastfeeding (a highly risky mode of infant feeding for transmitting HIV) by practicing exclusive breastfeeding.[28] By breastfeeding exclusively some mothers were at risk of scrutiny, suspicion, and criticism from family and their community. However, these mothers were able to maintain their intentions to breastfeed safely, primarily through creative means that shielded them from the gaze of their families and neighbors expecting traditional modes of breastfeeding (that is, mixed feeding). By employing creative means of reconfiguration of self, these mothers maintained their symbolic capital of motherhood. For example, one mother invented a satisfying explanatory story to avoid the social gaze of her mother and others and maintain her good-mother identity. Mothers repeatedly told us they were accustomed to finding "ways to make things work," particularly if they had some level of support. Our study confirmed that reconstruction of self-identity that fit into group cultural norms was possible when mothers were able to access personal support networks.[29]

Our empirical observations point to ways in which infant feeding decisions and maternal identity are linked, as well as the moral predicament such a connection imposes on women living in the margins. In the next section, we propose a paradigm shift to guide knowledge production in public health, in a way that could help diminish the moral underpinnings of public health discourse and practice.

Knowledge Exchange: Toward Harmonizing the Conflicting Social and Moral Orders of Breastfeeding

Women's lives include social, cultural, economic, political, and gendered dynamics. All these contextual elements, along with other discreet unidentified elements, continue to influence and shape infant feeding, as science and medicine continue to contribute to feeding decisions. These factors have often presented a challenge to the operational aspect of contextualized health promotion. We therefore propose a partnership between public health and the target population involved: namely, mothers and their communities.

The paradigm shift we propose involves, first, abandoning the connection between breastfeeding, morality, and good mothering both within social science literature and public health discourse, including policy, programming, promotion, intervention, and clinical communications. Second, to avoid victim blaming, future public health knowledge about breastfeeding needs to expand beyond the narrow confines of the mother/infant dyad to include the role of the diverse fields mothers navigate. To generate knowledge that is truly inclusive of mothers and their communities, future public health knowledge production should adopt a participatory action approach. This democratization of knowledge production should involve knowledge exchange between partners, namely, public health agents, mothers, and their communities. Such an approach recognizes that women are not empty vessels to be filled by biomedical knowledge, an underlying ontological postulate that has been ineffective in public health action. Use of maternal experiential knowledge as part of breastfeeding discourse is challenging because it requires power sharing, a difficult task for socially sanctioned bastions of power like health care and public health institutions, particularly when such sharing involves those living in the social margins. By recognizing the agency mothers exercise within their own social fields, public health has the potential of building both understanding of and respect for mothers' knowledge.

Taking up this challenge has the strong possibility of facilitating meaningful changes that would serve women at different levels of the socioeconomic structure. Moreover, such collaborations can effect change that is woman-centered and incorporates socially as well as culturally diverse women's voices.

We have suggested that some women exercise their power to enact their infant feeding decisions despite opposing forces. Vulnerable women's experiences of breastfeeding will be different from those of women with resources because of their social location. However, Foucault's assertion that power relations are not fixed means that regardless of social location, examination of women's sense of power is a useful process. Building an understanding of power relations and resistance to power dynamics will help provide insight into the differences and commonalities among women as they relate to breastfeeding practices.

Although our appeal to a paradigm shift sounds like a lofty ideal, it is important to keep in mind that social and cultural relationships are fluid and in constant movement. Through harmonized production of knowledge, destruction of the morally charged and overmedicalized breastfeeding discourse can take place, paving the way for a more supportive environment of breastfeeding as a woman's right, not a moral obligation.

Notes

1. Van Gennep, *Rites of Passage.*
2. Groleau, "Determinants culturels."

3. Groleau, Soulière, and Kirmayer, "Breastfeeding and the Cultural."
4. Jordan, *Birth in Four Cultures*; Kay, *Anthropology of Human Birth*.
5. A field is a setting, a place, a group, or a social class that determines access to power in specific ways and according to a specific position.
6. Van Gennep, *Rites of Passage*.
7. Habitus refers to the disposition of agents or "the mental structures through which they apprehend the social world, [and] are essentially the product of the internalization of the structures of that world" (see Van Gennep, *Rites of Passage*).
8. Sibeko et al., "Beliefs, Attitudes, and Practices."
9. World Health Organzation and UNICEF, "Protecting, Promoting and Supporting Breastfeeding"; World Health Organzation and UNICEF, "Global Strategy for Infant and Young Child Feeding."
10. Johnson et al., "Expressing Yourself."
11. Groleau and Cabral, "Reconfiguring"; Dykes, *Breastfeeding in Hospital*.
12. Riordan, *Breastfeeding and Human Lactation*.
13. Lee, "Living with Risk."
14. Wall, "Moral Constructions."
15. Eyer, "Mother-Infant Bonding"; Wall, "Moral Constructions."
16. Groleau and Rodriguez, "Breastfeeding and Poverty," 21. This study aims to understand the psychosocial processes involved in the low duration rates of breastfeeding amongst Canadian-born, low-income mothers. Ethnographic interviews were conducted with forty-two mothers that initiated breastfeeding; some breastfed for a few hours, a few days, or for many months. A critical approach was used to understand how mothers introduced and negotiated the cultural change of breastfeeding in the context of their social lives.
17. Marshall, Godfrey, and Renfrew, "Being a 'Good Mother.'"
18. Dykes, *Breastfeeding in Hospital*.
19. Crossley, "Breastfeeding as a Moral Imperative."
20. Ibid., 86.
21. Groleau and Cabral, "Reconfiguring."
22. Groleau and Rodriguez, "Breastfeeding and Poverty."
23. "Power/knowledge" is a Foucaultian term. It refers to knowledge that is embodied in discourse, which becomes a form of power. Understanding the underpinnings of discourse allows for power to be identified as it is exercised through epistemic forms of knowledge. See Foucault, *The History of Sexuality*.
24. Groleau and Cabral, "Reconfiguring"; Groleau, Souliere, and Kirmayer, "Breastfeeding and the Cultural"; Groleau and Rodriguez, "Breastfeeding and Poverty"; Groleau, Zelkowitz, and Cabral, "Enhancing Generalizability."
25. Groleau and Cabral, "Reconfiguring"; Groleau, Zelkowitz, and Cabral, "Enhancing Generalizability"; Groleau and Rodriguez, "Breastfeeding and Poverty."
26. Attree, "Low-Income Mothers."
27. Ryan, Bissell, and Alexander, "Moral Work."
28. Sibeko et al., "Mothers' Infant Feeding Experiences." This qualitative study seeks to explore challenges and factors enabling safe infant feeding practices by HIV-infected women residing in a resource-poor community in South Africa. Included are narratives of women's experiences of their encounters with barriers to breastfeeding, despite policies that promote safe breastfeeding practices for infected women choosing to breastfeed their infants.
29. Ibid.

Part VII

Media and Popular Culture

Reinstating Pleasure in Reality

Promoting Breastfeeding through *Ars Erotica*

Health Promotion and the Female Body

In 2010 the Department of Health and Aging in Canberra released a ten-point Australian National Breastfeeding Strategy for stakeholders and government agencies. The first point reads, "Monitoring and surveillance" and the last, "Education and awareness, including antenatal education." Between these are items relating to dietary guidelines, growth charts, the WHO's code of marketing, training in breastfeeding support for health professionals, research into milk banks, and other worthy projects.

In 2008 an Australian advertising firm released a tampon advertisement for U Tampons, manufactured by Kotex. In it an attractive young woman walks down the street with cheerful music in the background, carrying a pet beaver under her arm. They are on their way to have their hair and nails done, then head to the beach to sunbathe as young men wander admiringly past. Afterward they go out to lunch. Across the table at the restaurant, the woman presents a gift to her pet, who opens it to discover a box of U Tampons. The scene closes to a female voiceover: "You've only got one, so for the ultimate care down there, make it U."[1] Meanwhile, on late-night television, actress Toni Collette jokes about spraying her breast milk at the studio camera, and news of a New York chef creating cheese dishes from his partner's breast milk circulates in tabloid media.[2]

Although these texts target different audiences, the gap between them highlights the extent to which public health discourse fails, in contrast to popular culture, to acknowledge women's corporeal experience, as well as the need to embed knowledge within cultural as well as institutional contexts.

The conservative discourse of the public sector is unsurprising, yet its lack of recognition of these worlds suggests a lag in its conceptualization of intimate behavior and the processes of social change.

All health promotion addresses intimate behavior to some extent. The challenge is to balance scientific evidence of benefit or harm with a recognition of the complex and varied relationships people have with their bodies. In the case of breastfeeding, the scientific conceptualization of the practice of breastfeeding, together with the substance (milk) and the process (lactation), is at odds with a whole range of constraints outside clinical settings: partner expectations, sexuality, work, maternity leave, and architecture, to name a few. There exists a stark contrast between the clinical management of breast milk as a disembodied medicinal substance within a scarcity model of carefully measured protocols, risks and benefits, and the cultural celebration of a relational bodily process that engages with food, babies, and sex within a plenitude model of curiosity, irreverence, and pleasure.

A small number of health promotion campaigns developed by community breastfeeding organizations have included humor and a hint of sexuality. These include the 2002 Australian Breastfeeding Association television spot with a baby breastfeeding in close-up then speaking to the camera: "Get ahead in life. Suck up to the boss." Also in 2002 the New Zealand World Breastfeeding Week poster featured the actress Lucy Lawless breastfeeding while modestly attired in skirt and blouse, though revealing a curve of breast and legs in fishnet stockings.[3] These campaigns, including the U Tampon advertisement, attracted viewer complaints, as is not uncommon following advertising with sexual references.[4] While the respective governing bodies allowed them to continue, both the "suck up to the boss" and U Tampon ads were confined to mature audience viewing. The distance of these advertisements from official representations of lactation (and menstruation), as strictly the domain of the medical or asexually domestic, contributed to their shock value. In the case of the breastfeeding examples, the gap between institutional and popular culture approaches cannot be easily bridged unless advocacy discourse acknowledges that women's bodies are not only a medical responsibility—they also belong in the realm of play.

Occasional instances of irreverence in popular media cannot achieve a shift in values alone and may merely accentuate the polarization of the quirky from the proper. Given that mainstream coverage of breastfeeding rarely includes images of *any* kind, it is difficult to reassure women that breastfeeding is socially acceptable, even in its most decorous incarnation, particularly in public.[5] Adopting a more creative approach by canvassing a range of behavioral possibilities might assist health communicators to legitimize pleasure and reinforce the freer models that appear from time to time within popular culture.

The Repressive Hypothesis

In his *History of Sexuality, Volume I*, Foucault outlines his "repressive hypothesis," in which he argues that research into human sexuality proliferated throughout the nineteenth and twentieth centuries, creating a discourse that "speaks verbosely of its own silence." Rather than enabling a libertarian sexuality with increasing personal freedoms, as is understood to have occurred in the 1960s, Foucault sees knowledge of sexuality accumulating yet maintaining a medical and moral agenda consistent with Victorianism. He argues that postenlightenment writing about sexuality has had the effect of repression through analysis. Condemning Freud in particular, he writes that medico-scientific research was constrained by "medical prudence, a scientific guarantee of innocuousness, and so many precautions in order to contain everything, with no fear of 'overflow,' in that safest and most discrete of spaces, between the couch and discourse." Additionally, normative sexuality was defined in relation to reproduction, and anything that fell outside this "could [not] expect sanction or protection."[6]

Breastfeeding is not mentioned in Foucault's writing. However, if we substitute "sexuality" with "breastfeeding" in his argument, a similar picture emerges: the medicalization of breastfeeding, "in that safest and most discrete of spaces" between the scientific laboratory and maternity ward, with the confinement of lactation to the reproductive function of feeding infants. While scientific research is useful for understanding health benefits, and the accumulation of medical knowledge assists in promoting breast milk on health grounds, it provides neither a full nor engaging picture, any more than the blue fluid used to represent menses in advertisements for feminine hygiene products.

This is breastfeeding's "repressive hypothesis": a wealth of knowledge about immunoglobulins and mastitis proliferating as a "verbosity of discourse" within the echo chamber of the prenatal clinic. In response to the repressive hypothesis, Foucault proposes an "*ars erotica,*" which "is truth drawn from pleasure itself, understood as a practice and accumulated as an experience."[7] An *ars erotica* draws from a history of practices embedded in cultural traditions. Most important, Foucault points out that in an *ars erotica*, "pleasure is not considered in relation to an absolute law of the permitted and the forbidden, *nor by reference to a criterion of utility*, but first and foremost in relation to itself, its specific quality, its duration, its reverberation in the body and soul." An *ars erotica* is not interested in virtue, nor in holding the baby "correctly," but in exploring the mutually sensual, emotional, and psychological rewards of nurture. It is not about usefulness. This is not to say breastfeeding can't be learned, any more than any sexual behavior isn't learned, through its rich archive of sex manuals, research literature, and practice, within the context of the art of love.

As Foucault observed, repression, knowledge, and power are inextricably linked. Disentangling them is crucial to show how behavior has been regulated, and those regulations internalized, by different traditions, for different interests. He writes, "nothing less than . . . *a reinstating of pleasure within reality*" is needed; "one cannot hope to obtain the desired results simply from a medical practice, nor from a theoretical discourse, however rigorously pursued."[8] Breastfeeding needs its own Kama Sutra of positions and potentials for humans who lactate, based on cross-cultural practice throughout history, as we have nourished and loved our families with our milk.

Marketing Milk

Sociologist Deborah Lupton has written of the need for social marketing campaigns to learn from commercial advertising, not just by being slick, targeted, and expensive, but by using existing values, associations, and predispositions in the community, to represent health-enhancing behaviors as appealing. Rather than designing fear campaigns—attempting to persuade people to discontinue pleasurable but risky behaviors in favor of less pleasurable but healthy ones—Lupton argues that social marketing should focus on "only those health-related messages which fit readily into pre-existing popular and pleasurable values and activities . . . harnessing rather than competing with the promotional power of commercial commodities." Similarly, Lupton argues that promotional discourse needs to acknowledge "the ways in which the activities of everyday life are integral to the construction of identities." Because "promotional activities are most effective when they tap into a corpus of existing meanings, rather than attempting to create new ones," it follows that public discourse concerning breastfeeding and its relationship to identity might open up to broader meanings around pleasure, rather than relentlessly focusing on its health benefits. Although "advertising alone cannot create symbolic meanings around health protective lifestyle choices which do not already exist," there is a wealth of experiential material waiting to be tapped by social marketers, if only mothers were asked.

Lupton writes that there is also a lack of understanding of how "identities are produced" through personal choices, such as smoking, where the cultural signifiers associated with harmful activities may be equal to, or of greater importance than, their immediate psychoactive effects. We need to acknowledge, she says, the "shared symbolic codes of stylized behavior" that underlie behavioral and consumer choices. In relation to preferences around health, for example, "'good health' becomes a very minor component of people's reasons for engagement" and can be "superceded by concerns engendered by the powerful ideologies of morality, asceticism, self-discipline and control."[9] Reinforcing Lupton's point, Dean Whitehead proposes that social marketing works best when it acknowledges people's "desire to self-actualize and fulfill all capabilities," a point ripe for adoption in the breastfeeding context, where self-efficacy and empowerment underlie breastfeeding pleasures.[10]

The "shared symbolic codes" of breastfeeding have been limited in public health discourse to dutiful, scientized, and modest mothering. As a subject for promotion this presents opportunities to portray more nuanced and engaging versions of women's experiences in feeding their offspring. Forty years of liberationist discourse in scholarship, literature, magazines, advertising, film, and television could be mined in forging new associations between breastfeeding and modern femininity, from the insouciant mother breastfeeding in the shopping mall to the glamorous mother with her baby in a restaurant, and from the efficient mother pumping at work to the relaxed mother breastfeeding under a tree at lunchtime or luxuriously cuddled with her baby and partner through the night. These are only tame examples.

Additionally, Lupton argues that successful advertising does not focus on the use-value of its product, since there are too many competing products of equal use. Instead, advertisers seek to create symbolic and aesthetic differentiations between products by linking them "to certain archetypal lifestyles and abstract values." This argument applies to the promotion of breastfeeding, where formula acts as a competing "brand" of infant food, despite advocates' claims for breast milk's nutritional superiority. While the focus on health benefits may be persuasive to some, it might not outweigh evidence that formula is "good enough," especially if it's also more convenient and less disruptive to a woman's relationship to her workplace, body, partner, and family. The focus of breastfeeding advocates on health benefits can only be posed as relative in this context, whereas a focus on the uniquely emotional and embodied experiences around breastfeeding, while paying less attention to utility, may be more aesthetically and emotionally powerful. Once the similarities and differences between comparable products are set aside, the "aesthetics of commodities" persuade consumers to choose brands.[11]

Formula packaging may be attractive, and there may be consumer pleasure in acquiring bottles and storage tins, together with gratifying neatness, convenience, and containment. But as Robbie Kahn points out, "Bottle feeding releases the mother from a sensuous connection to her child; [and] like impeded birth, breaks apart the fusion of maternity and sexuality."[12] Associations to separation may be reassuring to mothers who fear connecting to their child's body, yet there exists a powerful set of competing associations to breastfeeding for the majority: the warmth of skin-to-skin contact; the rewards of empowerment and protection; the pleasures of drifting to sleep together; the tactile fun of being close, of being silly, of playing with milk. Celebrating connection by referring to the sensual, spiritual, and social potentials of breastfeeding could provide mothers with a range of inviting options.

With the expansion of the maternity wear market into more fashionable attire in the past two decades, photo opportunities for pregnant Hollywood actresses, the popularization of "yummy mommies," MILFs, and "cougars," it's not difficult to imagine a space for the humorous, hip mother who breastfeeds in public with confidence and style—or the father who puts his child to his own breast in an act of commensality. These are only two of many images that could be communicated through social marketing.

Breastfeeding, Health Promotion, and the Fear of Pleasure

Given the pervasiveness of the pleasure principle in commercial advertising, it is surprising that social marketing hasn't deployed this strategy for promotion to a greater extent. Partly this is because most health promotion campaigns seek to discourage populations from engaging in pleasurable activities that could be harmful to their health (such as smoking or unprotected sex). They instead see a need to appeal to reason to persuade populations that the long-term benefits to health and longevity will outweigh the short-term pain entailed in any act of self-denial. Apart from the implied pleasures of self-discipline, deferred gratification, and asceticism, which are rarely illustrated or even referred to explicitly, there is scarcely any mention of pleasure as a means to self-improvement or well-being. Yet critics of public health campaigns suggest that implicitly privileging asceticism may do more harm than good.[13] Within sex health education programs, there have been a small number of campaigns that promote pleasure as an outcome of safe sex. Whitehead writes of the need to acknowledge the pleasurable aspects of alcohol use in developing awareness and education campaigns for young people.[14]

In addition to pleasure being viewed as an obstacle to the prevention of harm, there has traditionally been an aversion to pleasure in public health discourse more generally. Coveney and Bunton comment that, "as researchers involved in social aspects of public health, nutrition, and of drug use, we are struck by the fact that pleasure is under-examined in public health research and practice." Providing a history of pleasure in philosophy, they write, "When Plato denounced the study of human emotions as inferior to the study of reason . . . he effectively extinguished an examination of pleasure as a serious academic subject. Thus, while classical literature is replete with references to the importance of 'good' or of 'happiness,' there is little coverage of pleasure, especially as a bodily experience."

Coveney and Bunton note that feminist theory offered a powerful critique of this discrimination against feeling through "an examination of the body and experiences such as pleasure and other emotions." Nevertheless, "the primacy given to thought over reason" continues to occupy the "heartland of mainstream philosophy," so that "in relation to health, theoretical and empirical studies of pleasure are very limited."[15]

Within political discourse the left has also been suspicious of pleasure, since it believes that pleasure leads to inaction. Like religion, it is the opiate of the people, particularly since it might encourage needless consumption.[16] Similarly, Warburton and Sherwood argue that the "Calvinist legacy in Europe and the Puritan tradition in the United States have had marked influence on attitudes to individual pleasure," so that governments have overlooked "the positive contribution of pleasure to the lives of ordinary people."[17]

Suspicions of pleasure as being less reasoned, less rigorous, less useful, and less moral have also been examined in relation to media and communication studies. Brian Ott argues how the focus on "method," particularly in the social sciences, has sidelined the pleasures of interpretation and the creation of new meanings.[18] As McKee notes in his critique of social scientific method, "Traditionally the sciences—and in particular the social sciences—have not been very good at recognizing the importance of fun."[19] In breastfeeding studies this tendency also dominates, especially where the social and natural sciences have favored evidence-based, utilitarian arguments at the expense of critical discourse analysis (such as this essay). The creation of new meanings, in particular, through interpretation and analysis of representations of breastfeeding, could be regarded as the task of social marketers as well as humanities academics.

Klaus and O'Connor similarly argue that by focusing on the ideological critique of public knowledge and popular culture, the communications discipline has diminished the status of theorists of pleasure in reception studies. In addition to the obvious link between breastfeeding and pleasure that has been overlooked in health promotion campaigns, there is therefore the potential for media to make use of the gendering of breastfeeding as public discourse, and build on the pleasures of media experienced by female audiences. Theorists of pleasure in communication studies may be useful in developing social marketing that appeals to women specifically—yet here, too, there has been ambivalence concerning the value of pleasure.

By developing social marketing that fits with the media women themselves favor, breastfeeding promotion could work with rather than against popular culture, enabling cultural change around breastfeeding—in particular, a broad acceptance in the community rather than just the nursery. That is, by reference to the emotional as well as rational narratives of women's lives, it then encompasses "all those everyday activities and communicative events through which people confirm their common culture, reconstruct their social identity and rework the norms and values regulating behavior."

It is beyond the scope of this chapter to consider entertainment education, but breastfeeding pleasures and dilemmas, as narratives contained in television drama, would also make sense. As O'Connor and Klaus put it, "Media offer the means for this ongoing endeavor in both their fictional and non-fictional program because social and cultural communication on all levels is media drenched."[20] Women identifying with breastfeeding characters on-screen could be a powerful means to normalize a range of nursing behaviors hitherto adrift in a cultural and ethical vacuum.[21]

Breastfeeding Pleasure and Maternal Sexuality

Resistance to pleasure in promoting breastfeeding is not only based on a privileging of rationality and scientific evidence. There is also a suspicion that maternal pleasure is the most problematic pleasure of all, not only because it celebrates the emotional life, but also because maternal sexuality might be a dangerous force. Iris Marion Young has written powerfully of the fear of maternal pleasure in her essay "Breasted Experience," where she speculates that the pleasures of the breast threaten a degree of auto-eroticism, implying that the mother needs no partner for her own pleasure, that she may be sexually independent.[22] Christina Traina argues that maternal pleasure is feared as a perverse erotic force within a relationship where there is an imbalance of power. Traina writes of the need to "stress the multidimensionality of women's sexuality, including its links to maternity," and argues that the "experience of maternity as erotically pleasurable is not categorically perverse—that it can be, in fact, a moral good—and that we must revise our ideals and norms of mothering in order to account for it."[23] As with Oxenhandler's work on the erotics of parenting, Traina seeks to demystify maternal sexuality so as to acknowledge its existence and to reduce moral panic concerning pedophilia or maternal neglect. This is no small task in a Christian culture that idealizes asexual motherhood through the iconography of the Madonna.[24]

As Susan Weisskopf similarly observes, "good mothers are generally asexual." Despite the secular impetus of medical research, the virtuous asexual mother has merely been replaced with the virtuous scientized mother, both marginalizing the interests of her body. This causes anxiety for women who do feel pleasure, sometimes sexual pleasure, when they breastfeed—an anxiety that extends to academics working in this area: "Both the lack of research on maternal sexuality and the fragmented quality of what is available attest to the ideology's impact on scholars." It is Weisskopf's view that many women have internalized this ideology and "as a result, experience consider-able psychological pain." While some women abandon breastfeeding due to pain, others give up due to pleasure, in both cases in distress and consumed by guilt.[25]

Thus, while ample evidence attests to the presence of normal sexual responses throughout conception, pregnancy, childbirth, and lactation, there is reluctance to recognize the sexual mother who experiences pleasure in the course of mothering. As research indicates, children, too, breastfeed for pleasure.[26]

Outlining the ways in which breastfeeding advice literature disembodies the milk for the baby at the expense of the mother, Saha notes, it is really the milk, not the breast, that is promoted as "best." That the mother may "actually desire breastfeeding for her own pleasure in becoming intimate with her baby—euphemistically referred to as bonding by much of the advice literature—is ignored." Arguing that "health professionals need to take on sexuality seriously and *critically* if they seek to promote an increasing acceptance of breastfeeding," Saha suggests a vital aspect of this project would entail "affirming the woman's autonomy over her own breasts." She sees this project specifically as a critique of the conservatism of health promotion campaigns: "We should not hesitate to demand a rethinking of the ethics of how medicine and public health continue to present their breastfeeding promotional messages as objective and scientifically rational while at the same time reflecting societal norms, especially with regard to gender and sexuality"—norms which reduce women's freedom, opportunity, support, and desire to breastfeed.[27]

Conclusion

Ambivalence toward pleasure within philosophy, politics, and public health has had far-reaching consequences, discouraging advocacy of healthful behavior as pleasurable and minimizing the value of pleasure in human sexuality. The fear of maternal pleasure in particular has stifled research into female sexuality and limited the autonomy of desiring mothers. Yet associating pleasure with breastfeeding could help to increase breastfeeding rates and permit mothers to openly enjoy breastfeeding. Social marketing might promote breastfeeding as sensually, psychologically, emotionally, and spiritually pleasurable, in addition to being good for babies. Pleasure is also valuable for its own sake: both the pleasure of health promotion that's entertaining and the pleasure of breastfeeding.

An *ars erotica* of breastfeeding and lactation invites a radical rethink of public health approaches, integrating the rational-sensual mother who is informed of the latest science, wise to her cultural legacy, and at ease with her body. Transcending the conflict between duty and pleasure, science and culture, permits the free expression of the maternal subject, breastfeeding for herself and her child within a reciprocal and relational playground of creativity.

Notes

1. YouTube, "U Tampon by Kotex."
2. YouTube, "Breast Is Best"; Cartwright and Olshan, "Wife's Baby Milk."
3. These may be found at YouTube, "Suck Up to the Boss"; and Breastfeeding Is Beautiful, "Best Role Ever."
4. Giles and Whelan, *Discrimination and Vilification.*
5. Hector, King, and Webb state that "only 1.3% of 334 articles were accompanied by photos of a baby being breastfed" (*Overview of Recent Reviews*, 13). See also Dyson et al., "Factors," 148.
6. Foucault, *History of Sexuality*, 8, 5, 4.
7. Promoting the pleasure of breastfeeding is not to deny that some women experience pain while breastfeeding, while others find it boring, tiring, or neutral—just as people do with other sexual behaviors.
8. Foucault, *History of Sexuality*, 57, 5 (emphasis added).
9. Lupton, "Consumerism," 117, 116, 116, 111, 113.
10. Whitehead, "In Pursuit," 223; Britton and Britton, "Maternal Self-Concept," 431–437.
11. Lupton, "Consumerism," 114.
12. Kahn, *Bearing Meaning,* 383.
13. McCormick, "Health Scares," 193.
14. See Philpott, Knerr, and Boydell, "Pleasure and Prevention"; Beasley, "Challenge of Pleasure"; Whitehead, "In Pursuit," 222, 223.
15. Coveney and Bunton, "In Pursuit," 161–163.
16. McKee, "Looking for Fun," 3.

17. Warburton and Sherwood, *Pleasure and the Quality of Life*, 8, 10.
18. Ott, "(Re)locating Pleasure," 202.
19. McKee, "Looking for Fun," 1.
20. O'Connor and Klaus, "Pleasure and Meaningful Discourse," 369–387.
21. Brodie et al., "Communicating Health Information." See also Foss, this volume.
22. Young, "Breasted Experience," 8, 84, 90.
23. Traina, "Maternal Experience," 370.
24. Kahn, "Lessons," 386. See also Sutherland, "Of Milk and Miracles," 1–20.
25. Weisskopf, "Maternal Sexuality," 768, 371.
26. Gribble, "Long-Term Breastfeeding," 5.
27. Saha, "Breastfeeding and Sexuality," 61, 66, 67, 71, 70.

Breastfeeding in the "Baby Block"

Using Reality Television to Effectively Promote Breastfeeding

The program *Bringing Home Baby* opens with a typical schedule for the first days after a baby is born. Title slides read: "First 36 hours"; then, "Day 1: Newborn baby," "Crying," and "Diapers." A second set of slides state: "Day 2: Feeding," "Sleeping." Images of real people performing these tasks accompany the slides. For the feeding slide, a father bottle-feeds his newborn. Similarly, the alternate opening of this program features baby items, including bottles, marching into a house. Because breastfeeding is not pictured, this opening presents bottle-feeding as the typical or default means of feeding a baby. This message is not unique to *Bringing Home Baby*. In 2005, the American Academy of Pediatrics criticized mainstream media for frequently presenting bottle-feeding as the normal means of feeding a baby, stating that these messages have likely hindered breastfeeding rates.[1]

Considering the health and social benefits lost when infants are not breastfed, the normalization of the bottle, perpetuated by media, is particularly alarming. And yet, little attention has been given to contemporary media representations of breastfeeding. This chapter examines these portrayals, using reality programming to explore what messages are conveyed on television and how this genre could be used as a tool to promote breastfeeding.

Media play a significant role in most people's health decisions, expanding knowledge, changing behavior, and shaping perceptions. Other than personal physicians, media outlets, especially websites, serve as most people's primary source for health information.[2] As news audiences continue to shrink, entertainment television has increasingly been recognized as an effective tool for disseminating information. For example, a 2008 Kaiser Family Foundation campaign on HIV and pregnancy found that many viewers could provide the statistic of healthy infants born to HIV-positive mothers after an episode of *Grey's Anatomy* covered the issue.[3] Entertainment programming has also been used to teach people about emergency contraception, designated driving, reproductive health, and other issues.[4] Given this recognized influence, it makes sense that people learn about infant feeding, including breastfeeding information, from magazines, websites, and television—an assumption that is supported by research. In a survey by Samir Arora and colleagues, many bottle-feeding mothers stated that they would have been more likely to breastfeed if television, magazines, or books had provided them with more information on breastfeeding.[5]

Media messages have also been shown to enact changes in health behavior. For example, in the 1980s media messages about the dangers of giving aspirin to children helped to dramatically reduce the incidence of Reye's syndrome.[6] And, following publicity of former First Lady Nancy Reagan's mastectomy, the frequency of breast-cancer patients choosing mastectomies over breast-conserving surgery (BCS) increased.[7]

Campaigns promoting behavior change are most effective if consumers believe that the benefits far outweigh the risk of not changing the behavior and if the behavior is somewhat easy to change.[8] With breastfeeding, it is not enough for women to know of the health benefits; they need to believe that not breastfeeding is risky enough to their infants to make it worthwhile. The recognized importance of focusing on risk prompted the Ad Council, as part of the National Breastfeeding Awareness Campaign, to create a series of public service announcements (PSAs) that featured pregnant women riding mechanical bulls or partaking in other dangerous activities, with a voiceover stating the risks of not breastfeeding. Unfortunately, fears about these messages being too effective prompted commercial formula manufacturers to protest.[9] And yet this campaign was a positive start toward framing breastfeeding as a healthy behavior with recognized risks if not practiced, similar to public health messaging concerning the risks of not immunizing children.

A key social institution, mass media help shape a person's meaningful reality, reinforcing or challenging dominant ideologies, including those held about breastfeeding.[10] The extent to which breastfeeding is perceived as the normal means of feeding an infant can impact breastfeeding success. For example, the attitudes of partners, family, physicians, and others have been shown to significantly influence breastfeeding initiation and duration.[11] Therefore, it is not just pregnant women or nursing mothers who are impacted by media messages about breastfeeding. These messages impact overall public perception of breastfeeding. According to cultivation theory, developed by communication scholar George Gerbner and colleagues, heavy television viewers tend to perceive the world as it is presented on television. For example, those who watch crime dramas are more likely to believe that crime is more prevalent than people who do not watch these programs.[12] Concerning infant feeding, cultivation theory suggests that consumption of shows that present formula-feeding as normal would lead viewers to believe that breastfeeding is uncommon or abnormal. Members of the general public may be less supportive of a breastfeeding woman, especially in a public space, if they perceive it as abnormal or unnecessary.

Historically, media products have influenced infant feeding decisions through advertising, medical books, popular literature, and other channels. In the 1800s newspapers advertised the services of wet nurses, marketing breasts as desirable commodities.[13] When commercial formula was developed in the mid-1800s, the emerging advertising industry quickly and successfully made this product popular and profitable to produce. By 1873 twenty-seven brands of infant formula had been patented.[14] Advertisements for commercial formula frequently appeared in women's and other popular magazines, as well as brochures.[15] Across class lines, formula use significantly increased.[16]

Since that time, media messages have continued to influence infant feeding decisions. Commercial formula companies still aggressively market their products, in magazines, television, and online, as well as through free samples in hospitals and directly to consumers.[17] Unlike the United Kingdom, no special regulations restrict formula marketing in the United States.[18] And while breastfeeding campaigns first emerged in the early 1900s, very little advertising has promoted breastfeeding.[19] As mentioned earlier, the PSAs in the National Breastfeeding Awareness Campaign of 2004–2006 linking not breastfeeding to risk hardly aired.[20] Products that aid breastfeeding are rarely advertised, except for the Medela breast pump commercials on cable networks. Since breastfeeding in itself is not commercially profitable, there are few direct methods of competing with formula industry messaging.

Given the problem with directly marketing breastfeeding, it is important to identify new ways, other than advertising and traditional public health campaigns, to promote breastfeeding. According to Jane Brown and Sheila Rose Peuchaud in "Media and Breastfeeding: Friend or Foe?," that media supports breastfeeding is questionable (even outside advertising), due to negative messages about breastfeeding disseminated by profit-driven media conglomerates.[21] Popular magazines tend to pay lip service to breastfeeding promotion while glossing over obstacles and solutions.[22] News stories tell of women who have been ridiculed for breastfeeding in public spaces, including airplanes, restaurants, and retail stores.[23] Media also impact breastfeeding rates indirectly, defining normal means of feeding babies as well as reinforcing social ideologies and policies that hinder breastfeeding rates, such as the sexualization of breasts and a dependency on experts for child-rearing advice.[24]

As summarized by Brown and Peuchaud, most studies on breastfeeding and media address magazine coverage of breastfeeding.[25] Little attention has been given to television depictions of breastfeeding, even though many people are uncomfortable with seeing breastfeeding in television. According to the 2001 Healthstyles survey, only 27.9 percent of respondents believed that "it is appropriate to show a woman breastfeeding her baby on TV programs."[26] This low percentage is alarming and suggests that perhaps television is underused in breastfeeding promotion. The wave of reality TV programs that feature new parents and their babies presents an opportunity to depict infant feeding decisions. In their call to action, Brown and Peuchaud argued that one means of effectively changing attitudes toward breastfeeding is to target a specific audience.[27] Certainly, reality programs on cable television exemplify such narrowcasting and thus could potentially shape viewers' health decisions, including infant feeding.

On the cable networks The Learning Channel (TLC) and Discovery Health Channel (DHC), the reality programs *A Baby Story*, *Bringing Home Baby*, and *Deliver Me: Home Edition* regularly follow real-life families as they experience labor, delivery, and caring for their new baby, including their child-rearing decisions. As these programs feature real women, they provide an opportunity to explore messages about infant feeding that are prevalent on television, especially given that these types of programs dominate these channels. For example, in one week, reruns of these programs constitute 27.5 hours of programming.[28]

A Baby Story (*ABS*) focuses on one couple in New York or New Jersey as they prepare for birth and experience childbirth. *Deliver Me: Home Edition* (*DMHE*), a spin-off from *Deliver Me*, which follows a group of obstetrician-gynecologists, centers on the relationship between a pregnant woman and her doctor in California, while *Bringing Home Baby* (*BHB*) follows the first thirty-six hours after a baby is brought home from the hospital. This latter program features a theme for each episode, conveyed in the title, such as "Panamanian Celebration" and "Stay at Home Dad." All three programs provide an update of the families within the baby's first year. Combined, these programs tell common stories of women prior to and during delivery, as well as an update a few months after birth. Since this process is documented, these programs often convey messages about breastfeeding initiation and duration—as indicated by the updates.

Nearly all of the breastfeeding images take place in the birthing center, hospital, or mother's home, conveying the idea that breastfeeding is a private activity.[29] For example, at the four-month update of the *DMHE* episode "Connie Kawai," Connie sits in a rocking chair breastfeeding her baby in the cradle position on a breastfeeding pillow. This image is repeated with different women in most of the episodes with breastfeeding depictions. Even in their own homes, most of the breastfeeding women sit alone with a blanket or discreet clothing to mask what they are doing. For example, in the *ABS* episode "Baby Frasca," the one-month update shows the mother holding her baby at the kitchen table. It is only when she pulls her shirt down afterward that it is clear that she was breastfeeding. Rarely are women shown breastfeeding around guests or even their spouses. Episodes also convey the idea that breastfeeding is limited to early infancy. The updates, which ranged from a few weeks to ten months, seldom show breastfeeding. Usually, babies are bottle-fed, or feeding is not mentioned. For example, at the ten-month update of the *DMHE* episode "First-Time Mom," the baby feeds from a bottle in the Pack 'n Play as the parents give their interview. No episodes addressed extended or tandem breastfeeding, or the breastfeeding of premature babies, multiples, or adopted children.

When they do breastfeed, mothers in the programs describe their experience as transforming from an initially difficult to a calm, wonderful activity. In *BHB* "Trainer's Baby," the mother admits that "breastfeeding was really hard at first, but it's getting a lot easier, and the bonding experience with breastfeeding is just so amazing." Likewise, in "Two Moms," the mother says: "Breastfeeding was my biggest concern. It was harder for us to learn to breastfeed than it was to actually deliver her." The mother breastfeeds as she continues, "We toughed it out and she learned to suck and it's like, it's the best feeling in the world." In the *DMHE* episode "Rachel McDermott," McDermott reflects, "My all-time favorite bonding experience is actually breastfeeding. I think that it's an automatic time-out during my day." At this point, the camera shows her breastfeeding her daughter as she gently strokes the baby's hair. McDermott continues: "To just spend time with her and it's something that I can give her. I love the fact that I can just hold her and look at her and she'll stay still. That's been one of the greatest things throughout my time with her so far is being able to have that time every day to breastfeed her. It's amazing." While mothers often mentioned the obstacles of early breastfeeding, no specific challenges were discussed. Also, no women specifically address how and why breastfeeding became easier.

When women weaned in the course of the episode, the mothers, their partners, or the program's narrator explained their decision. These stories are accompanied by visual images of the babies being fed commercial formula. For example, the *BHB* episode "Single Mom" features a twenty-one-year-old woman, Laura, who lives with her single mother. Soon after they arrive home, Laura bottle-feeds the baby. Grandma tells the camera that "Laura's milk is coming down, but it's very painful for her to breastfeed." Laura comments that it "feels like she has teeth and she's like biting me." Moments later, Grandma is outside her room, admitting that "I want to get in there and show her how, but I can't. She has to learn that for herself the same way I learned it for myself, so now we're doing the bottle and we're trying to give her breasts a break." Later, Laura explains, "I was breastfeeding her more in the hospital at first, you know. She was trying to latch on pretty good, but man, she hurt me." The camera shows a close up of the baby being fed from a Similac pre-filled formula bottle. Laura continues, "They're feeling really sore. I mean, that's why I have her on the bottle right now." Another close up of the Similac bottle is shown. That evening, Laura takes a shower to ease her engorged breasts and decides to give up breastfeeding, saying, "It's too much for me." Then Laura feeds the baby out of a pre-filled Similac formula bottle.

Likewise, in "Stay at Home Dad," the narrator explains, "Since Ariana's breast milk hasn't come in yet, she gets some formula to give to baby Aidan, whose weight is still a concern." The mother, Ariana, gives the baby premixed Similac. Later in the episode, the parents set up a breast pump and close the door. Afterward, the father, Eli, tells the camera that she failed to express milk, so the baby will have to have formula. Ariana does not attempt to breastfeed him. In the update teaser, the narrator asks: "Will Aidan switch to breast milk now that he's had nothing but formula since birth?" This question is accompanied by a close-up of Aidan getting a bottle. Not surprisingly, the answer is no. At the eight-week update, Ariana justifies why she switched to formula, as she bottle-feeds the baby: "I tried to breastfeed him and he wouldn't latch on. He took a bottle like that was what he was meant to do."

In two episodes of *BHB*, doctors recommend parents supplement with formula to help with a baby's jaundice. In "Headstrong Parents," the father mixes bottles as the narrator explains, "Because of the jaundice situation, the couple is feeding the baby a combination of breast milk and formula." In the interview, the mother admits, "It's disappointing to have him supplemented with formula because I wanted to do exclusively breast milk, because it's best for him for the first couple of months, but now, because the formula is so easy for him, it seems that's all he really wants. So, he's still latching on to the breast, but it's almost like he's using it as a pacifier to put himself to sleep. He really just wants the formula. But, he'll work through that. He'll be fine." In the ten-week update, the father feeds the baby a bottle. Breastfeeding is not mentioned. Similarly, in "Amber's Miracle" a doctor advises, over the phone, giving the baby formula for twenty-four hours. Despite the support of a lactation consultant, the ten-week update shows the baby being fed formula.

The clear product placement in these episodes indicates that the feeding decision story lines were likely devices to focus on the Similac bottles, especially because some of the products are also advertised during commercial breaks. Of course, the purpose of American television is to sell products and, because of increasingly fragmented audiences and technology allowing people to skip commercials, product placement marketing is rapidly growing. "The baby block" is not unique. *Survivor, American Idol, The Apprentice*, and other reality programs have included blatant product placement.[30] Nor is the product placement unusual for TLC. In 2007 four out of ten of the top cable programs for product placement aired on TLC.[31] *BHB* does not hide its product placement. Links on the show's webpage lead to an online marketplace in which viewers can learn more about the products.

The Implications of Media Messages on Breastfeeding

Extensive research has demonstrated the significant impacts that television has on people's knowledge, behavior, and perceptions. In fact, because of the recognition and fear of television's power over health, in the 1960s the U.S. Surgeon General created the Scientific Advisory Committee on Television and Social Behavior to study this relationship.[32] This committee's findings prompted the U.S. government to ban tobacco advertisements from television in 1971.[33]

How do television messages about breastfeeding influence viewers? The Social-Ecological Model (SEM) can illuminate the potential impact of media messages about breastfeeding, such as those in the "baby block." Women who lack information about breastfeeding from other resources may learn about infant feeding from these programs, which convey that only a certain type of child should be breastfed (a singleton, full-term infant). These programs also teach viewers that breastfeeding is private; therefore, by choosing to breastfeed, a woman binds herself to the home. Finally, because these programs do not present breastfeeding as the normal or dominant means of feeding infants, media messages like these suggest that formula is a more common choice. The normalization of formula-feeding is reinforced by the juxtaposition of the storyline with product placement of commercial formula in these programs, which sends three clear messages to women: breastfeeding is too difficult for most women, but look at how much easier formula is; doctors often recommend supplementing and here's the brand they recommend; and formula must be fine for babies, because these real women are giving it to their children on supposedly baby-friendly networks.

These programs could easily become more breastfeeding friendly, presenting breastfeeding as the dominant feeding choice, offering an array of experiences, and emphasizing the benefits of breastfeeding (and the risk of not breastfeeding) to consumers. As suggested by Brown and Peuchaud, media producers have the potential to positively impact breastfeeding perceptions and rates.[34] At each step of production, changes could be made to promote breastfeeding. Because a reality program is a contrived, packaged-for-television, media product, the program's producers, editors, and writers can shape the messages about breastfeeding.

In the screening process, casting agents can ask about infant feeding choices and select women who intend to breastfeed. During filming, the interviewers can ask mothers about breastfeeding. If they express concerns, lactation consultants can be provided (the visit could then be part of the show—which is not uncommon, as many episodes feature special outings, such as painting pottery or taking a birthing class). For the final package, footage can be edited to highlight successful breastfeeding and include more women talking about their experiences. Finally, the voiceover could support breastfeeding. In the episodes studied, narration only addressed breastfeeding if it was unsuccessful. Positive voiceovers could inform viewers about solutions to obstacles and reinforce success, with statements like, "Wanda treated her Thrush with Oregano Oil. Now, their breastfeeding relationship is back on track." The sponsorship of these programs should also be reconsidered, because the marketing of formula on television undermines pro-breastfeeding messages in television and is particularly problematic when placed into a reality program. Instead of providing commercial formula as part of product integration, producers can seek out breastfeeding-friendly products, such as Medela breast pumps or the My Brest Friend pillow.

Overall, television should be acknowledged as a vital tool for educating and encouraging breastfeeding. Government agencies should recognize this medium's influence on dissuading women from breastfeeding, and, as with tobacco ads in the 1970s, they should take action to ban the marketing of formula on television in the United States. While it is perhaps not possible for these particular reality programs to exist without formula advertisements, successful campaigns for other health issues have demonstrated that television can and should be used as a prosocial vehicle in improving the breastfeeding rates and experiences for its viewers.

Notes

1. American Academy of Pediatrics, "Policy Statement."
2. Hesse et al., "Trust and Sources of Health Information," 2618–2624. See also Arora et al., "Major Factors."
3. Rideout, "Television as a Health Educator."
4. Brodie et al., "Communicating Health Information," 192–199; Winsten, "Promoting Designated Drivers," 11–14; Folb, "Don't Touch That Dial!," 16–18.
5. Arora et al., "Major Factors," 67.
6. Soumerai, Ross-Degnan, and Kahn, "Effects of Professional and Media Warnings," 265–288.
7. Nattinger et al., "Effect of Nancy Reagan's Mastectomy," 762–767.
8. Hornik, "Public Health Communication," 1–22.
9. Ibid.
10. Berger and Luckmann, *Social Construction of Reality*; Gitlin, "Prime Time Ideology," 251–266.
11. Freed, Fraley, and Schanler, "Attitudes of Expectant Fathers," 224–227; Baranowski et al., "Social Support," 1599–1611; Littman, Medendorp, and Goldfarb, "Decision to Breastfeed," 214–219.
12. Gerbner and Gross, "Living with Television," 173–199.
13. Golden, *Social History*.
14. Baumslag and Michels, *Milk, Money, and Madness*.
15. Apple, *Mothers and Medicine*.
16. Wolf, *Don't Kill Your Baby*.
17. Apple, *Mothers and Medicine*; Wolf, *Don't Kill Your Baby*.
18. Faircloth, "Weak Formula for Legislation."
19. Ibid.
20. Wolf, "What Feminists Can Do," 397–424, 599.
21. Brown and Peuchaud, "Media and Breastfeeding."
22. Foss and Southwell, "Infant Feeding and the Media"; Young, "American Conceptions," 17–28; Potter, Sheeshka, and Valaitis, "Content Analysis," 196–203. See also Duckett, this volume.
23. Pheifer, "Breast-feeding Mother"; Raj, "Nursing Mom"; Seavey, "Mother Exposed"; McLean, "Breast-feeding Mom."
24. Wolf, *Don't Kill Your Baby*; Schanler, O'Connor, and Lawrence, "Pediatricians' Practices," e35.
25. Brown and Peuchaud, "Media and Breastfeeding."
26. Li et al., "Public Beliefs," 1162–1168.
27. Brown and Peuchaud, "Media and Breastfeeding."
28. I conducted a case study of reality TV programming exploring what messages are disseminated about infant feeding in this genre. One week of daytime programming was recorded, totaling 27.5 hours of programming: twenty-five episodes of *A Baby Story*, ten episodes of *Bringing Home Baby*, and ten episodes of *Deliver Me: Home Edition*. The programs were aired on TLC and DHC, and all originally aired between 2003 and 2010. I performed a textual analysis on the episodes studied. This qualitative method explores the meanings of texts as situated within a historical and

social context. The following questions guided the analysis: Is breastfeeding, bottle-feeding, or formula-feeding verbally addressed? During the episode, is the baby breastfed or bottle-fed? Is commercial formula mentioned or shown? What messages are conveyed about breastfeeding, by the narrator, parents, or family of the baby? Is infant feeding addressed in the update for the show? Is the woman still breastfeeding?

Overall, fifty-five episodes of the three programs were studied. Ten episodes of *ABS* did not address any method of infant feeding. Instead, the update focused on other aspects of child care, such as bathing or a walk in the stroller. Of the forty-five episodes with infant feeding, seventeen episodes visually and/or verbally depicted only breastfeeding. Eight episodes included both breastfeeding and an alternative (bottle- and/or formula-feeding). Twenty episodes addressed feeding without verbally addressing or visually depicting breastfeeding.

29. With the exception of the episode "Two Moms," about a lesbian couple, all breastfeeding takes place in the home.
30. Mittell, *Television*.
31. Saini, "U.S. Television."
32. U.S. Department of Health and Human Services, *Television and Behavior*, 9.
33. Eckard, "Competition."
34. Brown and Peuchaud, "Media and Breastfeeding."

Rethinking the Importance of Social Class

How Mass Market Magazines Portray Infant Feeding

Women go through intense role modification when they become pregnant and prepare for motherhood. From a sociological perspective, women typically begin a process of anticipatory socialization, or information-seeking practices, prior to giving birth. Women research the numerous aspects of pregnancy, childbirth, and childrearing.[1] Throughout this personal journey, women utilize widely varying sources of information, including popular and well-known texts like *What to Expect When You're Expecting*, obstetricians, mothers, print and television media, support networks like La Leche League, and what feminist psychoanalyst Suzie Orbach refers to as "visual muzak," the pervasive media that people encounter on a daily basis without consciously consuming it. Each resource is likely to provide differing facts and perspectives when it comes to what women should expect during their pregnancies and what society expects of them once they become mothers.[2]

The mass media have significant effects on human behavior and thought. The type of information that women receive regarding their bodies mediates behaviors and attitudes concerning breastfeeding. While some studies have examined the effectiveness of targeted health campaigns, and other studies have examined the effects of the media on body image, very few have tackled health messages in more popular forms of media.[3] This lack of attention is unfortunate given the fact that various scholars have found that women turn to magazines for general health information and that pregnant women, especially, use written media (including magazines) as their predominant source of information. Others have concluded that the vast majority of women who chose to bottle-feed with formula indicated that they would have been more likely to attempt and maintain breastfeeding if more information had been available through the media. Previous research has demonstrated the effects of the media on behavior. Low breastfeeding rates among working-class consumers of particular forms of media are not surprising in the context of information suggesting that working-class bodies are less capable of adequately nourishing an infant. This study examines those media messages to determine social class bias, as previous studies have already established the effect of media on mothers' behaviors.[4]

Social Class

For the purposes of this chapter, the term "social class" does not refer only to a calculation of approximate annual income or occupational prestige, although these measures are useful. Instead, I use "social class" to refer to the "set of experiences and strategies for approaching life that is carried into the home." This view of social class is common; studies point to the effects of social class as an "external force" that strongly influences individual decisions, family structure, child-rearing practices, and even "patterns of mass media behavior in the home."[5] Income difference is a shorthand method of categorizing people into different social classes: the amount of income a family brings in affects the number of luxuries they claim, the types of products (food and otherwise) they can afford, the quality of education they attain, and so on. In this sense, social class differences *become* cultural differences as life opportunities create income-defined subcultures.

This particular definition of social class is important in areas such as marketing and consumer research. In their study of "Yankee City," which examines the details of social life in a New England town, anthropologists W. Lloyd Warner and Paul Lunt discovered that members of different social classes spent their money differently, displayed different purchasing goals, and made purchases in distinctive ways. This finding demonstrates that social classes are not merely status groups; they are also "motivational groupings" that therefore "cause, not merely correlate, consumption choice."[6]

Social class mediates perceptions of fit mothers. Even a cursory examination of the ways in which the media portray motherhood shows a strong middle- and upper-class bias. Middle- and upper-class individuals as represented on television and in magazine articles and illustrations are prettier, taller, skinnier, happier, and seem to be more capable of taking care of their children and their children's problems than their working-class counterparts.[7] In her book discussing the commercial exploitation of the human body, Suzie Orbach points out the imperfections that affect ordinary people in relation to the perfectly lit, professionally trained, airbrushed ideals presented in mass media contexts. Although everyone experiences this sense of imperfection, access to resources allows some members of society to approach the ideal image more successfully than others. In addition, racial and class-based bodily characteristics have the potential to be stigmatizing if they mark the individual as disadvantaged.[8]

Lifestyle Choice

The concept of personal or lifestyle choice becomes important when social class is understood to influence the choices one makes. "Lifestyle choice" as a term suggests multiple equally viable options. Infant feeding debates highlight choice to indicate that each woman is able to weigh her options and make the decision that is best for her and her child. Literary scholar Helena Michie and legal theorist Naomi Cahn suggest that this perspective allows society to ignore the social constraints that can negatively affect women's supposedly free choices and lead to dire consequences. Philosopher Carolyn McLeod, in her examination of the ways women exert their autonomy in reproductive decision making, notes that class standing is important, but the perceptions of the stereotypes associated with class standing are of even greater importance.

McLeod gives the example of "Melissa," a twenty-five-year-old single, working-class woman who has little formal education. While Melissa is described as believing her pregnancy concerns are important, she does not voice her concerns to her doctor. In a private setting, "she is not normally shy . . . , she does not have a passive personality, nor does she lack confidence in her own judgment." Melissa is further described as being "eminently aware of the cultural stereotype of uneducated people as intellectually inferior"; she feels that her doctor will view her through that stereotypical lens. Because of this, Melissa does not express her opinions regarding any of the tests administered or prenatal diagnoses made by her doctor. She lacks the confidence to ask questions of her doctor or act upon her own choices. Melissa's doctor assumes that she is making an informed decision, when, in fact, Melissa is facing numerous social constraints that prevent her from feeling comfortable in questioning her doctor's authoritative voice.[9]

McLeod maintains that women frequently feel as though they are not perceived as smart, and therefore do not trust themselves enough to ask the necessary questions to make informed decisions. While many practitioners work from the perspective that women are making personal or lifestyle decisions regarding feeding their infants, they may be ignoring an entire spectrum of social constraints that affect how women make decisions and determine the kinds of decisions they make.

Popular Pregnancy Magazines

As part of a larger study on media and breastfeeding, I conducted a content analysis of three years' worth of the popular pregnancy magazines *American Baby*, *Parents*, *Parenting*, and *Working Mother*. The Magazine Publishers of America report that women of childbearing age read an average of 13.2 issues each month in 2006.[10] This statistic includes magazines that are skimmed in grocery stores, doctor's offices, and other venues. Each of the magazines listed above has a large readership, but *American Baby* is by far the most accessible to all women. A full 97 percent of its circulation is unpaid. Birthing hospitals and maternity clothing stores frequently provide a free yearlong subscription to *American Baby* to patients and customers. Additionally, *American Baby* is available in obstetric and pediatric offices around the country. The median income levels for readers of each magazine reveal that *American Baby* reaches more women with lower incomes than the other magazines.[11]

The study explores the messages that pregnancy and child-rearing magazines send to pregnant and nursing women, especially with respect to their abilities to adequately feed their children.[12] Between January 2007 and December 2009, there were 195 feature articles or monthly features that mentioned breastfeeding or bottle-feeding: 67 in *American Baby*, 54 in *Parents*, 53 in *Parenting*, and 21 in *Working Mother*. Overall, 91 segments (46 percent) advocated breastfeeding over bottle-feeding, 28 (14.36 percent) promoted or discussed exclusive bottle-feeding, and 32 (16.41 percent) discussed the two as equivalent options. The articles promoting breastfeeding were no more likely to appear in a more prominent (that is, earlier) position in the magazine than articles that discussed bottle-feeding or treated the two feeding methods as equivalent. Indeed, the placement of the articles (in the first, second, or third section of the magazine) did not demonstrate statistical significance.

Among the articles of interest, 96 articles (63.6 percent of the total number of articles contained in the magazines) presented breastfeeding as a lifestyle choice, coinciding with Bernice Hausman's comment that "the choice is personalized" and treated as though it occurs outside of the social structures that define that choice.[13]

Social-class differences emerged when I examined the articles with regard to their portrayal of formula as an equal or superior alternative to breastfeeding. *Parenting* was the most likely to present formula-feeding as equal to breastfeeding, although *Parents* and *American Baby* were not far behind.

Working Mother promoted breastfeeding as the natural and superior option, with less than a sixth of the relevant articles suggesting that formula-feeding was equivalent to breastfeeding. Where *Parenting*, *Parents*, and *American Baby* articles all provided ample advice concerning weaning within the first four to six months, *Working Mother* articles provided information and advice to help women continue breastfeeding even when they returned to work. This advice could well serve the readers of the other three magazines, but those assumed that women would want to transition their children to formula and then solid food well before the six-month mark.[14]

A common theme throughout the articles was anxiety over breastfeeding. Almost half of the articles in *American Baby* addressed anxiety, while less than a quarter of the articles in *Working Mother* followed this theme. Overall, *Working Mother* presented breastfeeding in the least problematic light. The articles in *Working Mother* displayed a strong emphasis on women in executive, upper-management positions. For example, one article quoted Gwen Stefani, a popular musician and celebrity, as saying, "My theory is that nursing gives you super powers. How else could I be doing all this?"[15] Other articles in *Working Mother* focused on the difficulty of pumping at work, particularly if the mother does not have a private office. The most common advice was to talk to a representative in human resources about establishing a lactation room. The fact that *Working Mother* assumes that women have enough power within their workplace to ask the workplace to cater to their needs shows that the magazine's readers enjoy elite status. As a result of their elite status, these women can at least imagine that they have the power to establish the necessary accommodations for breastfeeding or expressing milk at work.

Many *Working Mother* articles focused on the importance of family-oriented workplaces. One mother was quoted as saying, "Rather than pump, I'd drop by the center (which was on site) every day and nurse her." Another mother noted, "I'm a new mom, and my daughter Alicia, who attends the on-site child care facility, doesn't take a bottle. Thankfully, my company recognizes how important it is to keep your nursing infant close to you in the first year of life. When our senior management team recently convened off-site, my daughter and her caregiver accompanied me for the day—at no cost to me. I could fully participate in the meeting because I didn't have to worry about her. When I needed to feed her, I could just step outside."[16] Fourteen of the twenty-one articles that discussed breastfeeding anxiety in *Working Mother* focused either on whether or not to pump breast milk at work or on the benefits of having one's child at an on-site child care facility so that breastfeeding in public would not be necessary. Two other articles were celebrity profiles that discussed the benefits of breastfeeding. Two features were about notions of general child care, such as being aware of how one's baby responds to breast-feeding and the need for responding to the baby, through practices such as skin-to-skin contact and eye contact. A few other articles focused on the importance of nutrition, exploring the benefits of eating organic and local foods. The last article in the sample examined breastfeeding legislation and the associated facilities needed in the workplace, such as lactation rooms and on-site child care facilities, within the context of professional, white-collar jobs. These examples demonstrate that *Working Mother* promotes breastfeeding more readily than the other magazines in the sample.

Mass market magazines such as the ones analyzed here seem to encourage working-class women to switch to formula-feeding for their infants much more readily than their middle- and upper-class counterparts. Working-class women are not only targeted with more infant formula advertisements in the popular magazines they read; they are also starved of information regarding the benefits of breast milk and breastfeeding. The sheer number of articles dealing with anxieties regarding the physical and material aspects of breastfeeding found in *American Baby*, *Parents*, and *Parenting* suggests that their readers appear to suffer far more anxiety regarding their ability to nourish their infants naturally, or at least that their readers are concerned about the anxiety itself. The articles always seem to include a question-and-answer section, which distinguishes this group clearly and can be found consistently across many such features.

A full sixteen articles within *American Baby*, *Parents*, and *Parenting* were dedicated to issues of anxiety concerning the maternal body's ability to breast-feed, and included such topics as the transference of diet preferences (like Chinese food or broccoli) via breast milk, whether the baby is getting enough nutrients, whether the baby is getting enough food, and the need for vitamins or supplements while breastfeeding. The information regarding nutrients specifically noted that breastfeeding mothers should take Vitamin D and DHA supplements because breastfed babies will not receive as much of these nutrients as babies consuming formula. Five articles specifically noted that breastfed infants will not get enough Vitamin D and are probably not getting enough DHA if women are not taking at least 400 mg of a DHA supplement daily. For example, a mother wrote to *American Baby* with the following question: "My 12 month old is quite a picky eater and mostly breastfeeds when he's hungry. Is this okay?" The writers at *American Baby* responded, "Nurse as long as you like, but your child may not get enough of certain nutrients (specifically Vitamin D and iron)." Four articles dealt with the proper preparation of for-mula, with two of those giving tips for weaning four- to six-month-old infants onto formula. The other two discussed the effects of breastfeeding on the breast itself (one focusing on breast ptosis, or sagging, and the other on the benefits of wearing a bra with a larger cup size while breastfeeding).

Thirteen of the sixteen above-mentioned articles made clear the equivalency between breastfeeding and formula-feeding. One very explicit message read, "If you can breastfeed, great. If you cannot, great. Breastfeeding is not for everyone. You have the right to choose."[17] Instead of focusing on the importance of breastfeeding (and enforcing that importance with tips, message board postings, and information regarding low-cost lactation help), the message was clear: if breastfeeding is not easy for a woman, she should move quickly to formula-feeding, since generations of formula-fed children have grown up without any issues.

A full eleven articles discussed the hardships of breastfeeding, covering a full range that included painful ducts, cracked nipples, and infants who do not latch properly. The difficulty of breastfeeding in public was also discussed frequently. One article dealt with the workplace, and five suggested that formula was an easy alternative to feeling awkward while breastfeeding in public. The fact that breastfeeding was presented as equal to or, in some cases, less ideal than formula-feeding indicates that these magazines consider it a lifestyle decision—a woman may choose the option that better suits her personal preference without regard to the structural impediments she faces or the benefits of breastfeeding. In addition, the public health aspects of breastfeeding fell by the wayside in articles published in *American Baby*, *Parents*, and *Parenting*, in favor of lengthy discussions regarding the transference of substances and toxins through breast milk and whether the maternal body was capable of providing adequate and sufficient nutrition for infants.

Whether responding to questions from readers or offering advice, the shared message of three magazines was focused on formula equivalency. The literature most likely to be read by working-class and lower-middle-class mothers seems to say, "Congratulations if you can breastfeed," while portraying formula as an equal, if not better-suited, alternative, because it comes with the supplements and vitamins that breast milk lacks. Taken a step further, these popular magazines seem to be demonstrating distrust for the working-class mother's embodied ability to nurse while exalting the upper-class body as having "super powers." While numerous articles have appeared in *American Baby*, *Parents*, and *Parenting* regarding the need for supplements, ways to measure how much breast milk is produced, and the avoidance of particular foods, only one article appeared in *Working Mother* discussing food during the examined time period. It suggested eating organic foods for the health of the mother and baby and cited a study showing that moms whose dairy and meat consumption was at least 90 percent organic had conjugated linoleic acid levels 17 percent higher than women whose organic dairy and meat consumption was only 50 to 90 percent, and 30 percent higher than women who consumed less than 50 percent organic dairy and meat. *Working Mother* also addressed vegetarian and vegan diets in this article; in fact, of all of the articles examined, this was the only one that discussed vegetarianism or veganism and breastfeeding. *Working Mother*'s advice to all mothers was to eat as much organic food and drink as many organic beverages as possible, as both are "beneficial to baby and not a bad thing to do for yourself either."[18]

The social-class disparity is obvious in this case: the magazines aimed at working- and lower-middle-class women repeatedly discuss the need for women to add supplements to their assumedly inadequate diets, while upper-class women need not worry because they can afford to purchase and prepare more expensive organic meals. All of these examples show that mass media sources are actively working against public health efforts to increase breastfeeding rates, particularly among working-class women.

Conclusion

Parenting magazines continue to perpetrate the idea that middle- and upper-class women are better suited to breastfeeding. Given the cultural and logistical constraints discussed here and elsewhere in this volume, such a perspective serves to maintain the status quo. By limiting the information regarding breastfeeding in media readily available to and consumed by working-class women, these information sources directly conflict with public health efforts to raise awareness regarding the benefits of breastfeeding. Such messaging serves the interests of a capitalistic culture that does not offer maternity leave, mandate on-site day care for most employed mothers, or make it possible for breastfeeding women to express their milk at work.[19]

In their discussion of reproductive decisions as personal or lifestyle choices, Michie and Cahn suggest that viewing breastfeeding as a lifestyle choice allows society to ignore how the social constraints placed upon women affect the choices they are able to make.[20] While print media is not solely responsible for disparities in breastfeeding rates among women in the United States, magazines play into the notion of personal choice without ever recognizing that women of different social classes do not receive the same information regarding breastfeeding. This is evidenced by McLeod's discussion of lower self-trust and lack of information experienced by working-class women. By maintaining the notion of personal choice and formula equivalency, these magazines make it all too easy to overlook the social inequalities that exist among women attempting to breastfeed. While feminist philosopher Diana Meyers reminds us that, "in sum, a woman's motherhood decision [remains] crucial to her personal well-being, definitive of her social persona, and predictive of her economic horizons," her decisions are bound by social constraints that are left unnamed and unrecognized.[21] Researchers must bring attention to the information deficiencies working-class women face and recognize the social constraints that leave these women unable to make a *true* choice regarding infant feeding.

Notes

1. Bellamy, "Mother Love," 16–17.
2. Eisenberg, Murkoff, and Hathaway, *What to Expect*; Orbach, *Bodies*, 165–179; McKenzie, "A Model of Information Practices," 22–35; Steffensmeir, "A Role Model," 319–322; Pridham, "Transition to Being the Mother," 213–215.
3. Hornik, "Public Health Communication," 1–22; Galst, "Television Food Commercials," 935–938; Fortmann, Taylor, Flora, and Jatulis, "Changes in Adult Cigarette Smoking," 82–96; Orbach, *Bodies*, 1–17, 124, 137–138, 140–142, 167–169; Potter, Sheeshka, and Valaitis, "Content Analysis," 200–203; Andsager and Powers, "Framing Women's Health," 177–182; Frerichs et al., "Framing Breastfeeding," 110–113.
4. Warner and Procaccino, "Toward Wellness," 713; Lewallen, "Healthy Behaviors," 204; Wilson and Colquhoun, "Influences in the Decision," 190–191; Arora, McJunkin, Wehrer, and Kuhn, "Major Factors."
5. Jordan, "Social Class, Temporal Orientation," 376–377.
6. Warner and Lunt, *The Social Life,* provides an analysis of social class as a determinant for behavior; Coleman, "The Continuing Significance of Social Class," 265.
7. Thomas and Callahan, "Allocating Happiness," 186–190; Myers and Biocca, "Elastic Body Image," 131–133; Orbach, *Bodies*, 100–108; Gould, Stern, and Adams, "TV's Distorted Vision," 310–313; Jhally, "Image-Based Culture," 77–87.
8. Orbach, *Bodies*, 30–31.
9. Michie and Cahn, *Confinements,* 70–74; McLeod, *Self-Trust*, 150–151.
10. According to Magazine Publishers of America, "10-Year Magazine," magazine readership has remained relatively steady despite the steady growth and easy accessibility of nonprint media.
11. Magazine Publishers of America, "10-Year"; All You Can Read, "Top Parenting Magazines."
12. Lasswell, "The Structure and Function," 37. In my analysis, for each magazine issue I noted basic information such as the total number of advertisements and articles, then the number of advertisements and articles that dealt with breastfeeding or formula-feeding. I also noted the position of the author of each article (staff writer, expert guest writer, contributing mother) and the location of the article within the magazine. Location within the magazine is an important variable for both advertisements and articles. More expensive and more visible locations within the magazine (such as on the back cover and in the first third of the magazine) ensure that the article or advertisement has a greater chance of being seen.

    I paid special attention to articles that mentioned infant feeding. I noted possible social-class bias, coding as social-class bias any comment regarding breastfeeding that provided suggestions or examples clearly related to a particular social-class position. For example, advice concerning the use of lactation rooms assumes a particular kind of workplace more likely to be available to pink- and white-collar workers. In a study of British media and infant feeding, Henderson, Kitzinger, and Green noted that the media far more commonly depicted formula-feeding than breastfeeding. When breastfeeding was portrayed, it was shown as something done almost exclusively by middle- to upper-class women and celebrities ("Representing Infant Feeding," 1196–1198). In line with that study's methodology, I conducted my content analysis to understand the context and narratives surrounding depictions of infant feeding, including any special signifiers about the women, mention of jobs or lack of external employment, and language and imagery used alongside depictions of each type of infant feeding (Moriarty, "Content Analysis," 550–554). I also examined recurring segments, particularly the question-and-answer columns, to gain a greater understanding of the sorts of issues that readers faced and for which they sought advice.

13. Hausman, *Mother's Milk*, 106.
14. For examples, see Capetta, "Back to Work"; Riss, Palagano, and Ebron, "Fifty Best," 72.
15. Howard, "Newsbreak," 16.
16. Both quotes from *Working Mother,* "100 Best Companies," 76–80.
17. Estroff, "Dirty Looks," 109.
18. Lee, "Nursing? Eat Organic," 78.
19. The new Affordable Care Act has changed this scenario for women working in firms hiring more than fifty workers.
20. Michie and Cahn, *Confinements*, 70–74; further discussion can be found in Hausman, *Mother's Milk*.
21. Meyers, "The Rush to Motherhood," 735; McLeod, *Self-Trust*, 98–99, 110–113, 150–153.

Sexuality and Women's Bodies

Breastfeeding in Public

Women's Bodies, Women's Milk

Breastfeeding takes place within cultural contexts where women receive conflicting messages about their bodies, breastfeeding, and role as mothers. Although the public health message is "breast is best," cultural associations between women's bodily fluids, dirt, and pollution mean breastfeeding is often seen as dirty and not for public view. Women's difficulties with breastfeeding in public may be a barrier to exclusive and long-term breastfeeding. We synthesize the relevant public health and feminist literature, considering how women's understanding of their milk affects their experiences of breastfeeding in public so that public health practitioners may work to support them.

Breastfeeding in public raises issues of private and public places and how these are experienced, interpreted, and enforced. Drawing on the literature about the cultural construction of women's bodies, bodily fluids, and breastfeeding, we argue that ideas of normality and deviancy, as well as modernism and primitivism, shape public and private understanding of breastfeeding, and we illustrate how this influence impacts on women's experiences. Western cultures articulate significant tensions and conflicts around the nature and function of breasts (particularly the sexualization of breasts). Various public health approaches could address these issues, as a public health model would focus the issues around breastfeeding in public and help to identify solutions.

We adopt a broad social-ecological approach that "recognizes that behaviors and health are influenced at multiple levels from the individual to families to larger systems and groups and then to the broadest level, the population and ecosystem," to address the issue of breastfeeding in public.[1] Other feminists have used the Social-Ecological Model (SEM) to identify multiple layers of influence on women's decisions to initiate and continue breastfeeding.[2] We extend this discussion by exploring how the SEM may inform public health approaches to breastfeeding in public. The crux of our argument is that for women to be successful at breastfeeding, they have to be able to breastfeed in public.

Breastfeeding in Public

International and national health policy focuses on increasing breastfeeding initiation and maintaining duration rates so that babies have six months of exclusive breastfeeding.[3] Babies need frequent feeding due to the composition of human milk, but this requirement is not generally appreciated, and the implications of reduced feeding frequency are poorly understood. Unless women stay secluded at home and feed their babies alone, they have to face the fact that they must breastfeed when others are present. To be successful breast-feeders, women must feed their babies when they are hungry—wherever they are. Many women restrict their activities to avoid exposing their breasts to others, or schedule other activities to fit around breastfeeding. Others abandon their original intention and use formula milk or expressed breast milk in public. This may compromise lactation and baby health and cause maternal distress as well as reinforcing formula-feeding as normal.[4] Many women feel shame or embarrassment when breastfeeding in public, and when they do many strive to be invisible to reduce their anxiety. Where breastfeeding in public is more acceptable, initiation and duration rates appear to be higher, and there is evidence that social class and ethnicity indicate which women are most likely to breastfeed in public.[5]

Breastfeeding women face complicated decisions and negotiations about space and place. Understanding and thinking about how we experience spaces and places, and our location in terms of identity and power relationships, have been illuminated by insights from human geography.[6] Women experience places differently once they become mothers, as the distinction between private and public spaces becomes less clear. Women used to negotiating public space only for themselves may develop different meanings when they are "negotiating space and two bodies."[7] Breastfeeding in public is determined by the public space in which it happens and in turn changes the general understanding of that place. The public spaces occupied by women are predominantly spaces of consumption (shops and cafés); paradoxically, these are the very places where many women find it most difficult to breastfeed.[8]

Notions of private and public are interpreted and experienced differently by women at different times when they are breastfeeding. Breastfeeding has been constructed as a feminine, private activity, most appropriately done at home. However, in postindustrial society, women do not usually spend long periods of time at home with their babies, even if they are not in paid employment.[9] In Western urban settings there are easily recognizable public spaces; typically, these are parks or malls. However, for some, breastfeeding in front of relatives or friends in their own home may be experienced as "public" instead of private and therefore becomes a source of conflict.[10] The same place may be a supportive or a difficult breastfeeding environment depending on circumstances. A park may be a difficult public space when breastfeeding alone, but it can be redefined as supportive when women breastfeed together. Understanding and negotiating public and private boundaries is a complex task for breastfeeding women as they mediate between their feelings, experiences, and prevailing social norms.

Women's ability to access and use social spaces is compromised by their gender.[11] Power relationships about the ownership of space are identified and played out differently depending on the setting and on individual circumstances. Therefore, women negotiate and manage breastfeeding wherever they find themselves when their babies need to be fed.[12] Women breastfeeding in public may feel vulnerable, and being asked to leave a public space can be deeply distressing. The workplace is also culturally defined as a public space, and the difficulties of returning to work while breastfeeding are well documented. Breastfeeding often ends at this point, as it conflicts with the implicit expectation that women's bodily fluids should be contained within private spaces.[13]

There are various ways in which identity and power issues can be viewed in relation to breastfeeding in public. Stearns writes about women's confusion and conflict regarding the "good maternal body" and the sexual body.[14] How women feel about breastfeeding in front of men depends on various factors, with some women identifying different categories of men and constructing the experience (and its management) differently if they are strangers in public places, rather than male friends or family in the home. The fear is that public breast exposure will be read as sexual. When women feel the need to modify their behavior in these ways, we can be sure that gendered power imbalances are at play.[15]

For some women an audience of male relatives or friends (particularly fathers or fathers-in-law) transforms the home into a public space. This transformation may involve women's interpretation of the male gaze and the sexual nature of breasts, or it may be a response to overt control, such as being asked or expected to move elsewhere. Low-income women in poor or overcrowded housing may have few choices about where to breastfeed, while women living with violent partners may have difficulty asserting their right to feel comfortable when breastfeeding. Many women believe it is their responsibility to minimize the discomfort of others by covering themselves up or leaving the room.[16] Breastfeeding in "private" spaces (bedrooms or bathrooms) excludes women from social activity, reinforces beliefs that public breastfeeding is inappropriate, and emphasizes gendered power imbalances in intimate relationships.

One way of engaging and challenging these situations is to conceptualize them as discursive space. Discursive space is constructed via the attitudes and social conventions expressed by people in their everyday lives.[17] Breastfeeding women simultaneously manage their ideas and feelings about breastfeeding in public and their perceptions of people's responses to their breastfeeding. Recent research found that most women were happy to publicly breastfeed older babies and toddlers, but they were alert to the potential for others' negative reactions. This awareness was probably learned throughout the months in which they breastfed their younger babies. Women's breastfeeding management strategies included no eye contact with strangers, breastfeeding with friends, and careful positioning of themselves in public spaces. So strong was the expectation of negative reactions that women were shocked to receive positive comments. This response echoes Stearns's findings that many women anticipated being asked to leave public places when breastfeeding, and so left, although few were actually asked to do so.[18] Even where legal protection exists (such as in parts of the United States and Scotland), ambiguity and misunderstanding remain. Where breastfeeding in public was never illegal, legal clarification has nevertheless been unhelpful, leaving many breastfeeding women still unclear about their position. These difficulties for breastfeeding women mean that breastfeeding is not publically visible and is often absent from current discourse around maternity.[19]

Ideas of normalcy versus deviancy are also expressed in relation to breastfeeding in public. In many postindustrial countries breastfeeding rates decline sharply in the early weeks, and normal feeding is understood to be feeding formula from a bottle, despite long-standing initiatives such as the WHO Code and the Innocenti Declaration.[20] Media images of infant feeding are predominantly of formula-feeding, reinforcing its normalcy and the deviance of breastfeeding.[21] Science and modernity dominated many discourses during the twentieth century, including that of infant feeding. The development of formula milk and its association with science and the medical profession has been instrumental in the decline of breastfeeding in many cultures.[22] Breastfeeding is identified as natural, and with so-called primitive cultures, where science and modernity are prized, this association may be vilified.[23]

Women's Bodies and Bodily Fluids in Public

Cultural understandings of bodily fluids are complicated. There is a hierarchy of propriety: the way bodily fluids are seen in relation to each other varies between social and cultural contexts. Some fluids are seen as pure (tears, breast milk), whereas others are polluting or contaminating (genital secretions, vomit).[24] The degree of disgust about bodily secretions is greater for those associated with waste products (feces, urine, and menstrual blood) and is heightened when associated with sexual orifices (breast milk, lochia, and menstrual blood).[25] The combination of (leaking) breast milk and an exposed nipple is often seen as particularly difficult, even threatening.[26]

Menstrual blood and childbirth fluids are evidence of women's impurity in many cultures, influencing how women are viewed when menstruating and birthing, as well as how others behave toward them. In some societies women are ritually removed or hidden at these times and/or ritually cleansed afterward.[27] Milk and blood are often opposed; milk symbolizes purity and motherhood, but menstrual blood is seen as bad—draining and weakening.[28] Research in the United Kingdom into male and female attitudes to menstruation and breastfeeding suggests statistically significant relationships between the two.[29]

Breast milk is symbolically confusing—it is pure, life-giving, emblematic of motherhood, *and* is dirty.[30] Breastfeeding is associated with purity, but is also primitive, crude, and embarrassing; breasts remain sexual. Bottle-feeding with formula is perceived to be clean.[31] Although health promotion campaigns emphasize the natural goodness of human milk and the naturalness of breast-feeding, for some people breastfeeding is "indecent, disgusting, animalistic, sexual and even, for some, a perverse act."[32] These ambiguities coalesce around the idea of adults consuming breast milk or breast milk products.[33] Here breast milk is viewed as "matter out of place" and is taboo. The involuntary leakage of breast milk is "a powerful symbol of the 'distortion' to known body boundaries or borders. Leaking breast milk highlights the ambiguity of inside and outside, self and Other." Visible signs of women's lack of control are disturbing to both men and women.[34]

Breast milk's association with pollution has consequences for breast-feeding in public. Women in breastfeeding groups have been found to react negatively toward breast milk, behaving differently toward spilt breast milk and formula milk as well as the vomit of breast- and formula-fed babies.[35]

Breastfeeding in public can be seen as particularly disgusting in public eating places. Women are often asked not to breastfeed where people are eating, or are expected to breastfeed in washrooms.[36] Easily available private places for women to breastfeed outside the home are limited, and even specially allocated spaces (mother and baby rooms) may be unclean and nonseparate from diaper changing facilities.[37] The association with excretion or excreta is reinforced.

In all societies, children learn about public management of the body. In Western cultures, we learn that bodily functions are offensive and bodily fluids must be contained and disguised. Shame and guilt are associated with bodily functions and fluids, particularly those associated with sex or reproduction.[38] Young women learn from an early age to control and hide any body fluid leakage and to be ashamed when this fails.[39] The development and marketing of products intended to hide the evidence of menstruation (and of leaking breast milk) contributes to these cultural meanings. The stigma of loss of menstrual blood is evidence of women's lack of control over their bodies and interpreted as a threat to order.[40] Leakage is cited by some women as a reason for not breastfeeding in public in the early weeks after birth; women with stronger letdown reflexes may find this especially hard.[41]

Women's experience of breast milk leakage affects their experience of breastfeeding in public. Breast milk is expected to be controlled, although the flow is involuntary; visible evidence of leakage is embarrassing or even disgusting: a mother's body may be perceived as out of control. The internalization of cultural perceptions leads women to report experiencing letdown as stressful or revolting, saying that they feel dirty and unclean. Women talk about feeling compelled to hide and control breast milk leakage, feeling "sticky, messy, dirty, embarrassed and uncomfortable."[42] Babies may also draw attention to the presence of the milk in public by noisy feeding.[43] When breastfeeding in public, women have to practically and emotionally manage potential leakage. Many women are not prepared for this exigency (although some birth preparation classes give advice about containing breast milk when in public, as do other people).[44] Women's lack of preparation may be indicative of the absence of a breastfeeding culture combined with widespread discomfort in talking about any kind of bodily fluid leakage. Many women also experience difficulty with the body and breast changes that accompany breastfeeding and "objectify their lactating breasts and breast milk, noting that 'the stuff just pours out,' the breast 'deflated,' the breast milk had 'curdled.'"[45] Such objectification may be a means of coping with reality.

Given these complex and negative cultural constructions associated with breast milk, no wonder bottle-feeding may appear to be the solution. Changes in fertility and life expectancy mean that menstruation is a more openly discussed part of women's lives than breastfeeding (although this might change with women choosing to control their menstruation in novel ways).[46] Few people have seen breast milk leaking in public; fewer women have seen how others manage the milk in their bodies in public before they have their own babies. Women continue to "negotiate breastfeeding to cause least offence and embarrassment to themselves and others."[47]

Public Health Approaches

Social marketing is the application of commercial marketing techniques to achieve attitudinal and behavioral shifts in target audiences. These include "the design, implementation and control of programs calculated to influence the acceptability of social ideas and involving considerations of product, planning, pricing, communication, distribution and marketing research."[48] It is based on the idea of a mutually beneficial exchange, so it is important to know the target group's values and aspirations.[49] The marketing mix of product, price, place, and promotion may be applied to breastfeeding. The product is the breastfeeding behavior, including positive benefits of breast milk for both baby and mother. Negative connotations of breastfeeding need to be countered with positive attributes. Price refers to perceived costs (loss of time and possible embarrassment) rather than money, although there might be financial costs (inability to work). Place and promotion refer to how the marketing takes place—where and by what means.

Health professionals can support breastfeeding women and destigmatize issues around breastfeeding by being knowledgeable about breastfeeding. They can help to develop self-defense strategies with mothers, with practice at being assertive, and rehearse the application of principles to any situation unsupportive of breastfeeding. They can facilitate discussion about the interpersonal aspects of breastfeeding even before the baby is born and follow on through into the early weeks and beyond, offering practical ideas and support.[50]

Lay champions can be used as role models to contextualize the targeted desirable. Health professionals will need to tap into the target group's values, norms, and aspirations so that breastfeeding can be sold as desirable, normal behavior. One UK project used cardboard cutouts of breastfeeding mothers to raise awareness about breastfeeding in public. This technique had been used in California to raise awareness of public breastfeeding and overcome barriers to breastfeeding in public.[51]

Social marketing also includes four additional considerations—publics, partnerships, policy, and purse strings—which help clarify the target groups for the marketing intervention.[52] Publics are new mothers, their partners, and owners and managers of public facilities. Relevant partnerships could be created between health practitioners, women's groups, and the commercial sector, involving policies to support behavior shift (for example, local breastfeeding-friendly policies). Purse strings involves identifying sources of funding. A recent study investigated how to encourage teenage mothers to breastfeed, and the researchers identified three areas for social marketing strategies: creating a social norm, such as "breastfeeding welcome here" signs in shops, cafés, and public places; focusing on benefits for the mother—bonding, convenience, and program incentives (such as certificates or calendars); and training health staff to use empathy, facilitation, and peer supporters rather than a "we know best" attitude.[53] Social marketing may be applied to all new mothers to normalize breastfeeding. Mothers' perceived benefits of breastfeeding may vary from group to group, as will suitable incentives, but local research can identify which triggers would work for each subgroup of mothers to adopt breastfeeding. Embedding antenatal breastfeeding discussions in health workers' practice, and using empathy and facilitation rather than education and advice, appear to be universally appropriate strategies.

Social marketing ideas and techniques generate a range of opportunities to promote breastfeeding in public at individual, community, and societal levels. The interventions range from individual attitudinal and knowledge change to local policy initiatives, using key agencies to work on issues around public spaces and breastfeeding. Community public health campaigns have focused on social and public spaces so babies can breastfeed and eat in the best way possible. Techniques include posters on buses and in public venues, newspaper adverts, and radio and television broadcasts.[54] The societal level includes legislative action to protect the right to breastfeed in public and in workplaces, and is supported by the production by international agencies of breastfeeding-friendly policies and strategies.[55]

Conclusion

To support breastfeeding we should maximize the incidence and prevalence of women breastfeeding in public. Public health practitioners should focus on two major issues—women's experiences of spaces and places when breastfeeding, and women's experiences of the milk in their bodies in public. Prevailing social and cultural norms in postindustrial Western societies act as constraints on women's breastfeeding practices, but we urge colleagues to work to develop local solutions to local problems while supporting the creation of regional and national legislative infrastructures to challenge restrictive norms. Public health practitioners can draw on a wealth of research and knowledge for self-development and become key change agents and work in partnership with lay champions and lay organizations to make breastfeeding in public an unremarkable miracle. These working practices will help to challenge the way women's bodies are culturally explained and understood and create a virtuous circle impacting on women's breastfeeding behavior. A comprehensive list of answers cannot be generated to address every circumstance and place where breastfeeding in public is problematic. However, by taking a broad social-ecological approach in order to consider solutions at a number of levels, and by promoting the usefulness of social marketing, social change can be achieved, albeit slowly, for the benefit of women, their babies, and society.

Notes

1. Ockene et al., "Integrating Evidence-Based," 246. See also Dahlgren and Whitehead, *Policies and Strategies*; Dahlberg and Krug, "Violence."
2. See also Labbok, Smith, and Taylor, "Breastfeeding and Feminism"; Labbok, "Transdisciplinary."
3. For example, UK Department of Health, *Maternal and Infant Nutrition*; American Academy of Pediatrics, "Policy Statement"; National Health and Medical Research Council, *Dietary Guidelines*; World Health Organization and UNICEF, *Global Strategy*; Department of Health and Human Services, *Breastfeeding: HSS Blueprint*.
4. Stearns, "Breastfeeding," 311. See also Wolf, "Got Milk?"; Scott and Mostyn, "Women's Experiences"; Sheeshka et al., "Women's Experiences"; Pain, Bailey, and Mowl, "Infant Feeding"; Raisler, "Against the Odds"; Smyth, "Gendered Spaces."
5. See Stearns, "Breastfeeding"; Li, Fridinger, and Grummer-Strawn, "Public Perceptions"; Pain, Bailey, and Mowl, "Infant Feeding"; and Bolling et al., *UK Infant Feeding*, 289.
6. See Pain, Bailey, and Mowl, "Infant Feeding"; Smyth, "Gendered Spaces"; Mahon-Daly and Andrews, "Liminality and Breastfeeding"; and, more recently, Boswell-Penc and Boyer, "Expressing Anxiety?" and Boyer, "The Way."
7. Mahon-Daly and Andrews, "Liminality and Breastfeeding."
8. Smyth, "Gendered Spaces," 87; Bartlett, *Breastwork*.
9. Carter, *Feminism, Breasts and Breast-feeding*; Bartlett, *Breastwork*.
10. Pain, Bailey, and Mowl, "Infant Feeding"; Raisler, "Against the Odds."
11. Smyth, "Gendered Spaces."
12. Stearns, "Breastfeeding."
13. Discussed by Boswell-Penc and Boyer, "Expressing Anxiety," in the context of breast-pumping at work.
14. See Hurst, this volume.
15. Stearns, "Breastfeeding."
16. Dowling, "Women's Experiences"; Pain, Bailey, and Mowl, "Infant Feeding"; Stearns, "Breastfeeding."
17. See Teather, *Embodied Geographies*, 2–3.

18. Dowling, "Women's Experiences"; Stearns, "Breastfeeding."
19. Stearns, "Breastfeeding."
20. World Health Organization, *International Code*; World Health Organization and UNICEF, *Innocenti Declaration*.
21. Henderson, Kitzinger, and Green, "Representing Infant Feeding."
22. See Palmer, *Politics of Breastfeeding*; Apple, *Mothers and Medicine*.
23. Dowling, "Women's Experiences"; Faircloth, "What Science Says."
24. Shaw, "Virtues," 292; Grosz, *Volatile Bodies*, 195. See also Douglas, *Purity and Danger*.
25. Bramwell, "Blood and Milk," 92. See also Shaw, "Virtues," 292, as well as Grosz, *Volatile Bodies*, 192.
26. Smale, "Stigmatisation of Breastfeeding," 237; see also Susan Battersby, "Not in Public," 102.
27. See, for example, Bandyopadhyay, "Impact of Ritual Pollution."
28. Walker, cited in Bramwell, "Blood and Milk," 87, describes Aristotle's belief that menstrual blood was converted to breast milk. See also p. 89.
29. Bramwell, "Initial Qualitative Study."
30. Shaw, "Virtues," 292; Bramwell, "Blood and Milk."
31. Battersby, "Not in Public," 101.
32. Yalom, in Battersby, "Not in Public," 102.
33. See, for example, "Other People's Breastmilk," broadcast on Channel 4 in the United Kingdom, and *Today*, "Chef Dishes." See also Smale, "Stigmatisation of Breastfeeding."
34. Schmied and Lupton, "Blurring the Boundaries," 242. Douglas, *Purity and Danger*.
35. Mahon-Daly and Andrews, " Liminality and Breastfeeding ," 69.
36. Smale, "Stigmatisation of Breastfeeding."
37. Britton, "Natural Phenomenon," 305. Also Battersby, "Not in Public."
38. Battersby, "Not in Public," 102.
39. Britton, "Natural Phenomenon," 302; Battersby, "Not in Public," 102. See also Schmeid and Lupton, "Blurring the Boundaries," 245
40. Margrit Shildrick, *Leaky Bodies*, 34.
41. Britton, "Natural Phenomenon," 310.
42. Battersby, "Not in Public," 103. See also Mahon-Daly and Andrews, " Liminality and Breastfeeding ," 69; Schmied and Lupton, "Blurring the Boundaries," 242. Also discussed in Britton, "Natural Phenomenon."
43. Smale, "Stigmatisation of Breastfeeding"; Battersby, "Not in Public."
44. See Longhurst, "Pregnant Bodies," 81
45. Schmied and Lupton, "Blurring the Boundaries," 242.
46. See for example, Andrist et al., "Women's and Providers'"; Andrist et al., "Need to Bleed"; Johnston-Robledo et al., "To Bleed."
47. Mahon-Daly and Andrews, " Liminality and Breastfeeding ," 65.
48. Kotler and Zaltman, "An Approach," 5.
49. Lefebvre and Flora, "Social Marketing."
50. Smale, "Stigmatisation of Breastfeeding," 241–243.
51. Louise Condon et al., "'Cut Out for Breastfeeding.'"
52. Weinreich, "Social Marketing."
53. Bristol Social Marketing Centre, *Researching Social Marketing Solutions*.
54. Smyth, "Gendered Spaces," 89, 91.
55. For example, the different approaches supported and endorsed by the UNICEF Baby-Friendly Hospital and Community Initiatives.

Sexual or Maternal Breasts?

A Feminist View of the Contested Right to Breastfeed Publicly

Breastfeeding mothers must cope with the dominant notion of the sexual breast that pervades the culture of the United States.[1] Even though laws have been passed clarifying the right to breastfeed in public in forty-four states as well as on federal property, breastfeeding in public is still debated, sometimes discriminated against, and is commonly perceived as embarrassing for many mothers.[2] This chapter explores mothers' experiences of living with the sexual breast and the mother-led political struggle to establish a right to breastfeed. Ideological influences on individual and corporate behaviors are insidious, as most often they are not recognized on a conscious level.[3] Breastfeeding difficulties, especially around public breastfeeding, have prompted active resistance strategies from mothers. Demonstrating the impact of patriarchal ideology as a breastfeeding constraint can point public health strategy into new territory. Specifically, this chapter examines a central cultural dualism behind inhospitable attitudes toward public breastfeeding that is personified on one hand by the virginal Madonna and on the other by the seductive harlot. As women pick up the echoes of these polarized and moralistic views of women in the culture, they absorb a message implying that good mothers are not active sexual subjects. Re-membering mothers as fully embodied sexual beings suggests a possible transformation of public health advocacy of breastfeeding.

Breastfeeding in Cultural Context

Sexual connotations tied to breasts and breastfeeding constrain whether, where, and how long mothers breastfeed.[4] Mothers express concern about turning men on and feel vulnerable to social judgment when breastfeeding in public. Some women even express reluctance to breastfeed openly in their own homes due to their own codes of modesty or strictures placed on them by spouses, boyfriends, or significant others. Open breastfeeding, especially with older babies, is not yet a well-accepted cultural norm.[5] Some studies suggest that a mother's internal reticence to be subject to social judgment due to breastfeeding may be more constraining than actual experiences of negative interactions while in public.[6]

Choosing to breastfeed should not be understood as a simple act of individual volition, although breastfeeding promotion messages sometimes seem to imply that infant feeding is a simple choice. Feminist social critique maintains that economic and social structures impinge on women's freedom in many spheres; breastfeeding is one of them. Mothers do choose whether or not to breastfeed, yet this choice is conditioned by complex cultural understandings of the meaning of breastfeeding and mothering and of breasts and sexuality.[7] The choice to breastfeed is made within a net of relationship circumstances where the desirability of breastfeeding and a mother's prerogative to enact the practice may be disputed. Frequently, conflicting advice and expectations are placed on the mother. Opinions of her intimate partner, mother, sisters, and friends are influential.[8] Public health recommendations encouraging breastfeeding are filtered through primary support persons and professional helpers (nurses, midwives, doctors, and Women, Infants, and Children personnel). The choice to continue breastfeeding day to day, week to week, month to month, year to year is made by the mother only as she negotiates her way through this maze of advice and expectations, as well as her ongoing experience of success or frustration with what is occurring at the breast with her baby.

Mothers' rights to breastfeed are under continual negotiation, as well, in the broader milieu of society.[9] Skirmishes in the battle over breastfeeding in public have played out within the media; on buses, planes, and trains; in restaurants; on social networking sites like Facebook; and within state houses and Congress. Health recommendations to breastfeed exclusively for six months, to continue breastfeeding for a full year and beyond, and to meet Healthy People 2010 goals are tidy pronouncements on paper. It is messier by far to be the mother deciding how to explain herself—messier by far to claim an uncontested right to breastfeed wherever a mother and baby have a right to be in public.

Mothers' Voices

Mothers' own explanations of their situations can teach us about the impact of sexual perceptions of breasts and breastfeeding on mothers' perceived options.

The following short excerpts in mothers' own words show a range of experiences coping with the sexually defined breast in infant feeding. These excerpts are a data subset of a larger mixed-methods study of breastfeeding constraints.[10] They are arranged in an order beginning with those mothers least disposed to breastfeed, progressing through more ambivalent attitudes, and ending with mothers who demonstrate strong resolve to breastfeed despite sexual attributes placed on the practice by others. Mothers' words are preceded by identification of age, race or ethnicity, marital status, and the infant feeding experience of the speaker.

A twenty-five-year-old, single, Caucasian mother of two nonbreastfed children, the youngest six months old at the time of the interview: "Breastfeeding is nasty. I wouldn't do that. It would embarrass me."

A twenty-three-year-old, married, Caucasian mother of two nonbreastfed children, the youngest six weeks old at the time of the interview: "We were going to consider breastfeeding but health issues [complicated labor, then c-section] wouldn't let us. I was kinda relieved, 'cause I was okay with bottle-feeding, the convenience, you know. It is so much easier when you are in public. Then people aren't looking over and thinking that you are being gross."

A twenty-one-year-old, married, African American mother who breastfed her second baby three months: "I knew breastfeeding was healthy for her and she was premature so needed that. But I was really so-so about doing it. It was really difficult to go out in public. If she cried at all, I didn't want people looking at me with my shirt up. I liked it better at home. Breastfeeding got difficult because of this, formula is much easier when you go out."

A thirty-one-year-old, married, Caucasian mother who breastfed four older children for six months each and then decided to use formula after two weeks of nursing twins when she became fatigued and overwhelmed: "I kept working full time and breastfeeding with my oldest, but breastfeeding got to be too much with the twins and the other babies [a two-year-old and a three-year-old]. I know it is better for the baby and more natural, and helps with bonding, but I had to stop. My husband didn't like me to do it in front of anyone, too. Breastfeeding is such private behavior. So, then it is hard to be in public."

A twenty-one-year-old, single, Portuguese American mother still breastfeeding her first baby at five weeks old: "A friend of my mom was relentless about the need to breastfeed. It was really annoying at first, but then she helped me get through the hard time when I was engorged. We used cabbage leaves. It helped like magic! We talked about it—it's their problem, if some people don't like to see breastfeeding. A mother shouldn't have to hide it."

A thirty-six-year-old, married, African American mother who had seven children and was still breastfeeding her youngest at six months spoke in reference to her mother-in-law: "She would always be thinking that the baby was not getting enough milk. Always telling me some people might not understand it. But I didn't listen to her, and I kept breastfeeding all seven of my children."

A twenty-four-year-old, partnered, African American mother who breastfed her first child two years and was still breastfeeding her second child at eight months: "My sisters would say stuff that might make a weak-minded person feel uncomfortable or ashamed of breastfeeding. Like 'you're going to take out your bosom and feed your baby in the mall? It's going to upset everyone if you do that.' And, 'Doesn't that feel awkward or gross? How can you sit there and let the baby suck on your breast?'"

An eighteen-year-old, married, Mexican immigrant who breastfed her first baby six months: "I liked it. It was easy, great. I only stopped because I went back to work full time a month ago. I don't agree that breastfeeding interferes with sex, for my husband it turned him on."

These excerpts reveal that sexual perception plays a role in many individual mothers' experiences of infant feeding, and that pubic breastfeeding is an especially problematic prospect for many. These examples show mothers attending to the relational context of their infant feeding. Some mothers were accommodating to the opinions of their significant others, while other mothers followed their own lights, persevering with breastfeeding in spite of disapproval. These excerpts speak to how mothers experience pressure to conform to ideological constraints concerning mothering and the use of the female body.

Demonstrating Ideological Impacts

Ideology is communicated ubiquitously, through story, art, media, and typical commonplace social relationships and cultural patterns, as a structuring influence on everyday life.[11] Ideology has historical roots with modern-day manifestations that help people make sense out of the inputs they receive and the expectations society places on their behavior. An ideological constraint placed on mothering is a common distancing of maternity and sexuality. Culturally, a dichotomy exists between the ideal, virtuous, pure mother and her potential rival—the evil temptress or sexually seductive woman.

Beginning with Plato, through Augustine and Descartes, up until our time, prominent philosophers have divided the mind from the body.[12] Women have been associated with the body, with sexual activity viewed as antithetical to the life of the mind and spirit. Ideal motherhood, ironically, becomes desexualized.[13] The Virgin Mary may be the purest cultural image of the supposedly asexual mother. The image of the breastfeeding Madonna is among the oldest of Christian icons and became a starring subject in medieval art. Paradoxically, part of the power of these images may be their ability to subvert a puritanical ideological standard visually, as much of this art actually communicates sensuality and wholeness. For living women, virginity is miraculous and unattainable. The route to motherhood must pass through sex in some form.

Wives, too, ironically, have an asexual image as mothers; they may be slotted as mild-mannered, domesticated, and focused on their offspring.[14] Relentless media coverage of sexual scandals within prominent marriages, like that of Bill and Hillary Clinton, Elliot and Silda Spitzer, Mark and Jenny Sanford, John and Elizabeth Edwards, or Tiger Woods and Elin Nordegren, captivate the public's attention. These stories are the retelling of a patriarchal morality tale pitting the wronged wife against the sexual temptress, both of whom vie for the man's devotion. Whether an individual onlooker sympathizes with the wife or feels for the sexually uninhibited temptress, the stories reinforce a cultural message that real mothers aren't sexual.

Public health breastfeeding advocacy trips over this polarizing ideology dichotomizing women as pure or seductive and viewing mothering as divorced from sexuality. Breastfeeding promotion downplays the sexual significance of women's breasts in order to claim the breast as nurturing and maternal. When breastfeeding is claimed by the asexual mother side of this cultural dichotomy, the normalcy and decency of breastfeeding is championed and the rightness of breastfeeding in public seems obvious. Desexualizing breasts, however, may make breastfeeding less attractive. It certainly misses the reality of many women's lives in a sexually charged culture where women's breasts and bodies are used ubiquitously to sell commodities.

The sexually unavailable breast perceived in public breastfeeding may be the most offensive transgression of dominant ideology within a jealous patri- archy. The feminist pro-choice abortion argument echoes in this definitional tug-of-war over breast meaning and use. Instead of whose body is it, the ques- tion becomes whose breasts are they? Are breasts supposed to be sexually available for heterosexual men or are they for babies? A feminist answer to this question: Neither. A woman's breasts belong to the woman herself. A mother has a reproductive right to use her breasts *both* for her own pleasure and for a procreative breastfeeding purpose as it pleases her.

Mothers' sexual agency needs re-memberment in breastfeeding promotion. Too often the sexual may be skirted, ignored, and not talked about as an important and motivating aspect of mothers' identities and concerns.[15] Mothers need their professional helpers, their lactation consultants, counselors, social workers, doctors, nurses, and midwives to see them as fully sexual beings. Conversations regarding what sexual meanings and issues a mother may have about her own breastfeeding experience may be crucial. Conversations regarding how her significant others understand this use of her breasts, and what pressures she may feel about where and when she breastfeeds, may be pivotal to her breastfeeding success. A mother who is fully available in her body, who is acting as an executive within the family she calls her own, who is responsible for nurturing care of her children, and who is free to participate in a playful, sexually fulfilling adult relationship is a powerful woman.

A Political Struggle

Emerging from women's experiences of subjugation, feminist theory is critical and activist, seeking to bring greater power and possibility to women and in so doing improve social life for everyone.[16] Women's and mothers' domestic contributions have for too long been invisible in economic calculations, been taken for granted, or been dismissed, even while the service women provide in family roles, such as breastfeeding, is crucial to the well-being of society.[17] A feminist vision of power makes individual capacity and capability central to what power is, including the ability to create, the capability to think for oneself, and the ability to be self-disciplined and possess the will to resist.[18] The excerpts presented earlier represent separate personal experiences of breastfeeding constraint. Some of the mothers were able to use their power to think critically for themselves and to resist nonsupport for their breastfeeding. Philosopher Hannah Arendt also describes power *with* others, "the human ability not just to act but to act in concert."[19] When individuals act together, personal resistance can become political power.

Over the last two decades, breastfeeding activism, or lactivism, has brought breastfeeding mothers and supporters together to fight for laws protecting public breastfeeding. Coordinated efforts in different states to pass breastfeeding laws are often sparked by the experience of a mother whose breastfeeding at a public location was not welcomed. Following a mother's breastfeeding discrimination experience in a museum, Florida in 1993 passed the first state law exempting breastfeeding from laws against indecent exposure.[20] These laws frequently make reference to public health and the need to increase the practice of breastfeeding. At the federal level, law now allows a mother to nurse her child in any location on federal property where she otherwise has a right to be. As of March 2010, the Affordable Care Act requires employers to allow unpaid break time for lactating employees to pump for as long as one year after the baby's birth.[21] Currently, forty-four states also have laws with wording allowing breastfeeding in any public or private location, while twenty-eight states have laws specifically stating that breastfeeding in public is not indecent exposure.[22]

Despite the technical legality of breastfeeding in public, mothers breastfeeding in places like malls, pools, restaurants, and stores, or while traveling on buses or planes have continued to experience problems with being asked to leave, go to the restroom to nurse, or cover themselves with blankets. Social change on this front is led by mothers' resistance efforts. Mothers like Kerry Madden-Lunsford in California, Amy Swan in Kansas, Lorig Charkoudian in Maryland, Emily Gillette in Vermont, and Brooke Ryan in Kentucky have responded to personal experiences of being asked to stop their breastfeeding or cover up with organized resistance. Letters have been written, legislators have been lobbied, and legal action has been brought against the offending stores, restaurants, and corporations over incidents.[23] Breastfeeding discrimination incidences communicated to other mothers willing to act have resulted in organized groups of mothers staging nurse-in protests, with their babies in tow, at locations where incidents have occurred. These events usually reap public interest and media coverage. In 2005 Barbara Walters stated on her talk show *The View* that she felt uncomfortable sitting next to a breastfeeding mother during an airplane flight. Viewers organized protests over the Internet that resulted in a nurse-in protest staged outside of ABC's New York headquarters by two hundred breastfeeding mothers.[24]

Lactivist mothers discover that along with positive support, their public resistance has made them the target of harsh criticism from strangers. One organizing mother, Lorig Charkoudian, said, "I was amazed at how many of the responses . . . about the nurse-in have really been trying to shame me for my choices, and make these really personal attacks on me and my choices as a mother."[25] People have opined that breastfeeding mothers should just stay at home, that their breastfed children will have sexual complexes, and that the mother is really doing some other thing, like drinking caffeine, that is actually "bad" for the child. Public breastfeeding as a cause has also been belittled as petty and relatively unimportant.[26]

Interestingly, as technology continues to push the frontiers of the public world, controversy over public breastfeeding has arrived on the Internet as well. And the fight is ugly. With anonymity as a cover, blogs about nurse-ins reveal discussions of public breastfeeding with a shocking lack of civility. Postings include name-calling, crass sexual language and innuendo, and personal attacks on the character of the activists.[27] In defense of breastfeeding in response to such postings, other writers appeal rationally to breastfeeding recommendations from the American Academy of Pediatrics or the World Health Organization—as if allying public breastfeeding with public health puts this mothering behavior back in the province of good mother actions. The real offense of empowered mothers standing up for breastfeeding rights may be the transgression of an outdated status quo.

Controversy simmered for months in 2009 over Facebook removing breastfeeding photos uploaded by mothers to share with family and friends. Facebook claimed that the photos violated their decency code by showing exposed breasts. A petition to Facebook was organized, as well as a Facebook group titled "Hey Facebook, breastfeeding is not obscene!"[28]

Breastfeeding rights have come a long way since Florida codified the first law providing protection for public breastfeeding in 1993.[29] Mothers seeking information regarding public breastfeeding can find many Internet sites with helpful information. Such sites link a new mother to efforts that mothers before her have made. Now when an individual mother experiences discrimination she is not alone. She can communicate the incident to a breastfeeding advocacy organization like FirstRight or the National Alliance of Breastfeeding Advocacy (NABA).[30] FirstRight aims to correspond with the organization in question to support the implementation of a more breastfeeding-friendly policy. NABA collects statistics on breastfeeding discrimination incidents.

Yet in order to make more safe space in society for breastfeeding, personal, political, and social resistance will need to continue. Breastfeeding mothers, individually and in concert, as owners of the lactating potential of society, will decide if, when, where, and how long breastfeeding happens. Many mothers, as the excerpts in this chapter attest, feel cowed when their breastfeeding is distasteful to others. Other breastfeeding mothers suckle their babies proudly, openly, and even defiantly, refusing calls for discretion.

One breastfeeding advocacy strategy is to increase the sensual or sexual marketing of breastfeeding itself. Best for Babes is an organization with an Internet site and an aim to make breastfeeding more accessible and attractive to mothers. Their work can be seen as one exemplar of re-membering mothers with sexual agency. Danielle Rigg and Bettina Forbes launched Best for Babes "to help moms beat the 'booby traps,' the cultural and institutional barriers, that prevent moms from achieving their personal breastfeeding goals."[31] This is done, in part, by transgressing the tired good mother–bad mother, pure-seductive dualisms in dominant ideology about being a mother and a woman. Aiming to inspire, prepare, and empower mothers, Best for Babes intends "to give breastfeeding a makeover."[32] The makeover includes raising money to support a pro-breastfeeding ad campaign. Celebrity mothers have been recruited to pose as models in the campaign. Breastfeeding photos and graphics are making their way into print magazines and other advertising venues. One of their pictures charts new ground for breastfeeding awareness in the culture by picturing a naked mother and baby as a sensual and beautiful image. Advertising posters, including one graphic portraying breasts as "life-saving devices," have been proffered in public with pro-bono public service advertising space. Best for Babes images do re-member, and even exploit, the connection between sexuality and motherhood.[33] Their pictures make mothering glamorous and sexually attractive.

A peaceful public consensus concerning public breastfeeding is doubtful in the near future. In spite of vitriol and attack from some quarters against public breastfeeding, cultural change is proceeding incrementally. While brave women have done much to resist dominant ideological breastfeeding constraint and secured a right to breastfeed in public in the United States, it is still a controversial right in need of further advocacy. This struggle for breastfeeding rights takes its place alongside other struggles for justice and dignity. As more mothers are able to claim breastfeeding, enjoy it, and bring it into the public sphere, dividends will be won for maternal and child health.

Notes

1. Wolf, "Got Milk?"
2. National Conference of State Legislatures, "Breastfeeding Laws."
3. See Hausman, this volume.
4. Stearns, "Breastfeeding and the Good Maternal Body," 308–325.
5. Li, Fridinger, and Grummer-Strawn, "Public Perceptions," 227–235.
6. Sheeshka et al., "Women's Experiences Breastfeeding," 31–38.
7. Forbes et al., "Perceptions of the Woman," 379–388.
8. Rempel and Rempel, "Partner Influence," 92–111; Dykes et al., "Adolescent Mothers," 391–400; Earle, "Factors Affecting the Initiation," 205–214.
9. Li et al., "Public Beliefs," 1162–1168; Scott and Mostyn, "Women's Experiences," 270–277.
10. Hurst, "Constraints on Breastfeeding Choices," discusses study methodology in detail, 64–92. This data subset was collected in a larger mixed-methods study using a cross-sectional survey design to explore breastfeeding constraints of mothers participating in the Women, Infants, and Children (WIC) program in central Virginia. WIC is a federal supplemental food program for low-income mothers and children. In Virginia it is provided through local health department regions. Mothers and children are eligible to receive supplemental food, and formula, if family income is 185 percent of the poverty level.

    In the study, a questionnaire was completed through survey or structured interview, first with forty mothers with a baby between birth and eighteen months in a pilot study, and later with an additional 140 mothers with a baby between six and eighteen months of age. Some open-ended qualitative questions were asked to give mothers the opportunity to provide their personal viewpoints in this intimate area of inquiry. The eight vignettes included here represent mothers who responded to the open-ended queries regarding their feeding choice (breast or formula) and regarding their support or discouragement experiences with that feeding method by spontaneously making reference to public breastfeeding or sexual perceptions of breastfeeding. While these qualitative vignettes provide a composite view of mothers' perceptions, they cannot be generalized to the entire sample.

Multiple regression analysis using the entire sample did show that increased public breastfeeding discomfort, measured on a quantitative scale, was a significant predictor both of not initiating breastfeeding and of shorter breastfeeding duration for those who did breastfeed (120, 124).

11. For a comprehensive discussion of ideology, see Hausman, this volume.
12. Bordo, *Flight to Objectivity*; Grosz, "Refiguring Bodies," 3–24.
13. Rodgers and Chase, "Mothers, Sexuality, and Eros," 115–134.
14. Ibid.
15. See Mulford, this volume, for a detailed discussion of mothers' roles.
16. Lengermann and Neibrugge-Brantley, "Contemporary Feminist Theory," 307–355.
17. Galtry, "Suckling and Silence," 1–23; Smith and Ingraham, "Mother's Milk," 41–62.
18. Allen, "Rethinking Power," 21–41.
19. Arendt, *On Violence*, 44.
20. Weimer, "Summary of State Breastfeeding Laws."
21. National Conference of State Legislatures, "Breastfeeding Laws."
22. Ibid.
23. See Fraley, "Booby Juice"; Regales, "Nursing at Starbucks"; Kang, "Mothers Rally," D1; Birth without Borders, "Breastfeeding Supporters."
24. Harmon, "Lactivists Taking Their Cause."
25. Regales, "Nursing at Starbucks."
26. Ibid.; Maher, "Bill Maher on Breastfeeding."
27. "Writer Doesn't Want."
28. *San Jose Mercury News,* "Protests Mount."
29. Weimer, "Summary of State Breastfeeding Laws," 6–7.
30. Female Intelligence Agency, "Breastfeeding in Public."
31. Forbes and Rigg, "Mission."
32. Ibid.
33. Ibid.

Chapter 23

Intersections

Child Sexual Abuse and Breastfeeding

At the 2010 Breastfeeding and Feminism Symposium, I asked the attending feminist scholars, activists, and clinicians, "How many of you practice with the assumption that mothers who were sexually abused as children will be difficult patients, for whom the best therapy is likely to give 'permission' to not breastfeed?" Not surprisingly, nearly all the clinicians in the room indicated that this was the case. I then argued, as I do in this chapter, that these assumptions are not based in fact. We can learn from women about the complex relationship between child sexual abuse (CSA) and breastfeeding, which includes opportunities for healing and empowerment, as well as struggle.

The belief that mothers with a history of childhood sexual abuse may be vulnerable while breastfeeding is based in more general research that found CSA survivors experience certain challenges more frequently than women who were not abused. These challenges include traumatic memory triggers, avoidance, dissociation, low interdependency, decreased self-efficacy, self-distain, and vulnerability to messaging from health care institutions and corporations.[1] However, there has been only one published study investigating the effect of CSA survivorship on women's breastfeeding experiences, which found that mothers who experienced CSA are 2.5 times as likely to breastfeed their children as women who do not report having been sexually abused.[2] The research presented in this chapter can help us understand how CSA may impact breastfeeding experiences. I highlight mothers' own representations of their experiences in order to model the feminist practice of *listening to women* and privileging their direct commentary on their struggles and solutions.

Child Sexual Abuse, Feminism, and Public Health

One in four girls in the United States report having been sexually abused before their eighteenth birthday, and millions more may endure this trauma and never disclose at all.[3] Rates of child sexual abuse continue to rise, as do attempts to quantify the violence so commonly inflicted upon girls in the United States.[4] Despite the epidemic prevalence of CSA, most existing treatment and prevention frameworks are highly individualized and private.[5]

Since the 1960s, feminists have called upon women and girls to "break the silence" that enshrouds their experiences with childhood sexual abuse.[6] Speaking out, feminists contend, will empower the speakers and increase potential for healing. Speaking out is also intended to raise community consciousness of the issue.[7] Consciousness-raising is a fundamental feminist approach to motivating social change, but it cannot achieve this objective until oppositional *actions* are in effect.

Public health professionals are ideally suited to take action by helping to situate this epidemic within our models of population-level (primary, secondary, and tertiary) prevention. Public health has a responsibility to respond to epidemics, and often does so by creating and supporting social change. To date, public health has responded to CSA by characterizing the population of victims and articulating some of the risk factors for CSA and its outcomes.[8] We can move toward fulfilling the public health responsibility by implementing three fundamental feminist ideals: listening to women, politicizing their stories, and complementing theory with practice.

Survivor Mothers and Breastfeeding

In this chapter, I present direct quotations from a qualitative, exploratory study I conducted in winter 2010. Women were recruited via informal social networks and wrote about their experiences with CSA and breastfeeding in a structured, open-ended questionnaire. The ten themes that emerged stand alone but also intersect, reflecting survivor mothers' propensity to persevere through adversity to success. The primary themes identified include strong intention to breastfeed, difficulty in getting started, fear of becoming perverted, being triggered during feedings, dissociation during feedings, public breastfeeding evoking shame response and inciting a familiar cycle of feeling abused, determination, therapeutic processes, globalized sense of healing and empowerment, and reclamation of self.

Strong Intention to Breastfeed

Supporting Prentice et al.'s finding about high breastfeeding initiation rates, 89 percent of respondents to this qualitative study asserted strong intentions to breastfeed, saying specifically that it seemed "integral to pregnancy," and "natural," and that they "never doubted" this choice both before and after giving birth. One woman wrote, "There was never any doubt in my mind that I wanted to breastfeed, despite how nervous I was that I would be able to be comfortable doing it. . . . It was a choice very opposite of what I was taught and what my experiences would have dictated, but I was determined to do it. I knew that it was the right thing for my baby, and I was not going to let my abuser take that away from my child."

Significant Difficulty Getting Started

While the female body is designed to breastfeed following childbirth, the early days of feeding are marked by a steep learning curve for most mothers.[9] For some women in this study, birth activates a sense of powerlessness that they associate with their abuse. Survivor mothers suggest that this association may make getting started with breastfeeding difficult:

> First of all, I was re-traumatized by giving birth, especially in a hospital where I did not feel safe. This state of feeling like you have to fight for your very own survival is a difficult place from which to begin caring for someone so helpless. Fighting through the trials of early breastfeeding, engorgement, improper latch, I struggled to stay present and keep from dissociating or being triggered. I remember several times that while trying to endure the pain of nursing my son, I suddenly had to remove him quickly and plop him on the bed away from me. We would both be screaming when my husband came running into the room. But what could he do? What could anyone do?
>
> It was a nightmare to breastfeed my son and I had no support getting started. I managed to tough through it because I believed in it so strongly, but it was hard. I had [postpartum depression] and [post-traumatic stress disorder] from a traumatic cesarean birth (that I later learned was unnecessary) and post partum period. I left the hospital with bleeding nipples and my son was diagnosed as failure to thrive.

Public Breastfeeding Evoking Shame Response and Inciting a Familiar Cycle of Abuse

Breastfeeding scholars from various fields have long noted the sexualization of breasts as a barrier to breastfeeding in the United States, especially when doing so in public spaces. It follows that a survivor of CSA may feel acute discomfort with breastfeeding in public. This seems to be the case for many survivor mothers: "I was told on a couple occasions to not publically breastfeed, and my immediate reaction was shame.... I was really angry, knew I had been wronged, but had walked away in silence . . . quite similar to the abuse cycle I went through."

Others suggested that their experience as survivors fortified their convictions that they would not allow negative responses to their public breastfeeding to shame them:

> I almost think that the abuse has helped me realize that I never have to be under somebody's control. I am a breastfeeding advocate and nurse in public openly. I am deathly tired of the pornographizing of women's breasts. Why should I cover my breast? My son is eating. It is not my problem that some people have a problem of sexualizing everything. And that is directly from my abuse. Everything I did, every move I made was perverted in my dad's eyes. He felt that everything I did beckoned sexual attention. Breastfeeding is a way to feed a baby, and I will not let somebody sexualize the most innocent event.

Fear of Becoming Perverted

The response to breastfeeding in public is complicated by the frequently referenced fear of either becoming perverted or being perceived as such:

> I have also worried that if someone found out that I was molested and now breastfeeding that they would think that I was a pervert about it by proxy or something. Like my abuse was contagious because no one has ever talked about abuse and breastfeeding to me.
>
> It wasn't my own internal feelings however that convinced me to give up after only two weeks, it was the rest of the world's disapproval of breastfeeding, which reinforced this false feeling of breastfeeding being wrong and sexual. It was through my own perseverance that with subsequent children, I was able to overcome that feeling, and my ability to nourish and nurture my children became a most significant source of empowerment. Neither I nor my breasts were dirty, or disgusting, or solely for sexual purposes.

In addition, survivors of CSA (especially when perpetrated by a parent) often report fears that they will be bad parents, with the worst possible scenario of becoming a predator. While becoming a perpetrator is rare in sexual abuse survivors, especially females, it is common for survivor mothers to overprotect or dissociate from (neglect) their children, which may result from a fear of crossing the line between intimacy to inappropriate behavior.[10] Some women reported feeling that breastfeeding is inappropriate because the infant is unable to consent or even be offered a conscious choice.[11]

> I didn't realize breastfeeding activates chemical processes all over your body that you may have been repressing all of these years because any rushing of oxytocin and adrenaline feels similar to the panic and unwanted arousal that happens with molestation. I have heard, and also felt like, "if I feel this way, does it mean I am a predator?" and the answer is, no, it doesn't mean that. . . . I remember feeling just "aroused" all over my body, like, tingly everywhere, and feeling my face get hot, and feeling angry about it, and feeling angry with my baby because I was so uncomfortable, and sad. I felt like such a weirdo, and so gross.

> The whole idea of having a little person suck on my breasts was very disconcerting—especially because we are culturally trained to view breasts as sexual objects and not as feeding devices. It was also disconcerting because in my relationship with my husband, my breasts are used in sexual stimulation. So I imagine I pondered the same questions that other moms do: Will I feel aroused? Will I think about sex? (and for someone with a history of sexual abuse, I wondered if I thought about sex if I would in any way start to go down that road of sexual abuse either in thoughts or actions).

Becoming Triggered during Feedings

Challenges unique to CSA survivors may lead to premature cessation (as defined clinically and according to mothers' intentions).[12] Perhaps the most commonly noted cause of premature cessation is "triggering" (flashbacks and other reminders of their abuse). This may occur with the sensation of suckling (especially when abuse occurred during or after breast development), playful feeding of older infants and younger children, nighttime feeding, or cluster feedings when mothers commonly report feeling "touched out."

> Physical sensations at night were very triggering, and I remember sometimes feeling very alone and scared. Those nights brought up some of the most intense feelings I've ever had about being sexually abused. I felt like the difficulty with breastfeeding did impact my ability to feel close to and bonded with my first born; I felt very numb. After I quit, we established a closer relationship. With my second child, I felt clearer about what was happening, but too ashamed to talk about it. . . . After talking to a friend who also had some difficulty with nursing at night

(she was sexually abused as a child, too) I decided that nighttime was too triggering. We made the decision to supplement, and by six months, I was done breastfeeding.

Nearly one in four lactating women report sexual arousal during breastfeeding, but for survivor mothers this fairly normal occurrence may feel particularly threatening.[13]

> Around 14 months with each of my kids, my baby hormones were fading and my period was coming back. I was feeling more like a sexual being, and the sensations of nursing were very disturbing then. I had a lot of flashbacks . . . I [breastfed] for 21, 18, and 23 months, just putting up with it, but eventually those feelings would overcome my intentions. I feel good about what I did give my kids, but I always wished I could have done child-led weaning. I just couldn't.
>
> I remember being alone in the house with my son and I had the strongest urge to give him everything that I could. At the same time, the stimulation (baby suckling) of breastfeeding felt totally triggering. There were times when I felt like I was being molested all over again. The long feedings or strong suckling were hard at first. Very quickly, I decided that something had to change if I was going to give the gift of breastfeeding to my baby. This may sound strange, but I did a kind of meditation and prayer where I left my body for a time.

Many women in this study mentioned that they breastfed despite triggers with the support and advice of other survivor mothers. Common coping mechanisms included ending feedings early, limiting touching of infant hands, night weaning, feeding expressed milk, and distracting themselves.

Dissociation during Feedings

Avoidance and dissociation are common long-term effects of CSA and have been noted to be "at the heart of serious sequelae."[14] Dissociation is thought to be a learned coping mechanism children use to separate themselves from the ongoing trauma. Many survivor mothers report higher levels of intimate parenting anxiety than women who were not abused, and say they use dissociation to endure related discomfort.[15] Many report working actively on "remaining present" (not dissociating) in order to create healthy, meaningful relationships with their children.

> I think, looking back from a very different altitude now, that I was unaware of most of the physical sensations of breastfeeding. It was

something I endured for the sake of a healthy baby. I didn't like thinking of the physical sensations because I had had to numb myself so significantly for years and years. To wake up to those sensations would be to unlock Pandora's box of body-feelings. Like pregnancy, I approached it all very mechanically, keeping my reason and logic and problem-solving and planning mind in the forefront. . . . It's the numbing that kept me from being present for breastfeeding with both children. The numbing is how I'd coped for years, and breastfeeding came closer than anything to breaking through it. But in the end, I kept the wall up and didn't register what my body was doing. But I still remember their eyes looking up at me, and their fingers grabbing their toes as they nursed, a leg perched high in the air, a milky smile forming around the nipple. There are a few images of them in my mind like that. Treasures.

Determination

Lactation consultants and other health professionals report having been taught that the CSA survivor will often present as the mom who refuses to breastfeed or whines over small struggles, takes up more than their share of our precious professional time, fail to do what they are told to resolve their breastfeeding issues, and whose pain is not real but rather psychosomatic. This representation has not been demonstrated in any study to date, and perpetuating it is unlikely to be productive in supporting mothers. It is possible that breastfeeding supporters are seeing some of the determination, self-reliance, and discomfort with interpersonal power-differentials that many survivor mothers speak about.

> [Breastfeeding] was a nightmare due to my birthrape and forced section. We struggled for months because of it. I finally was able after 4 months of frustrations, pain and determination to BF for 2 years. . . . In my case and due to my hatred of most in the medical community, I was more determined to BF. I was going to do it in spite of them.
>
> I ignored the barriers and breastfed anywhere and everywhere. I learned to ignore authority as part of my upbringing and survival. I also learned to be defiant about my wants and desires as part of my upbringing; breastfeeding became part of that.

Rather than interpreting such expressions as "being difficult," we can learn valuable lessons by listening and responding accordingly. In these quotations, I read the potential for re-victimization *or* healing. This potential is an overwhelming, even intimidating, force that may compel survivor mothers to present to providers with unyielding, sometimes rebellious, determination to breastfeed. Or survivor mothers may appear noncompliant with providers' instructions due to a sense of self-sacrifice for their babies (for example, ignoring breast damage due to poor latch in order to meet a baby's needs), discomfort with providers, or reflexive rebellion against the perceived control of a person in a position of power.

Therapy

CSA survivors often embark on a formal therapeutic process to heal from their trauma and prevent unhealthy, lifelong sequelae of their abuse. This process typically involves resolving emotional consequences (powerlessness, shame, distrust), building healthy interpersonal relationships, and grieving the experience of abuse. In essence, the therapeutic ideal is to shift from victim to survivor, a goal which many women feel they are able to achieve. In this study, therapy is commonly referenced as a key facilitator of breastfeeding initiation, as well as satisfaction and self-awareness in the mothering role:

> It wasn't until I started to seek therapy as a young mom in my early 20s that I realized . . . that the way I felt about my body, my right to privacy, my sexuality, everything, came from that mixture of total fear, and being so uncomfortable, and sad, and feeling so, so, gross. Nothing about my body or sexuality was comfortable to me, I just was so ambivalent, like, I had to prove my body was mine, and I could choose what I wanted for it, and so I chose to be slutty, and pierce and cut myself, just to prove it was mine. Then, when my son was born, I had to prove he was mine, too, and that I could care for him with NO help. If I had been able to, I think I'd have given birth in the woods, just to prove I didn't need anyone or anything to validate me.

Healing and Empowerment

Empowerment is a shared goal of feminist and public health work, known to aid in the healing process and promote wellness for women and, consequently, children, families, and communities. The violence and betrayal of trust involved in CSA often leaves victims feeling disempowered and struggling with issues of power, control, and personal boundaries. Many women expressed their belief that breastfeeding was an opportunity to heal and regain power lost in their victimization: "I actually felt empowered by breastfeeding. I felt like I was taking back my breasts from all the perverts. That I was using them for what they were meant for, and that all those men were crazy and I am fine. Breastfeeding my firstborn changed my life, it empowered me in a way that allowed me to start a business, write several books, raise my children the way I believed was right, re-negotiate the power structure of my marriage, which not only survived but became happier."

Reclamation

Extensive research demonstrates the high prevalence and long-term impact of several consequences of CSA, including risk of self-harm, self-disdain, low interdependency, and low self-efficacy.[16] Feminist scholars note potential for reclamation of self-worth and possession of one's own body through childbirth and breastfeeding with minimal technologic intervention.[17] Survivors are sometimes aware of this potential prior to pregnancy and birth, which may explain some of their strong intentions to breastfeed: "I think as a result of my very dysfunctional family, I decided long before I had children that I would be the very best mother I could be and that my children would come first. I always knew I would breastfeed. I was a little concerned about how it might make me feel, but I once heard someone say that birthing a baby as naturally as possible and breastfeeding were ways to reclaim your body, I felt strongly that this would be true for me. It was a way to take back my body and for it to do what it was meant to do."

Having experienced extremely violent sexual abuse by a trusted family member consistently from ages four to fifteen, and having breastfed all four of her children, one mother had this to offer about the power of breastfeeding toward reclaiming a body and sense of self previously marked by victimization:

> I think [having been abused] made me more committed [to breastfeeding]. Breastfeeding was me taking back my body. It was something only I controlled. It was sacred, an expression of the fact that I am NOT damaged, that I can love, and nurture and give life, that my body can bring me and my child something besides pain. It makes me feel valuable, worthwhile, deserving. It has helped me to love and bless myself. It helped me to believe that I could succeed at something worthwhile. It made me love my breasts, that before I had hated because my [abuser] watched them as they grew in and commented on them constantly. He owned them, and even other men owned them, until I gave them to my child, and now they belong to me! . . . The peace and quiet contentment that I feel while nursing my child is a gift of healing and joy that the Goddess has given me. . . . And I know that it is right; I'm not doing something shameful. It is, in a way, the first time and way that I really

felt clean, pure. I felt like an expression of the Goddess herself, blessed, worthy, whereas before I had always felt like a worthless dirty slut. My milk washed me clean.

Conclusion

In the United States, victims of child sexual abuse most frequently find support from private therapists, detectives, social workers, and support groups. By binding their stories in confidential contexts, we may perpetuate the secretive nature of the experience. With this limitation, the feminist ideal of achieving consciousness raising through speaking out falls flat. All too often, public discourse on child sexual abuse (and breastfeeding, too) is promulgated through experts and professionals. With respect to CSA, the discourse often seems sterile, watered down with numbers and scientific terminology that fail to convey the experience of survivors—both the damage and their wisdom. If we can manage to blend these two powerful voices, to incorporate survivor mothers' voices into expert discourse about the epidemic of child sexual abuse, we may have greater ability to politicize, publicize, and change the problem.

In this chapter, I present direct quotations to demonstrate the complexity and diversity of women's experiences. The stories are characterized by "survivor discourse": the speakers reference empowerment, healing, transformation, and other concepts from self-help and psychosocial therapy.[18] By integrating their discourse into a complex collective voice, I hope to clarify the opportunities and challenges for breastfeeding inherent in their stories and contribute to survivor-centered practices for feminist health care workers involved with breastfeeding programs or primary support.

Survivor mothers who breastfeed may face particular challenges and should be commended on finding whatever balance helps them to feel safe and continue breastfeeding. Still, some of these coping mechanisms (especially night weaning and exclusively feeding expressed milk) lead to premature cessation and other suboptimal health outcomes. When premature cessation is perceived as yet another failure of the body and self, or even as a symbol of continued enslavement to one's abuser, survivor mothers may experience additional trauma. Survivor mothers need and deserve to have their needs and boundaries honored in order to heal.

Many people require reassurance that they are capable of being healthy, positive parents. For survivors, this reassurance may be paramount given their unique fears and the potential for healing. And yet, with our most common assumptions and efforts to support survivor mothers, we risk reinforcing the belief that they are incapable. The stories presented here demonstrate how child sexual abuse survivors may have the potential for tremendous vulnerability, but also for resilience and empowerment. Breastfeeding may play a vital role in helping women redefine and normalize their embodied experiences. We must set aside our assumptions about this population and embrace the idea that many survivor mothers want to breastfeed and will work hard to make that happen.

Notes

1. Spataro et al., "Impact of Child Sexual Abuse"; Martin et al., "Sexual Abuse and Suicidality"; Ohene et al., "Sexual Abuse History"; Noll et al., "Sleep Disturbances"; Bergen et al., "Sexual Abuse"; Noll, Trickett, and Putnam, "Prospective Investigation."
2. Prentice et al., "Association."
3. U.S. Department of Health and Human Services, Centers for Disease Control and Prevention, "Adverse Childhood Experiences."
4. Ibid.
5. Naples, "Deconstructing and Locating."
6. Dobash and Dobash, *Rethinking Violence*; Profitt, *Women Survivors*.
7. Gerson and Peiss, "Boundaries."
8. Sedlak et al., *Fourth National*.
9. Blum, *At the Breast*.
10. Kendall-Tackett, "Breastfeeding and the Sexual."
11. Weichert, "Sexual Arousal," 99.
12. Prentice et al., "Association."
13. Weichert, "Sexual Arousal," 99.
14. Klingelhafer, "Sexual Abuse and Breastfeeding."
15. Douglas, "Reported Anxieties."
16. U.S. Department of Health and Human Services, Centers for Disease Control and Prevention, "Adverse Childhood Experiences"; Naples, "Deconstructing and Locating;" Gerson and Peiss, "Boundaries"; Sedlak et al., *Fourth National*.
17. Simkin, *When Survivors Give Birth*.
18. Survivor discourse uses the term "survivor mothers," and I use that phrase here, as opposed to "victims of CSA"; Naples, "Deconstructing and Locating."

**Paige Hall Smith, Bernice L. Hausman,
and Miriam Labbok**

Conclusion

Beyond Health, Beyond Choice:
New Ways Forward in Public Health

The collected chapters in this work make it clear that pushing women to breastfeed for health reasons alone is a weak strategy. Such encouragement does not address the complexity of decision making that is created by the constraints and realities of women's lives. In continuing to discuss breastfeeding as a *choice*, we fail to appreciate that most women do not have a source of unbiased information, or the economic, social, and clinical support and resources needed to freely choose whether or not they will breastfeed beyond the first few weeks of their babies' lives. In and of itself, this is not news. Nevertheless, the injunction to mothers to breastfeed because "breast is best" or because it is good for baby's health are the default messages that leave public health workers, clinicians, and mothers frustrated. This volume presents the argument that the way forward involves a more concerted focus on reducing the constraints in women's lives formed by gender inequalities in institutions (including health care), labor, power, and sexuality.

Today most women are physically separated from their babies shortly after birth and are not offered economic, social, or even emotional support for being together, let alone for breastfeeding. Yet much of the health promotion discourse enjoins women to breastfeed (since that is what "good mothers" do), making infant feeding a moral minefield that has the potential to undermine not only breastfeeding but also women in their roles as mothers and as paid laborers. Political, economic, and social constraints undermine women's choices by creating and sustaining structural forces outside their individual control. Indeed, if those opposed to women's equality had schemed to devise a socioeconomic and political milieu to undermine breastfeeding, they might have devised the environment that most women in the United States find themselves in today.

This volume argues that unless we refocus attention on how women experience breastfeeding, motherhood, and their own lives, and use these experiences to create and support new public policy, health promotion, and clinical services, breastfeeding rates and practices in this country will not improve. Indeed, the backlash by both feminists and others against breastfeeding that is created by lack of attention to such constraints further suggests that initiation and continuation rates may decline, because, in the current situation, breastfeeding often exacerbates tensions that continue to plague mothers seeking to integrate their multiple roles into one whole life.

Lactation is a biological capacity of female mammals that, in humans, is often associated with traditional gender roles and exclusive maternity. Some could, and have, argued that it is precisely the changing roles of women— changes that lead women toward employment and away from full-time mothering—that are the cause of limited breastfeeding. Such critics might further argue that women do not want to breastfeed, and public health efforts to promote it are flying in the face of women's new roles and, perhaps, indirectly seeking to reengage women in a full-time, sometimes constraining motherhood role.

We see lactation and breastfeeding as different phenomena. While lactation is the biological action of milk production, breastfeeding also involves a social practice and a skill. Historically, breastfeeding was normative in human communities, practiced by most parturient women (mothers), as well as by other women who cared for both their own and other children. As a social practice, breastfeeding is affected by the social norms, values, expectations, and standards held for mothers, paid workers, children, and social institutions. Infant feeding decisions are affected not just by women's preferences for feeding or how they want to use their bodies, but also by the support they receive for breastfeeding or formula-feeding, as well as for the full range of their multiple roles as mothers, workers, and individuals. Our analysis demonstrates that women receive very little support for their mothering practices in general, let alone for breastfeeding. This lack of support for mothers is compounded by the extraordinary forces (both material and ideological) working against successful breastfeeding. The sociocultural, economic, and institutional forces that work against the biology of breastfeeding astonish us, and we have to ask why that is so.

There are potentially numerous answers to this question, and we put forward two that represent overarching themes that emerge from the chapters in this book. The first is that women's breastfeeding patterns are adversely affected not by women's paid employment per se, but by their continued lower, relative to men, economic, social, and political status. Essentially, women who have less power and control over their bodies and their social environments use more formula. This finding interweaves with a second key theme: although health messages may assert that formula use has risks, for many women breastfeeding is the riskier and more costly option. Messaging about the benefits of breastfeeding is based on a medical conceptualization of risk. Women tend to experience the risks of breastfeeding as social, and sometimes personal, risks to their well-being as workers, wives, mothers, and members of diverse communities. Hence, for most women the risks of breastfeeding are *social risks*, and feminist analysis is necessary to uncover and investigate them.

Several authors in the book describe, both theoretically and empirically, how low status is implicated in less than optimal rates of breastfeeding initiation and very short durations of breastfeeding. The low status of women is reinforced by the pervasiveness of gender-based personal and structural violence, the sexualization of women's bodies and their breasts as objects of male desire, and by continued gender inequities in labor, power, and social relationships. For minority women, racism further contributes to low status. The continued rigidity of gender roles results in a society-wide failure to support mothers regardless of whether or not they combine motherhood with paid employment. We fail to support caregivers for their labor and devalue their contributions, but at the same time we fail to support the employed mothers' needs for maternity leave, flex time, child care, and workplace breastfeeding support. In addition, the use of women's bodies and breasts to sell all manner of goods and services reinforces the belief that, as Germaine Greer puts it, "a husband takes precedence over his children in enjoying access to his wife's body." Essentially, women's bodies are still not fully their own to control. Society is pervaded by a powerful ambiguity about what women and mothers *should* do. The ambiguity leaves women psychologically and socially vulnerable to fickle messages about what "good mothers" do, justifies a labor force that continues to be organized about the needs that "ideal" men have historically required, and provides space for socially conservative voices to paint government support for breastfeeding as coercive governmental intrusion into the private domain.

These constraints to gender equity increase the social risks and the direct, indirect, and opportunity costs of breastfeeding. Breastfeeding women risk being vulnerable to unwanted sexual attention, are asked to leave public space, and are judged less competent or worthy as paid workers. The direct costs of breastfeeding increase because many women need to buy high quality pumps to sustain a good milk supply for exclusive breast milk feeding. Since many workplace and community settings make it difficult or uncomfortable for women to breastfeed in those spaces, pumping is becoming the default method by which both employed and nonemployed mothers navigate breastfeeding constraints and realities. Health care professionals, including lactation consultants, also increase the cost of breastfeeding both indirectly and directly. Indirect costs stem from failure of physicians and nurses to learn and follow through with established best practices in lactation management and breast-feeding education, a failure that leads to reduced milk supply, pain, and difficulty managing breastfeeding. Direct costs include hiring professional lactation support and other health care visits women need to help them manage problems that stem from inadequate medical care and health educa-tion. In addition, as several authors point out, the values and commercial interests of formula companies interweave with health care responses to infant feeding in ways that privilege both medical authority and commercial interests over the public's health. However, public health discourse in industrialized countries does not systematically address these issues.

The decision concerning method of infant feeding is one, but only one, of the choices mothers face as they decide how much of their own time they can invest in their children and how much they want to allocate to paid labor, partners, family, friends, and their own leisure. Women have the option to breastfeed, to express milk and have a caretaker give it to the baby in a bottle, to use formula, or to use some combination of these methods. With manufactured infant formulas readily available, breastfeeding may well be seen as an optional investment by mothers as they seek to achieve money and status in a workplace that is still designed around the norm of a male worker with a wife at home, especially when such mothers must manage their domestic and child care responsibilities with limited help. Employed mothers must also mediate the demands of lactation as a physiological process with the demands of work in public settings.

Since the problem of breastfeeding is not located in women's bodies but in political, economic, and social structures that shape women's practices and experiences, solutions must also reside in those contexts. We need to work toward the creation of environments that enhance the ability of women to function as free and equal people, supported and valued for the ways they choose to express their reproductive and productive capabilities. Breastfeeding "success or failure" should move away from being a normative judgment of maternal goodness or moral strength and toward being a gauge for evaluating social support and equality for mothers.

In our vision of a society in which the needs of mothers are taken seriously and breastfeeding capacity is a measure of social equality, there must be broad-based societal support for breastfeeding. Such social and civic support will only emerge when interests merge and partnering of concerns takes place. For working mothers to be able to calibrate their bodies in relation to the bodies of their babies, they must have more control over their work environment, flexibility in their working hours and conditions, and control over domestic resources. This scenario requires that mothers be near their babies or, if working away, have access to milk expression technologies that meet their needs. In public spaces, mothers and babies must be accepted as free citizens with rights to feed as needed, without censure based on discriminatory perceptions of women's bodies as men's possessions. Such freedom means both legal rights for women who choose to breastfeed openly, as well as other spaces set aside for nursing mothers who need more privacy to accommodate their babies' needs. To achieve these rights, we must seek and find the partners in all sectors who would join in this struggle.

The chapters in this volume raise awareness of a wide variety of gender inequities, social risks, public interests, and real costs associated with breast-feeding. Our hope is that public health and breastfeeding researchers, advocates, practitioners, and policy makers, and feminists in all these fields will engage with the perspectives and experiences of women presented here to pave a new way forward in the protection, promotion, and support of breastfeeding mothers. Public policy must emerge from this effort as well. There are a number of recent actions in the United States that are encouraging: the 2010 Patient Protection and Affordable Care Act P.L. 111-148 requires employers to provide a decent place and reasonable break time for women to express milk. In addition, the 2011 *Surgeon General's Call to Action to Support Breastfeeding* underscores the need for everyone—families, friends, communities, clinicians, health care leaders, employers, and policy makers—to help make breastfeeding easy. These recent federal actions, alongside the messages and ideas presented in pages of this book, suggest that an important part of the way forward is to recognize both the value of breastfeeding for the public's health *and* the important contributions that women make to human communities.

Bibliography

Abbett, Mandy. "Expressing." *A Mother's (and Others) Guide to Breastfeeding* 8 (2008): 20–22. http://www.mothersguide.co.uk/mothersguidesample.pdf.

Abbott, Stephen, Mary J. Renfrew, and Alison McFadden. "'Informal' Learning to Support Breastfeeding: Local Problems and Opportunities." *Maternal and Child Nutrition* 2 (2006): 232–238.

Abt, Isaac A. *Baby Doctor.* New York: McGraw-Hill Book Co., 1944.

Acker, Joan. "Hierarchies, Jobs, Bodies: A Theory of Gendered Organizations." *Gender and Society* 4, no. 2 (1990): 139–158.

Advertisement for Similac Early Shield Advance Infant Formula. *People*, September 2008.

Agency for Healthcare Research and Quality. "Guide to Clinical Preventive Services, 2010–2011." AHRQ Publication No. 10–05145. Rockville, MD: Agency for Healthcare Research and Quality, 2010. http://www.ahrq.gov/clinic/pocketgd.htm.

Ahluwalia, Indu B., Brian Morrow, and Jason Hsia. "Why Do Women Stop Breastfeeding? Findings from the Pregnancy Risk Assessment and Monitoring System." *Pediatrics* 116 (2005): 1408–1409.

Albanesi, Stefania, and Claudia Olivetti. "Gender Roles and Medical Progress." Working Paper 14873. Cambridge, MA: National Bureau of Economic Research, 2009.

Alcabes, Philip. "Epidemiologists Need to Shatter the Myth of a Risk-Free Life." *Chronicle of Higher Education* 49, no. 37 (2003): B11–12.

Allen, Ann. "Rethinking Power: Feminists and Power." *Hypatia* 13, no. 1 (1998): 21–41.

Alliance for Work-Life Progress. "About National Work and Family Month." *Work and Life.* WorldatWork, 2008. http://www.awlp.org/awlp/nwfm/nwfm-history.jsp.

All You Can Read. "Top 10 Parenting Magazines." *All You Can Read.* http://www.allyoucanread.com/magazines/.

Altorki, Soraya. "Milk-Kinship in Arab Society: An Unexplored Problem in the Ethnography of Marriage." *Ethnology* 19, no. 2 (1980): 233–244.

American Academy of Pediatrics. "Policy Statement: Breastfeeding and the Use of Human Milk." *Pediatrics* 115, no. 2 (2005): 496–506.

American Academy of Pediatrics Work Group on Breastfeeding. "Breastfeeding and the Use of Human Milk." *Pediatrics* 100, no. 6 (1997): 1035–1039.

American College of Obstetricians and Gynecologists. "Trends in Out-of-Hospital Births." In *Manpower Planning in Obstetrics and Gynecology.* Washington: American College of Obstetricians and Gynecologists, 1991.

American Psychological Association. "Task Force on the Sexualization of Girls." *Report of the APA Task Force on the Sexualization of Girls.* Washington, DC: American Psychological Association, 2007.

Amin, Sarah. "A Brief History of the Breastfeeding Movement." In *The Breastfeeding Movement: A Sourcebook*, edited by Lakshmi Menon, Anwar Fazal, Sarah Amin, and Susan Siew, 1–21. Penang, Malaysia: World Alliance for Breastfeeding Action, 2003.

Anderson, Erin, and Elizabeth Geden. "Nurses' Knowledge of Breastfeeding." *Journal of Obstetrical Gynecologic, and Neonatal Nursing* 20 (1990): 58–64.

Bibliography

288

Andrist, Linda C., Raquel D. Arias, Deborah Nucatola, Andrew Kaunitz, Lynn B. Mussleman, Suzanne Reiter, Jennifer Boulanger, Linda Dominguez, and Steven Emmert. "Women's and Providers' Attitudes towards Menstrual Suppression with Extended Use of Oral Contraceptives." *Contraception* 70 (2004): 359–363.

Andrist, Linda C., Alex Hoyt, Dawn Weinstein, and Chris McGibbon. "The Need to Bleed: Women's Attitudes and Beliefs about Menstrual Suppression." *Journal of the American Academy of Nurse Practitioners* 16, no. 1 (2004): 31–37.

Andsager, Julie L., and Angela Powers. "Framing Women's Health with a Sense-Making Approach: Magazine Coverage of Breast Cancer and Implants." *Health Communication* 13, no. 2 (2001): 163–185.

Anonymous. "Question: How Do I Handle My Feelings of Failure for Not Breastfeeding?" *Mom Answers.* Babycenter, August 24, 2004. http://www.babycenter.com/400_how-do-i-handle-my-feelings-of-failure-for-not-breastfeeding_500721_1001.bc.

———. "Question: How Do I Handle My Feelings of Failure for Not Breastfeeding?" *Mom Answers.* Babycenter, October 9, 2006. http://www.babycenter.com/400_how-do-i-handle-my-feelings-of-failure-for-not-breastfeeding_500721_1001.bc.

Apple, Rima D. "'To Be Used Only under the Direction of a Physician': Commercial Infant Feeding and Medical Practice, 1870–1940." *Bulletin of the History of Medicine* 54 (1980): 402–417.

———. "The Medicalization of Infant Feeding in the United States and New Zealand: Two Countries, One Experience." *Journal of Human Lactation* 10, no. 1 (1994): 31–37.

———. *Mothers and Medicine: A Social History of Infant Feeding, 1890–1950.* Madison: University of Wisconsin Press, 1987.

———. *Perfect Motherhood: Science and Childrearing in America.* New Brunswick, NJ: Rutgers University Press, 2006.

"Approved Residencies and Fellowships for Veteran and Civilian Physicians." *Journal of the American Medical Association* 131 (August 17, 1946): 1322–1354.

Arendt, Hannah. *On Violence.* New York: Harcourt Brace, 1968.

Armstrong, Helen C. "Breastfeeding as the Foundation of Care." *Food and Nutrition Bulletin* 16, no. 4 (1995): 299–312.

Arney, William Ray. *Power and the Profession of Obstetrics.* Chicago: University of Chicago Press, 1982.

Arnold, Lois D. W. "Becoming a Donor to a Human Milk Bank." *Leaven* 36, no. 2 (April–May 2000): 19–23. http://www.llli.org//llleaderweb/LV/LVAprMay00p19.html.

Arnold, Sandra. Telephone interview by Linda Fentiman. July 31, 2007.

Arora, Samir, Cheryl McJunkin, Julie Wehrer, and Phyllis Kuhn. "Major Factors Influencing Breastfeeding Rates: Mother's Perception of Father's Attitude and Milk Supply." *Pediatrics* 106, no. 5 (2000): 67.

Artis, Julie. "Breastfeed at Your Own Risk." *Contexts* 8, no. 40 (2009). http://contexts.org/articles/fall-2009/breastfeed-at-you-own-risk/.

Attree, Pamela. "Low-Income Mothers, Nutrition and Health: A Systematic Review of Qualitative Evidence." *Maternal and Child Nutrition* 1, no. 4 (2005): 227–240.

Auerbach, Kathleen G. "The Role of the Nurse in Support of Breast Feeding." *Journal of Advanced Nursing* 4, no. 3 (1979): 263–285.

Austin, Marsha. "Sides Clash over Putting Price on Mothers' Milk." *Denver Post*, March 26, 2006, sec. A.

Avishai, Orit. "Managing the Lactating Body: The Breast-Feeding Project and Privileged Motherhood." *Qualitative Sociology* 30 (2007): 135–152.

"Baby Food—US." *Euromonitor International,* October 2008. Database, Pace University Law Library.

Badinter, Elisabeth. *Le Conflit: La Femme et la Mère.* Paris: Flammarion, 2010.

Baer, Edward. "Promoting Breastfeeding: A National Responsibility." *Studies in Family Planning* 12, no. 4 (1981): 198–206.

Bailey, Doraine. "ILCA: 20 Years of Building a Profession." *Journal of Human Lactation* 21, no. 3 (2005): 239–242.

Bailyn, Lotte. *Breaking the Mold: Women, Men and Their Time in the New Corporate World.* New York: Free Press, 1993.

Bainbridge, Jay, Marcia K. Meyers, and Jane Waldfogel. "Child Care Policy Reform and Employment of Single Mothers." *Social Science Quarterly* 84, no. 4 (2003): 771–791.

Bandyopadhyay, Mridula. "Impact of Ritual Pollution on Lactation and Breastfeeding Practices in Rural West Bengal, India." *International Breastfeeding Journal* 4 (2009). http://www.internationalbreastfeedingjournal.com/content/4/1/2.

Baranowski, Tom, David E. Bee, David K. Rassin, C. Joan Richardson, Judy P. Brown, Nancy Guenther, and Philip R. Nader. "Social Support, Social Influence, Ethnicity and the Breastfeeding Decision." *Social Science Medicine* 17, no. 21 (1983): 1599–1611.

Barclay, Linda, and Deborah Lupton. "The Experience of New Fatherhood: A Socio-Cultural Analysis." *Journal of Advanced Nursing* 29, no. 4 (1999): 1013–1020.

Barker, Kristin. "A Ship upon a Stormy Sea: The Medicalization of Pregnancy." *Social Science and Medicine* 47, no. 8 (1998): 1067–1076.

Bartick, Melissa, and Arnold Reinhold. "The Burden of Suboptimal Breastfeeding in the United States: A Pediatric Cost Analysis." *Pediatrics* 125, no. 5 (2010): 1048–1056.

Bartky, Sandra Lee. *Femininity and Domination: Studies in the Phenomenology of Oppression.* New York: Routledge, 1990.

Bartlett, Alison. "Breastfeeding as Headwork: Corporeal Feminism and Meanings for Breastfeeding." *Women's Studies International Forum* 25 (2002): 373–382.

———. "Breastfeeding Bodies and Choice in Late Capitalism." *Hecate* 29, no. 2 (2003): 153–165.

———. *Breastwork: Rethinking Breastfeeding.* Sydney, Australia: University of New South Wales Press, 2005.

Bateson, Gregory, and Margaret Mead. *Balinese Character.* New York: New York Academy of Sciences, 1942.

Battersby, Susan. "Not in Public Please: Breastfeeding as Dirty Work in the UK." In *Exploring the Dirty Side of Women's Health,* edited by Mavis Kirkham, 101–114. New York: Routledge, 2007.

Baumslag, Naomi, and Dia L. Michels. *Milk, Money, and Madness: The Culture and Politics of Breastfeeding.* Westport, CT: Bergin & Garvey, 1995.

Beal, Anne C., Karen Kuhlthau, and James M. Perrin. "Breastfeeding Advice Given to African American and White Women by Physicians and WIC Counselors." *Public Health Reports* 118, no. 4 (2003): 368–376.

Beasley, Chris. "The Challenge of Pleasure: Re-imagining Sexuality and Sexual Health." *Health Sociology Review* 17, no. 2 (2008): 151–163.

Belkin, Lisa. "Equally Shared Breast-Feeding." *New York Times—Motherlode Blog,* March 16, 2009. http://parenting.blogs.nytimes.com/2009/03/16/equally-shared-breast-feeding.

Bellamy, Elizabeth. "Mother Love Gone Wrong." *Weekend Australian Review,* March 21–22, 1998.

Bennhold, Katrin. "In Sweden, Men Can Have It All." *New York Times*, June 15, 2010, sec. A, 6.

Benoit, Cecilia, Robbie Davis-Floyd, Edwin van Teijlingen, Jane Sandall, and Janneli Miller. "Designing Midwives: A Comparison of Educational Models." In *Birth by Design: Pregnancy, Maternity Care, and Midwifery in North America and Europe*, edited by Raymond DeVries, Cecilia Benoit, Edwin van Teijlingen, and Sirpa Wrede, 139–165. New York: Routledge, 2001.

Bentley, Margaret E., Deborah L. Dee, and Joan L. Jensen. "Breastfeeding among Low-Income, African-American Women: Power, Beliefs and Decision Making." *Journal of Nutrition* 133 (2003): s305–s309.

Bergen, Helen A., Graham Martin, Angela A. Richardson, Stephen Allison, and Leigh Roeger. "Sexual Abuse, Antisocial Behaviour and Substance Use: Gender Differences in Young Community Adolescents." *Australian and New Zealand Journal of Psychiatry* 38, nos. 1–2 (2004): 34–41.

Berger, Peter L., and Thomas Luckmann. *The Social Construction of Reality: A Treatise in the Sociology of Knowledge*. Garden City, NY: Anchor Books, 1966.

Bernhard, Blythe. "Human Milk Now for Sale in O.C." *Orange County Register*, May 3, 2006. http://www.ocregister.com/articles/human-milk-now-1128779-vbfor-sale-in-oc#.

Best for Babes. "Breastfeeding on the Job." http://www.bestforbabes.org/breastfeeding-on-the-job.

Betancourt, Joseph R., Alexander R. Green, J. Emilio Carrillo, and Owusu Ananeh-Firempong. "Defining Cultural Competence: A Practical Framework for Addressing Racial/Ethnic Disparities in Health and Health Care." *Public Health Reports* 118 (2003): 293–301.

Bhopal, Raj. "Glossary of Terms Relating to Ethnicity and Race: For Reflection and Debate." *Journal of Epidemiology and Community Health* 58, no. 6 (2004): 441–445.

———. "Race and Ethnicity: Responsible Use from Epidemiological and Public Health Perspectives." *Journal of Law, Medicine, and Ethics* 34, no. 3 (2006): 500–507.

Bianchi, Joyce, Lynn Casper, and Rosalind Berkowitz King. "Complex Connections: A Multidisciplinary Look at Work, Family, Health, and Well-Being Research." In *Work Family, Health and Wellbeing*, edited by Suzanne M. Bianchi, Lynne M. Casper, and Rosalind Berkowitz King, 329–341. Mahwah, NJ: Lawrence Erlbaum Associates, 2005.

Bianchi, Suzanne M., John P. Robinson, and Melissa A. Milkie. *Changing Rhythms of American Family Life*. New York, NY: Russell Sage Foundation, 2006.

Binns, Colin W., Nwet N. Win., Yun Zhao, and Janet A. Scott, "Trends in the Expression of Breast Milk 1993–2003." *Breastfeeding Review* 14, no. 3 (2006): 5–9.

Birth without Borders. "Breastfeeding Supporters Gather Nationwide." News release, September 9, 2007. http://www.birthwithoutboundaries.com/applebees.htm.

Black, Robert E., Lindsay H. Allen, Zulfi qar A. Bhutta, Laura E. Caulfield, Mercedes de Onis, Majid Ezzati, Colin Mathers, Juan Rivera. "Maternal and Child Undernutrition 1: Global and Regional Exposures and Health Consequences." *Lancet* 371 (2008): 243–260.

Black Robert E., Saul S. Morris, and Jennifer Bryce. "Where and Why Are 10 Million Children Dying Every Year?" *Lancet* 361 (2003): 2226–2234.

Blum, Linda. *At the Breast: Ideologies of Breastfeeding and Motherhood in the Contemporary United States*. Boston: Beacon Press, 1999.

———. "Mothers, Babies, and Breastfeeding in Late Capitalist America: The Shifting Contexts of Feminist Theory." *Feminist Studies* 19, no. 2 (1993): 291–311.

Bolling, Keith, Catherine Grant, Becky Hamlyn, and Alex Thornton. *UK Infant Feeding Survey 2005: Final Report.* The Information Centre for Health and Social Care. new.wales.gov.uk/topics/statistics/headlines/health-2007/hdw20070514/?lang=en.

Bonuck, Karen A. "Country of Origin and Race/Ethnicity: Impact on Breastfeeding Intentions." *Journal of Human Lactation* 21 (2005): 320–321.

Booker, W. D. "The Early History of the Summer Diarrhoeas of Infants." *Transactions of the American Pediatric Society* 13 (1901): 7–35.

Bordo, Susan. *The Flight to Objectivity: Essays on Cartesianism and Culture.* Albany: State University of New York Press, 1987.

Boulware, L. Ebony, Lisa A. Cooper, Lloyd E. Ratner, Thomas A. LaVeist, and Neil R. Powe. "Race and Trust in the Health Care System." *Public Health Reports* 118 (2003): 358–364.

Bourgois, Philippe. *In Search of Respect: Selling Crack in El Barrio.* New York: Cambridge University Press, 1995.

Boswell-Penc, Maia, and Kate Boyer. "Expressing Anxiety? Breast Pump Usage in American Wage Workplaces." *Gender, Place and Culture* 14, no. 5 (2007): 551–567.

Boyer, Kate. "'The Way to Break the Taboo Is to Do the Taboo Thing': Breastfeeding in Public and Citizen Activism in the UK." *Health and Place* 17, no. 2 (2011): 430–437. http://www.sciencedirect.com.

Bramwell, Ros. "An Initial Qualitative Study of the Relationship between Attitudes to Menstruation and Breastfeeding." *Journal of Reproductive and Infant Psychology* 26, no. 3 (2008): 244–255.

———. "Blood and Milk: Constructions of Female Bodily Fluids in Western Society." *Women and Health* 34, no. 4 (2001): 85–96.

Braveman, Paula, Catherine Cubbin, Kristen Marchi, Susan Egerter, and Gilberto Chavez. "Measuring Socioeconomic Status/Position in Studies of Racial/Ethnic Disparities: Maternal and Infant Health." *Public Health Reports* 116 (2001): 449–463.

Breastfeeding Is Beautiful. "Breastfeeding—My Best Role Ever." *World Breastfeeding Week,* August 1–7, 2002. Archive for the Lucy Lawless category. http://www.bfino .wordpress.com/category/lucy-lawless/.

Brennemann, Joseph. "Periods in the Life of the American Pediatric Society: Adolescence, 1900–1915." *Transactions of the American Pediatric Society* 50 (1938): 56–67.

Bridges, Catherine B., Deborah I. Frank, and John Curtin. "Employer Attitudes toward Breastfeeding in the Workplace." *Journal of Human Lactation* 13 (1997): 215–219.

Bristol Social Marketing Centre. *Researching Social Marketing Solutions to Encourage Breastfeeding amongst Teenage Mothers in Hard to Reach Communities.* NHS Bristol, University of the West of England, 2009.

Britton, Cathryn. "Breastfeeding: A Natural Phenomenon or a Cultural Construct?" In *The Social Context of Birth,* edited by Caroline Squire, 297–310. Abingdon, UK: Radcliffe Medical Press, 2003.

Britton, John R., and Helen L. Britton. "Maternal Self-Concept and Breastfeeding." *Journal of Human Lactation* 24 (2008): 431–438.

Brodie, Mollyann, Ursula Foehr, Vicky Rideout, Neal Baer, Carolyn Miller, Rebecca Flournoy, and Drew Altman. "Communicating Health Information through the Entertainment Media. *Health Affairs* 20, no. 11 (2001): 192–199.

Brotman, Barbara. "Natural Wonder: Scientists Explore Using Breast Milk as Medicine." *Chicago Tribune,* November 17, 1999, sec. 1.

Brown, George W., and Patricia M. Moran, "Single Mothers, Poverty and Depression." *Psychological Medicine* 27 (1997): 31–33.

Brown, Jane, and Sheila R. Peuchaud. "Media and Breastfeeding: Friend or Foe?" *International Breastfeeding Journal* 3 (2008). http://www.internationalbreastfeeding journal.com/content/3/1/15.

Browne, Irene, ed. *Latinas and African-American Women at Work*. New York: Russell Sage Foundation, 1999.

Browner, Carol, and Nancy Press. "The Production of Authoritative Knowledge in American Prenatal Care." *Medical Anthropology Quarterly* 10, no. 2 (1996): 141–156.

Bryder, Linda. "Breastfeeding and Health Professionals in Britain, New Zealand and the United States, 1900–1970." *Medical History* 49 (2005): 179–196.

Buckley, Kathleen M. "A Double-Edged Sword: Lactation Consultants' Perceptions of the Impact of Breast Pumps on the Practice of Breastfeeding." *Journal of Perinatal Education* 18, no. 2 (2009): 13–22.

Budlender, Debbie. "A Critical Review of Selected Time Use Surveys." Geneva: United Nations Research Institute for Social Development, 2007.

Bulletin of the Chicago School of Sanitary Instruction, June 3, 1911.

Bullough, Colin H. W., Rose S. Msuka, and Lucy Karonde. "Early Suckling and Postpartum Haemorrhage: Controlled Trial in Deliveries by Traditional Birth Attendants." *Lancet* 334, no. 8662 (1989): 522–525.

Burman, Erica. *Deconstructing Developmental Psychology*. 2nd ed. London: Routledge, 2008.

Burton, Thomas M. "Spilt Milk: Methods of Marketing Infant Formula Land Abbott in Hot Water—It Pushed Baby-Food Rivals to Bar Ads, Limiting a New Player's Chances—A Big Antitrust Settlement." *Wall Street Journal*, May 25, 1993, sec. A.

Butte, Nancy, and Janet King. "Energy Requirements of Lactation." In *Human Energy Requirements*, Report of a Joint FAO/WHO/UNU Expert Consultation, 2001. http://www.fao.org/docrep/007/y5686e/y5686e0b.htm.

Cahill, Mary Ann. *Seven Voices, One Dream*. Schaumburg, IL: La Leche League International, 2001.

Calnen, Gerald. "Paid Maternity Leave and Its Impact on Breastfeeding in the United States: An Historic, Economic, Political, and Social Perspective." *Breastfeeding Medicine* 2, no. 1 (2007): 34–44.

Cantrill, Ruth M., Debra K. Creedy, and Marie Cooke. "An Australian Study of Midwives' Breast-feeding Knowledge." *Midwifery* 19, no. 4 (2003): 310–317.

Capetta, Amy. "Back to Work." *Parents*, April 2007, 137–138.

"The Care of Infants: Historical Data." *Journal of the American Medical Association* 59, no. 7 (1912): 542–543.

Carroll, Katherine, and Kerreen Reiger. "Fluid Experts: Lactation Consultants as Postmodern Professional Specialists." *Health Sociology Review* 14, no. 2 (2005): 101–110.

Carter, Pam. *Feminism, Breasts, and Breast-Feeding*. New York: St. Martin's Press, 1995.

Cartwright, Lachlan, and Jeremy Olshan. "Wife's Baby Milk in Chef's Cheese Recipe." *New York Post*, March 9, 2010. http://www.nypost.com/p/news/local/manhattan/nurse_made_JQlMRBr5ZgO6iD07AX83MJ.

Casemore, Stephanie. "Exclusively Pumping: A Resource Site for Exclusively Pumping Moms." *Exclusively Pumping*. 2011. http://www.exclusivelypumping.com/.

Chantry, Caroline J., Peggy Auinger, and Robert S. Byrd. "Lactation among Adolescent Mothers and Subsequent Bone Mineral Density." *Archives of Pediatrics and Adolescent Medicine* 158, no. 7 (2004): 650–656.

Chapman, Donna J., and Rafael Pérez-Escamilla. "U.S. National Breastfeeding Monitoring and Surveillance: Current Status and Recommendations." *Journal of Human Lactation* 25, no. 2 (2009): 139–150.

Chen, Aimin, and Walter J. Rogan. "Breastfeeding and the Risk of Postneonatal Death in the United States." *Pediatrics* 113, no. 5 (2004): 435–439.

Cheney, Rose A. "Seasonal Aspects of Infant and Childhood Mortality: Philadelphia, 1865–1920." *Journal of Interdisciplinary History* 14 (1984): 561–585.

Chicago Daily News. "Scarcely Any Pure Milk." September 1, 1892, 2.

Chicago Lying-In Hospital Dispensary. *First Annual Report, 1895–96.* Northwestern Memorial Hospital Archives, Chicago.

———. *Second Annual Report, 1896–97.* Northwestern Memorial Hospital Archives, Chicago.

———. *Thirteenth Annual Report, 1906–07, 1907–08.* Northwestern Memorial Hospital Archives, Chicago.

Chicago Tribune. "Stop the Bogus Milk Traffic." September 23, 1892, 4.

Child Trends Data Bank. "Birth and Fertility Rates." 2011. http://www.childtrendsdata bank.org/pdf/79_PDF.pdf.

Chin, Ashley C., Leann Myers, and Jeanette H. Magnus. "Race, Education, and Breastfeeding Initiation in Louisiana, 2000–2004." *Journal of Human Lactation* 24, no. 2 (2008): 175–185.

Chin, Nancy P., and Anna Solomonik, "INADEQUATE: A Metaphor for the Lives of Low-Income Women?" *Journal of Breastfeeding Medicine* 4 (2009): S41–43.

Christup, Henry Wyatt. "Litigating a Breast-feeding and Employment Case in the New Millennium." *Yale Journal of Law and Feminism* 12 (2000): 263–282.

Clarke, Edward H. *Sex in Education; or, A Fair Chance for Girls.* Boston: James R. Osgood, 1873.

Clark-Hitt, Rose, Jennifer Malat, Diana Burgess, and Greta Friedemann-Sanchez. "Doctors' and Nurses' Explanations for Racial Disparities in Medical Treatment." *Journal of Health Care for the Poor and Underserved* 21 (2010): 386–400.

Clemons, Sarah N., and Lisa H. Amir. "Breastfeeding Women's Experience of Expressing: A Descriptive Study." *Journal of Human Lactation* 26, no. 3 (2010): 258–265.

Coalition for Improving Maternity Services. "Ten Steps of the Mother-Friendly Childbirth Initiative for Mother-Friendly Hospitals, Birth Centers, and Home Birth Services." http://www.motherfriendly.org/MFCI.

Code, Lorraine. *Ecological Thinking.* New York: Oxford University Press, 2006.

Coleman, Richard P. "The Continuing Significance of Social Class to Marketing." *Journal of Consumer Research* 10, no. 3 (1983): 265–280.

Collins, Patricia Hill. *Black Feminist Thought: Knowledge, Consciousness, and the Politics of Empowerment,* 2nd ed. New York: Routledge, 2000.

———. "Moving beyond Gender: Intersectionality and Scientific Knowledge." In *Revisioning Gender,* edited by Judith Lorber, Myra Marx Ferree, and Beth Hess, 261–284. Thousand Oaks, CA: Sage, 1999.

Colson, Suzanne. "Maternal Breastfeeding Positions: Have We Got It Right?" *Practising Midwife* 8, no. 10 (2005): 24–27.

Condon, Louise, Clare Tiffany, Nicki Symes, and Ruth Bolgar. "'Cut Out for Breastfeeding': Changing Attitudes to Breastfeeding." *Community Practitioner* 83, no. 4 (2010): 29–31.

Connell, R. W. *Gender and Power: Society, the Person, and Sexual Politics.* Stanford: Stanford Press University Press, 1987.

Convery, Kelly M., and Diane L. Spatz. "Sexuality and Breastfeeding: What Do You Know?" *American Journal of Maternal/Child Nursing* 34, no. 4 (2009): 218–223.

Conway, M. Margaret, David W. Ahern, Gertrude A. Steuernagel. *Women and Public Policy: A Revolution in Progress.* Washington: CQ Press, 1999.

Coreil, Jeannine, Carol Bryant, Bonita Westover, and Doraine Bailey. "Health Professionals and Breastfeeding Counseling: Client and Provider Views." *Journal of Human Lactation* 11, no. 4 (1995): 265–271.

Countryman, Betty Ann, Heidi S. Roibal, and JoAnne Scott. "The LLL Leader and the IBCLC—A Partnership in Breastfeeding History." *Leaven* 36, no. 3 (2000): 52–53.

Coveney, John, and Robin Bunton, "In Pursuit of the Study of Pleasure: Implications for Health Research and Practice." *Health: An Interdisciplinary Journal for the Social Study of Health, Illness, and Medicine* 7, no. 2 (2003): 161–179.

Cragin, Edwin. B., J. Clifton Edgar, Charles M. Green, Edward P. Davis, J. Whitridge Williams, J. Clarence Webster, and Barton C. Hirst. "Report of the Committee of the American Gynecological Society on the Present Status of Obstetrical Education in Europe and America and on Recommendations for the Improvement of Obstetrical Teaching," ca. 1910, Rush University Medical Center Archives, Chicago.

Creedy, Debra K., Ruth Cantrill, and Marie Cooke. "Assessing Midwives' Breastfeeding Knowledge: Properties of the Newborn Feeding Ability Questionnaire and Breastfeeding Initiation Practices Scale." *International Breastfeeding Journal* 3 (2008). http://www.internationalbreastfeedingjournal.com/content/3/1/7.

Crenshaw, Kimberlé W. "Demarginalizing the Intersection between Race and Sex: A Black Feminist Critique of Antidiscrimination Doctrine, Feminist Theory and Antiracist Politics." *University of Chicago Legal Forum* (1989): 139–167.

Cricco-Lizza, Roberta. "Black Non-Hispanic Mothers' Perceptions About the Promotion of Infant-Feeding Methods by Nurses and Physicians." *Journal of Obstetric, Gynecologic and Neonatal Nursing* 35, no. 2 (2006): 173–180.

Crossley, Michele L. "Breastfeeding as a Moral Imperative: An Autoethnography Study." *Feminism and Psychology* 19, no. 1 (2009): 71–87.

Cutler, Bob D., and Robert F. Wright. "The U.S. Infant Formula Industry: Is Direct-to-Consumer Advertising Unethical or Inevitable?" *Health Marketing Quarterly* 19 (2002): 39–55.

Dahlberg, Linda L., and Etienne G. Krug. "Violence—A Global Public Health Problem." In *World Report on Violence and Health*, edited by Etienne G. Krug, Linda L. Dahlberg, James A. Mercy, and Anthony B. Zwi, 1–56. Geneva, Switzerland: World Health Organization, 2002.

Dahlgren, Gören, and Margaret Whitehead. *Policies and Strategies to Promote Social Equity in Health*. Stockholm: Institute of Future Studies, 1991.

Daly, Mary, and Guy Standing. *Care Work: The Quest for Security*. Geneva: International Labour Organization, 2001.

Dankwa-Mullan, Irene, Kyu B. Rhee, David M. Stoff, Jennifer R. Pohlhaus, Francisco S. Sy, Nathaniel Stinson, and John Ruffin. "Moving toward Paradigm-Shifting Research in Health Disparities through Translational, Transformational, and Transdisciplinary Approaches." *American Journal of Public Health* 100, no. 1 (2010): s19–s24.

Davis, Effa V. "Breast Feeding." *Bulletin Chicago School of Sanitary Instruction* 13 (1901): 2.

Davis-Floyd, Robbie. *Birth as an American Rite of Passage*. Austin: University of Texas Press, 1992.

———. "Mutual Accommodation or Biomedical Hegemony? Anthropological Perspectives on Global Issues in Midwifery." *Midwifery Today* 53 (2000): 12–17; 68–89.

Declercq, Eugene R., Carol Sakala, Maureen P. Corry, and Sandra Applebaum. *New Mothers Speak Out: National Survey Results Highlight Women's Postpartum Experiences*. New York: Childbirth Connection, 2008. http://www.childbirthconnection.org/pdf.asp?PDFDownload=new-mothers-speak-out.

Deigh, John. "Shame and Self-Esteem: A Critique." *Ethics* 93, no. 2 (1983): 225–245.

De Lauretis, Teresa. *Technologies of Gender: Essays on Theory, Film, and Fiction.* Bloomington: Indiana University Press, 1987.

DeLee, Joseph B. "Mother's Day Address." May 12, 1940, Joseph B. DeLee Papers, Northwestern Memorial Hospital Archives, Chicago.

———. "Motherhood: An Address before the Women's Society of Isaiah Temple January 4th 1898." Joseph B. DeLee Papers, Northwestern Memorial Hospital Archives, Chicago.

———. "The Prophylactic Forceps Operation." *American Journal of Obstetrics and Gynecology* 1 (October 1920): 34–44.

"Discussion of 'The Early Recognition of Impending Obstetric Accidents' by Joseph Lee." *Chicago Medical Recorder* 24 (1903): 440–442.

Dobash, R. Emerson, and Russell P. Dobash. *Rethinking Violence Against Women.* California: Sage, 1998.

Dodgson, Joan E. "A History of African American Infant Feeding Practices in Durham, North Carolina, and the Influences of Social Policy and National Legislation." Abstract. Proceedings, 16th International Nursing Research Congress, Sigma Theta Tau International, 2005, 66.

Dodgson, Joan E., and Roxanne Struthers. "Indigenous Women's Voices: Marginalization and Health." *Journal of Transcultural Nursing* 16, no. 4 (2005): 339–346.

Dodgson, Joan E., Amanda L. Watkins, and Myunghan Choi. "Evaluation of Supportive Breastfeeding Hospital Practices: A Community Perspective." *Avances En Enfermería (Advances in Nursing)* 28, no. 2 (2010): 17–30.

Dorfman, Lori, and Heather Gehlert. *Issue 18: Talking about Breastfeeding: Why the Health Argument Isn't Enough.* Berkeley, CA: Berkeley Media Studies Group, 2010. http://www.bmsg.org/pdfs/BMSG_Issue_18.pdf.

Doucet, Andrea. *Do Men Mother? Fathering, Care, and Domestic Responsibility.* Toronto: University of Toronto Press, 2006.

Douglas, Anne R. "Reported Anxieties Concerning Intimate Parenting in Women Sexually Abused as Children." *Child Abuse and Neglect* 24 (2000): 425–434.

Douglas, Mary. *Purity and Danger.* New York: Routledge, 1966.

Dowling, Sally. "Women's Experiences of Long-term Breastfeeding." Ph.D. diss., University of the West of England, Bristol, forthcoming.

Drago, Robert, Jeffrey Hayes, and Youngmin Yi. "Better Health for Mothers and Children: Breastfeeding Accommodations under the Affordable Care Act." Institute for Women's Policy Research, 2010. http://www.iwpr.org/pdf/B292.pdf.

Draper, Susan B. "Breast-Feeding as a Sustainable Resource System." *American Anthropologist* 98, no. 2 (1996): 258–266.

Duffy, Elizabeth P., Patricia Percival, and Esme Kershaw. "Positive Effects of an Antenatal Group Teaching Session on Postnatal Nipple Pain, Nipple Trauma and Breast Feeding Rates." *Midwifery* 13 (1997): 189–196.

Dunn, Laurie, and Sue Evans. Interview by Linda Fentiman, Wakemed Mother's Milk Bank, Raleigh, NC, August 29, 2008.

Durfee, Alicia, and Marcia K. Meyers. "Who Gets What from Government? Distributional Consequences of Child Care Assistance Policies." *Journal of Marriage and Family* 68 (2006): 733–748.

Dykes, Fiona. *Breastfeeding in Hospital: Mothers, Midwives and the Production Line.* New York: Routledge, 2006.

———. "Education of Health Practitioners Supporting Breastfeeding Women: Time for Critical Reflection." *Maternal and Child Nutrition* 2 (2006): 204–216.

———. "'Supply' and 'Demand': Breastfeeding as Labour." *Social Science and Medicine* 60, no. 10 (2005): 2283–2293.

———. "Western Medicine and Marketing: Construction of an Inadequate Milk Syndrome in Lactating Women." *Health Care for Women International* 23, no. 5 (2002): 492–502.

Dykes, Fiona, Victoria Hall Moran, Sue Burt, and Janet Edwards. "Adolescent Mothers and Breastfeeding: Experiences and Support Needs." *Journal of Human Lactation* 19, no. 4 (2003): 391–400.

Dyson, Lisa, Josephine Green, Mary Renfrew, Brian McMillan, and Mike Woolridge. "Factors Influencing the Infant Feeding Decision for Socioeconomically Deprived Pregnant Teenagers: The Moral Dimension." *Birth: Issues in Perinatal Care* 37, no. 2 (2010): 141–149.

Earle, Sarah. "Factors Affecting the Initiation of Breastfeeding: Implications for Breastfeeding Promotion." *Health Promotion International* 17, no. 3 (2002): 205–214.

———. "Why Some Women Do Not Breastfeed: Bottle Feeding and Fathers' Role." *MIDAS Midwifery Digest* 11, no. 2 (2001): 237–242.

Earp, Jo Anne, and Susan T. Ennett. 1991. "Conceptual Models for Health Education Research and Practice." *Health Education Research* 6 (2): 163–171.

Eaton, P. J. "A Few of the Things a Pediatrician Should Teach." *Transactions of the American Pediatrics Society* 21 (1909): 40–47.

Eckard, E. Woodrow, Jr. "Competition and the Cigarette TV Advertising Ban." *Economic Inquiry* 29, no. 1 (1991): 119–133.

Ehrenreich, Barbara, and Deirdre English. *Witches, Midwives, and Nurses: A History of Women Healers.* 2nd ed. New York: Feminist Press, 2010.

Eichner, Maxine. "Parenting and the Workplace: The Construction of Parenting Protections in United States Law." *International Breastfeeding Journal* 3 (2008): 14.

Eisenberg, Arlene, Heidi Murkoff, and Sandee Hathaway. *What to Expect When You're Expecting.* 2nd ed. New York: Workman, 1991.

Eisenstein, Zillah R. *The Female Body and the Law.* Berkeley: University of California Press, 1988.

Else-Quest, Nicole M., Janet Shibley Hyde, and Roseanne Clark. "Breastfeeding, Bonding, and the Mother-Infant Relationship." *Merrill-Palmer Quarterly* 49, no. 4 (2003): 495–517.

Ely, Robin, and Irene Padavic. "A Feminist Analysis of Organizational Research on Sex Differences." *Academy of Management Review* 32, no. 4 (2007): 1121–1143.

Engelmann, George J. "Birth- and Death-Rate as Influenced by Obstetric and Gynecologic Progress." *Boston Medical and Surgical Journal* 146 (1920): 505–508.

England, Paula, and Nancy Folbre. "Contracting for Care." In *Feminist Economics Today: Beyond Economic Man,* edited by Marianne A. Ferber and Julia A. Nelson, 61–79. Chicago: University of Chicago Press, 2003.

Epstein, Laura. "Women and Children Last: Anti-Competitive Practices in the Infant Formula Industry." *American University Journal of Gender and Law* 5, no. 1 (1996): 21–56.

Ertman, Martha M. "What's Wrong with a Parenthood Market? A New and Improved Theory of Commodification." In *Rethinking Commodification: Cases and Readings in Law and Culture,* edited by Martha M. Ertman and Joan C. Williams, 303–323. New York: New York University, 2005.

Estroff, Sharon. "Dirty Looks, Dirty Bathrooms. Every Credible Medical Organization Recommends Nursing. So Why Are Women Who Breastfeed in Public Made to Feel as if They're Doing Something Wrong?" *Parents,* July 2007, 106–109.

Eyer, Diane E. "Mother-Infant Bonding: A Scientific Fiction." *Human Nature* 51, no. 1 (1994): 69–94.

Ezramomma. "Breast or Bottle: What's the Right Choice for You?" *Similac Strong Moms,* November 20, 2008. http://similac.com/community/boards/forums/p/29/29.aspx.

Faircloth, Charlotte. "A Weak Formula for Legislation: How Loopholes in the Law Are Putting Babies at Risk." United Kingdom: UNICEF UK, Save the Children, and the National Childbirth Trust, nd. http://www.savethechildren.org.uk/en/docs/report-formula_legislation.pdf.

———. "'What Science Says Is Best': Parenting Practices, Scientific Authority and Maternal Identity." *Sociological Research Online* 15, no. 4 (2010). http://www.socresonline.org.uk/15/4/4.html.

Fallon, Anthony B., Desley Hegney, Maxine O'Brien, Wendy Brodribb, Maree Crepinsek, and Jackie Doolan. "An Evaluation of a Telephone-Based Postnatal Support Intervention for Infant Feeding in a Regional Australian City." *Birth* 32 (2005): 291–298.

Farmer, Paul. "Chapter One: Women, Poverty, and AIDS." In *Women, Poverty, and AIDS: Sex, Drugs, and Structural Violence,* edited by Paul Farmer, Margaret Connors, and Janie Simmons, 3–38. Monroe, ME: Common Courage Press, 1996.

Fein, Sara B., Bidisha Mandal, and Brian E. Roe. "Success of Strategies for Combining Employment and Breastfeeding." *Pediatrics* 122 (2008): s56–s62.

Feldman, Ruth, Aron Weller, Orna Zagoory-Sharon, and Ari Levine. "Evidence for a Neuroendocrinological Foundation of Human Affiliation: Plasma Oxytocin Levels across Pregnancy and the Postpartum Period Predict Mother-Infant Bonding." *Psychological Science* 18, no. 11 (2007): 965–970.

Female Intelligence Agency. "Breastfeeding in Public and Discreet Nursing." *007 Breasts.* http://www.007b.com/breastfeeding_public.php.

Fentiman, Linda C. "Organ Donation as National Service: A Proposed Federal Organ Donation Law." *Suffolk University Law Review* 27, no. 4 (1993): 1593–1612.

———. "Marketing Mothers' Milk: The Commodification of Breastfeeding and the New Markets for Breast Milk and Infant Formula." *Nevada Law Journal* 10, no. 1 (2010): 29–81.

Fildes, Valerie A. *Breasts, Bottles, and Babies: A History of Infant Feeding.* Edinburgh: Edinburgh University Press, 1986.

Fisher, Irving. "Address." *Transactions of the American Association for the Study and Prevention of Infant Mortality: First Annual Meeting, 1910,* 38–42. http://www.archive.org.

Fletcher, Joyce. "Gender Perspectives on Work and Personal Life Research." In *Work, Family, Health and Wellbeing,* edited by Suzanne M. Bianchi, Lynne M. Casper, and Rosalind Berkowitz King, 325–338. Mahwah, NJ: Lawrence Erlbaum Associates, 2005.

Flores-Paniagua, Veronica. "Office Support for Nursing Moms, About Time." *San Antonio Express-News,* April 6, 2010.

Florida ex rel. Butterworth v. Abbott Laboratories, Inc. No. 91–40002-MP, 1993 WL 216099, (N.D. Fl. 1993).

Folb, Kate L. "'Don't Touch That Dial!' TV as a—What!?—Positive Influence." *SIECUS Report* 28, no. 5 (2000): 16–18.

Folbre, Nancy. *The Invisible Heart: Economics and Family Values.* New York: New Press, 2001.

Forbes, Bettina, and Danielle Rigg. "Mission." *Best for Babes,* 2011. http://www.bestforbabes.org/.

Forbes, Gordon B., Leah E. Adams-Curtis, Nicole R. Hamm, and Kay B. White. "Perceptions of the Woman Who Breastfeeds: The Role of Erotophobia, Sexism, and Attitudinal Variables." *Sex Roles* 49, nos. 7–8 (2003): 379–388.

Forste, Renata, Jessica Weiss, and Emily Lippincott. "The Decision to Breastfeed in the United States: Does Race Matter? *Pediatrics* 108 (2001): 291–296.

Fortier, Corinne. "Blood, Sperm and the Embryo in Sunni Islam and Mauritania: Milk Kinship, Descent and Medically Assisted Procreation." *Body and Society* 13, no. 3 (2007): 15–36.

Fortmann, Stephen P., C. Barr Taylor, June A. Flora, and Darius E. Jatulis. "Changes in Adult Cigarette Smoking Prevalence after 5 Years of Community Health Education: The Stanford Five-City Project." *American Journal of Epidemiology* 137, no. 1 (1983): 82–96.

Foss, Katherine A., and Brian G. Southwell. "Infant Feeding and the Media: The Relationship between *Parents* Magazine Content and Breastfeeding, 1972–2000." *International Breastfeeding Journal* 1 (2006). http://www.biomedcentral.com/content/pdf/1746-4358-1-10.pdf.

Foucault, Michel. *The History of Sexuality.* Vol. 1: *An Introduction.* Translated by Robert Hurley. Middlesex, UK: Penguin, 1981.

———. "The Politics of Health in the Eighteenth Century." In *Power/Knowledge: Selected Interviews and Other Writings, 1972–1977*, edited by Colin Gordon, 166–182. New York: Pantheon, 1980.

Fox, Mary Kay, William Hamilton, and Biing-Hwan Lin, eds. "Effects of Food Assistance and Nutrition Programs on Nutrition and Health." Vol. 3, *Literature Review.* Food Assistance and Nutrition Research Report No. 19-3.

Fraley, Amber. "Booby Juice." *Op Ed News*, July 26, 2008. http://www.opednews.com/a/64921?show=votes.

Frampton, Edith. "'You Just Can't Fly on Off and Leave a Body': The Intercorporeal Breastfeeding Subject of Toni Morrison's Fiction." *Women: A Cultural Review* 16, no. 2 (2005): 141–163.

Fraser, Gertrude J. "Modern Bodies, Modern Minds: Midwifery and Reproductive Change in an African American Community." In *Conceiving the New World Order: The Global Politics of Reproduction*, edited by Faye Ginsburg and Rayna Rapp, 42–58. Berkeley: University of California Press, 1995.

Freed Gary, Sarah Clark, Robert Cefalo, and James Sorenson. "Breast-feeding Education of Obstetrics-Gynecology Residents and Practitioners." *American Journal of Obstetrics and Gynecology* 173, no. 5 (1995): 1607–1613.

Freed, Gary L., J. Kennard Fraley, and Richard J. Schanler. "Attitudes of Expectant Fathers Regarding Breast-Feeding." *Pediatrics* 90 (1992): 224–227.

Frerichs, Leah, Julie L. Andsager, Shelly Campo, Mary Aquilino, and Carolyn Stewart Dyer. "Framing Breastfeeding and Formula-Feeding Messages in Popular U.S. Magazines." *Women and Health* 44, no. 1 (2006): 95–118.

Fried, Mindy. *Taking Time: Parental Leave Policy and Corporate Culture.* Philadelphia: Temple University Press, 1998.

FTC v. Abbott Laboratories, 853 F. Supp. 526, 526–27 (D.D.C. 1994).

Fuller, Alison, Vanessa Beck, and Lorna Unwin. "The Gendered Nature of Apprenticeship: Employers' and Young People's Perspectives." *Education and Training* 47, no. 4–5 (2005): 298–311.

Furber, Christine, and Ann M. Thompson. "Breaking the Rules in Baby-Feeding Practice in the UK: Deviance and Good Practice?" *Midwifery* 22 (2006): 365–376.

Furth, Charlotte, and Ch'en Shu-yueh. "Chinese Medicine and the Anthropology of Menstruation in Contemporary Taiwan." *Medical Anthropology Quarterly* 6, no. 1 (1992): 27–48.

Galst, Joann P. "Television Food Commercials and Pro-Nutritional Public Service Announcements as Determinants of Young Children's Snack Choices." *Child Development* 51, no. 3 (1980): 935–938.

Galtry, Judith. "Extending the 'Bright Line': Feminism, Breastfeeding and the Workplace in the United States." *Gender and Society* 14, no. 2 (2000): 295–317.

———. "'Sameness' and Suckling: Infant Feeding, Feminism, and a Changing Labour Market." *Women's Studies Journal of New Zealand* 13, no. 1 (1997): 65–88.

———. "Suckling and Silence in the USA: The Costs and Benefits of Breastfeeding." *Feminist Economics* 3, no. 3 (1997): 1–24.

Galtung, Johann. "Violence, Peace, and Peace Research." *Journal of Peace Research* 6, no. 3 (1969): 167–191.

Gatrell, Caroline Jane. "Secrets and Lies: Breastfeeding and Professional Paid Work." *Social Science and Medicine* 65 (2007): 393–404.

Geddes, Donna T. "Ultrasound Imaging of the Lactating Breast: Methodology and Application." *International Breastfeeding Journal* 4 (2009). http://www.internationalbreast feedingjournal.com/content/4/1/4.

Genna, Catherine Watson, and Lisa Sandora. "Breastfeeding: Normal Sucking and Swallowing." In *Supporting Sucking Skills in Breastfeeding Infants*, edited by Catherine Watson Genna, 1–41. Sudbury, MA: Jones & Bartlett, 2008.

Georges, Eugenia. "Fetal Ultrasound Imaging and the Production of Authoritative Knowledge in Greece." *Medical Anthropology Quarterly* 10, no. 2 (1996): 157–175.

Gerbner, George, and Larry Gross. "Living with Television: The Violence Profile." *Journal of Communications* 26 (1976): 173–199.

Gerson, Judith M., and Kathy Peiss. "Boundaries, Negotiation, Consciousness: Reconceptualizing Gender Relations." *Social Problems* 32, no. 4 (1985): 317–331.

Gerstel, Naomi, and Katherine McGonagle. "Job Leaves and the Limits of the Family and Medical Leave Act: The Effects of Gender, Race, and Family." *Work and Occupations* 26, no. 4 (1999): 510–534.

Giles, Fiona. *Fresh Milk: The Secret Life of Breasts*. New York: Simon & Schuster, 2003.

———. "Reimagining Breastfeeding: Return to the Lactating Subject." Paper presented at the Society for Literature and Science Conference, Pasadena, CA, October, 2002.

Giles, Fiona, and Jenni Whelan. *Discrimination and Vilification in Advertising: A Report Produced by the Advertising Standards Bureau*. Canberra, Australia: Advertising Standards Bureau, 2009.

Gillespie, Brenda, Hannah d'Arcy, Kendra Schwartz, Janet Kay Bobo, and Betsy Foxman. "Recall of Age of Weaning and Other Breastfeeding Variables." *International Breastfeeding Journal* 1 (2006). http://www.internationalbreastfeedingjournal.com/content/1/1/4.

Gitlin, Todd. "Prime Time Ideology: The Hegemonic Process in Television Entertainment." *Social Problems* 26, no. 3 (1979): 251–266.

Glass, Thomas A., and Matthew J. McAtee, "Behavioral Science at the Crossroads in Public Health: Extending Horizons, Envisioning the Future." *Social Science Medicine* 62 (2006): 1650–1671.

Glendon, Mary Ann. *Rights Talk: The Impoverishment of Political Discourse*. New York: Free Press, 1993.

Glynn, Keva, Heather Maclean, Tonia Forte, and Marsha Cohen. "The Association between Role Overload and Women's Mental Health." *Journal of Women's Health* 18 (2009): 217–223.

Golden, Janet L. *A Social History of Wet Nursing in America: From Breast to Bottle*. Cambridge: Cambridge University Press, 1996.

Goodman, Elissa Aaronson. "Breastfeeding or Bust: The Need for Legislation to Protect a Mother's Right to Express Breast Milk at Work." *Cardozo Women's Law Journal* 10 (2003): 146–174.

Goodwin, Michele. *Black Markets: The Supply and Demand of Body Parts.* New York: Cambridge, 2006.

———. "The Body Market: Race Politics and Private Ordering." *Arizona Law Review* 49, no. 3 (2007): 599–636.

Gottlieb, Scott. "When Population-Wide Politics and Personal Medical Care Collide: The Campaign to End Infant Formula in Developing Countries." Position Paper 502. New York: Independent Women's Forum, 2005. http://www.aei.org/docLib/20050513_IWF.pdf.

Gould, Christopher, Dagmar C. Stern, and Timothy D. Adams. "TV's Distorted Vision of Poverty." *Communication Quarterly* 29, no. 24 (1981): 309–314.

Green, Lawrence W. "Public Health Asks of Systems Science: To Advance Our Evidence-Based Practice, Can You Help Us Get More Practice-Based Evidence?" *American Journal of Public Health* 96 (2006): 406–409.

Green, Marina. "The Medicalization of Breastfeeding." Master's thesis, University of British Columbia, 2002.

Green, Tiffany L., and William A. Darity Jr. "Under the skin: Using Theories from Biology and the Social Sciences to Explore the Mechanisms behind the Black-White Health Gap." *American Journal of Public Health* 100 (2010): S36–S41.

Greenberg, Judith G. "The Pregnancy Discrimination Act: Legitimating Discrimination against Pregnant Women in the Workforce." *Maine Law Review* 50 (1998): 225–250.

Greiner, Ted. "How Can We Increase the Father's Involvement in Childcare?" Paper presented at the WABA International Workshop Breastfeeding Women and Work: From Human Rights to Creative Solutions," Quezon City, Philippines, June 1, 1998. *Childbirth Solutions.* http://www.childbirthsolutions.com/articles/daddy/fatherchild.php.

———. "Ideas for Action Programmes for Promoting Breastfeeding." In *The Breastfeeding Movement: A Sourcebook*, edited by Lakshmi Menon, Anwar Fazal, Sarah Amin, and Susan Siew, 61–65. Penang, Malaysia: World Alliance for Breastfeeding Action, 2003.

———. "Infant and Young Child Nutrition: A Historic Review from a Communication Perspective." In *Communication Strategies to Support Infant and Young Child Nutrition*, edited by Peggy Koniz-Booher, 7–15. Cornell International Nutrition Monographs 24–25, 1993.

Gribble, Karleen. "Long-term Breastfeeding: Changing Attitudes and Overcoming Challenges." *Breastfeeding Review* 16, no. 1 (2008): 5–15.

Groleau, Danielle. "Determinants culturels et l'approche ecologique: Le cas de la promotion de l'allaitement chez les immigrantes Vietnamiennes." Ph.D. diss. Department of Social and Preventive Medicine, Faculty of Medicine, University of Montreal, 1998.

Groleau, Danielle, and Ivone E. Cabral. "Reconfiguring Insufficient Breast Milk as a Sociosomatic Problem: Mothers of Premature Babies Using the Kangaroo Method in Brazil." *Maternal and Child Nutrition* 5, no. 1 (2009): 10–24.

Groleau, Danielle, and Charo Rodriguez. "Breastfeeding and Poverty: Negotiating Cultural Change and Symbolic Capital of Motherhood in Québec, Canada." In *Infant and Young Child Feeding: Challenges to Implementing a Global Strategy*, edited by Fiona Dykes and Victoria Hall Moran, 80–98. Oxford: Wiley-Blackwell, 2009.

Groleau, Danielle, Margot Souliere, and Laurence J. Kirmayer. "Breastfeeding and the Cultural Configuration of Social Space among Vietnamese Immigrant Woman." *Health and Place* 12, no. 4 (2006): 516–526.

Groleau, Danielle, Phyllis Zelkowitz, and Ivone E. Cabral. "Enhancing Generalizability: Moving from an Intimate to a Political Voice." *Qualitative Health Research* 9, no. 3 (2009): 416–426.

Gross, Leon. "Statistical Report of the 2009 IBLCE Examination." *Journal of Human Lactation* 26, no. 2 (2010): 201.

Grosz, Elizabeth. "Refiguring Bodies." In *Volatile Bodies: Towards a Corporeal Feminism*, 3–24. Bloomington: Indiana University Press, 1994.

———. *Volatile Bodies: Towards a Corporeal Feminism*. Bloomington: Indiana University Press, 1994.

Grummer-Strawn, Lawrence, Kathleen S. Scanlon, Natalie Darling, and Elizabeth J. Conrey. "Racial and Socioeconomic Disparities in Breastfeeding—United States, 2004." *Morbidity and Mortality Weekly Report* 55, no. 12 (2006): 335–339.

Grzywacz, Joseph G., Shari McMahan, Janet R. Hurley, Daniel Stokols, and Kimari Phillips. "Serving Racial and Ethnic Populations with Health Promotion." *American Journal of Health Promotion* 18, no. 5 (2004): s8–s12.

Guendelman, Sylvia, Jessica L. Kosa, Michelle Pearl, Steve Graham, Julia Goodman, and Martin Kharrazi. "Juggling Work and Breastfeeding: Effects of Maternity Leave and Occupational Characteristics." *Pediatrics* 123 (2009): e38–e46.

Guerrina, Roberta. "Equality, Difference and Motherhood: The Case for a Feminist Analysis of Equal Rights and Maternity Legislation." *Journal of Gender Studies* 10, no.1 (2001): 33–42.

Guthrie, Doug, and Louise Marie Roth. "The State, Courts, and Maternity Policies in U.S. Organizations: Specifying Institutional Mechanisms." *American Sociological Review* 64 (1999): 41–63.

Halpern, Sydney A. *American Pediatrics: The Social Dynamics of Professionalism, 1880–1980*. Berkeley: University of California Press, 1988.

Handwerker, Lisa. "The Consequences of Modernity for Childless Women in China: Medicalization and Resistance." In *Pragmatic Women and Body Politics*, edited by Margaret Lock and Patricia A. Kaufert, 178–205. Cambridge: Cambridge University Press, 1998.

Hankivsky, Olena, Colleen Reid, Renee Cormier, Colleen Varcoe, Natalie Clark, Cecilia Benoit, and Shari Brotma. "Exploring the Promises of Intersectionality for Advancing Women's Health Research." *International Journal for Equity in Health* 5 (2010). http://www.equityhealthj.com/content/9/1/5.

Haraway, Donna J. *Simians, Cyborgs, and Women: The Reinvention of Nature*. London: Free Association Books, 1991.

———. "Situated Knowledges: The Science Question in Feminism and the Privilege of Partial Perspective." In *Simians, Cyborgs, and Women*, 183–201. New York: Routledge, 1991.

Harmon, Amy. "Lactivists Taking Their Cause, and Their Babies, to the Streets." *New York Times*, June 7, 2005. http://www.nytimes.com/2005/06/07/nyregion/07nurse.html?_r=1.

Harris, Cheryl I. "Finding Sojourner's Truth: Race, Gender, and the Institution of Property." *Cardozo Law Review* 18, no. 2 (1996): 309–410.

Hausman, Bernice L. "Contamination and Contagion: Environmental Toxins, HIV/AIDS, and the Problem of the Maternal Body." *Hypatia* 21, no. 1 (2006): 137–156.

———. "The Feminist Politics of Breastfeeding." *Australian Feminist Studies* 19, no. 45 (2004): 273–285.

———. "Motherhood and Inequality: A Commentary on Hanna Rosin's 'The Case Against Breastfeeding.'" *Journal of Human Lactation* 25, no. 3 (2009): 266–268.

———. *Mother's Milk: Breastfeeding Controversies in American Culture*. New York: Routledge, 2003.

————. *Viral Mothers: Breastfeeding in the Age of HIV/AIDS.* Ann Arbor: University of Michigan Press, 2011.

————. "Women's Liberation and the Rhetoric of 'Choice' in Infant Feeding Debates." *International Breastfeeding Journal* 3 (2008). http://www.internationalbreastfeeding journal.com/content/3/1/10.

Hawkins, Summer, Lucy J. Griffiths, Carol Dezateux, Catherine Law, and the Millennium Cohort Study Child Health Group. "Maternal Employment and Breast-Feeding Initiation: Findings from the Millennium Cohort Study." *Pediatric and Perinatal Epidemiology* 21 (2007): 242–247.

Heck, Katherine, Paula Braveman, Catherine Cubbin, Gilberto F. Chavez, and John L. Kiely. "Socioeconomic Status and Breastfeeding Initiation among California Mothers." *Public Health Reports* 121 (2006): 51–59.

Hector, Debra, Lesley King, and Karen Webb. *Overview of Recent Reviews of Interventions to Promote and Support Breastfeeding.* Sydney: NSW Centre for Public Health Nutrition, 2004.

Heird, William. "Progress in Promoting Breast-Feeding, Combating Malnutrition, and Composition and Use of Infant Formula 1981–2006." *Journal of Nutrition* 137 (2007): s499–s500.

Hellings, Pam, and Carol Howe. "Assessment of Breastfeeding Knowledge of Nurse Practitioners and Nurse-Midwives." *Journal of Midwifery and Women's Health* 45, no. 3 (2000): 264–270.

Henderson, Ann M. "Mixed Messages about the Meanings of Breast-Feeding Representations in the Australian Press and Popular Magazines." *Midwifery* 15 (1999): 24–31.

Henderson, Lesley, Jenny Kitzinger, and Josephine Green. "Representing Infant Feeding: Content Analysis of British Media Portrayals of Bottle Feeding and Breast Feeding." *British Medical Journal* 321 (2000): 1196–1198.

Henry, Shannon. "Banking on Milk." *Washington Post,* January 16, 2007, sec. F.

Hesse, Bradford W., David E. Nelson, Gary L. Kreps, and Robert T. Croyle. "Trust and Sources of Health Information. The Impact of the Internet and Its Implications for Health Care Providers: Findings from the First Health Information National Trends Survey." *Archives of Internal Medicine* 105 (2005): 2618–2624.

Himmelweit, Susan. "Can We Afford (Not) to Care: Prospects and Policy." New Working Paper Series 15. London: London School of Economics Gender Institute, July 2005.

Hoddinott, Pat, and Roisin Pill. "Nobody Actually Tells You: A Study of Infant Feeding." *British Journal of Midwifery* 7, no. 9 (1999): 558–565.

Holmes, Alison V., Nancy Chin, Janusz Kaczorowski, and Cynthia R. Howard. "A Barrier to Exclusive Breastfeeding for WIC Enrollees: Limited Use of Exclusive Breastfeeding Food Package for Mothers." *Breastfeeding Medicine* 4 (2009): 25–30.

Hornik, Robert. "Public Health Communication: Making Sense of Contradictory Evidence." In *Public Health Communication: Evidence for Behavior Change,* edited by Robert Hornik, 1–22. Mahwah, NJ: Lawrence Erlbaum Associates, 2002.

Horta, Bernardo L., Rajiv Bahl, José Carlos Martinés, and Cesar G. Victora. "Evidence on the Long-Term Effects of Breastfeeding: Systematic Reviews and Meta-analysis." World Health Organization, 2007. http://www.who.int/child_adolescent_health/ documents/9241595230/en/index.html.

"Hospital Grows in Popularity as Family Birthplace." *Presbyterian Hospital of the City of Chicago Bulletin* 32 (1940).

"Hospitals Approved for Residencies in Specialties." *Journal of the American Medical Association* 107, no. 9 (1936): 703–715.

Howard, Caroline, ed. "Newsbreak." *Working Mother*, April 2007, 16.

Howard-Grabman, Lisa, Cynthia P. Willis, Elizabeth Arteaga, Carla Queierolo And Ccolla, and Sejas Perez. "A 'Dialogue of Knowledge' Approach to Better Reproductive, Sexual and Child Health in Rural Andean Communities." In *Realizing Rights: Transforming Approaches to Sexual and Reproductive Well-Being*, edited by Andrea Cornwall and Alice Welbourn, chap. 21. London: Zed Books, 2002.

Huber, Joan. *On the Origins of Gender Inequality*. Boulder, CO: Paradigm Publishers, 2007.

Hulko, Wendy. "The Time- and Context-Contingent Nature of Intersectionality and Interlocking Oppressions." *Journal of Women and Social Work* 24 (2009): 44–55.

Human Milk Banking Association of North America. "ALERT: Milk Donors are URGENTLY NEEDED." February 11, 2011. http://www.hmbana.org/.

———. "Donate Milk." http://www.hmbana.org/index/donatemilk.

Hurley, Kristen M., Maureen M. Black, Mia A. Papas, and Anna M. Quigg. "Variation in Breastfeeding Behaviours, Perceptions, and Experiences by Race/Ethnicity among a Low-Income Statewide Sample of Special Supplemental Nutrition Program for Women, Infants, and Children (WIC) Participants in the United States." *Maternal and Child Nutrition* 4, no. 2 (2008): 95.

Hurst, Carol Grace. "Constraints on Breastfeeding Choices for Low Income Mothers." PhD diss., Virginia Commonwealth University, 2007.

Hylton, Maria O'Brien. "'Parental' Leaves and Poor Women: Paying the Price for Time Off." *University of Pittsburgh Law Review* 52 (1991): 475–493.

Institute of Medicine of the National Academies. Board on Health Sciences Policy. *Preterm Birth: Causes, Consequences and Prevention*. Consensus Report, July 13, 2006. http://www.iom.edu/en/Reports/2006/Preterm-Birth-Causes-Consequences-and-Prevention.aspx.

International Board of Lactation Consultant Examiners. "Facts and Figures about IBCLCs in the Americas." 2011. http://americas.iblce.org/factsandfigures.php.

———. "IBLCE Exam Blueprint." March 8, 2008. http://www.iblce.org/upload/downloads/IBLCEExamBlueprint.pdf.

———. "Number of IBCLCs in the World." January 2011. http://www.iblce.org/upload/downloads/NumberIBCLCsWorld.pdf.

International Breast Milk Project. "Donation Process." 2010. http://www.breastmilk project.org/hiw_donationdiagram.php.

International Labour Organization. *Maternity at Work: A Review of National Legislation*. 2nd ed. Geneva: International Labour Office, 2010.

International Lactation Consultant Association. "Mission and Vision." http://www.ilca .org/i4a/pages/index.cfm?pageid=3281.

———. "Position on Breastfeeding, Breast Milk, and Environmental Contaminants." October 2001. http://www.ilca.org/files/resources/ilca_publications/EnvironContiPP.pdf.

International Lactation Consultant Association and La Leche League International. "Women's Human Rights and the Elimination of Violence: Where Does Breastfeeding Fit In?" In *The Breastfeeding Movement: A Sourcebook*, edited by Lakshmi Menon, Anwar Fazal, Sarah Amin, and Susan Siew, 199–200. Penang, Malaysia: World Alliance for Breastfeeding Action, 2003.

International MotherBaby Childbirth Initiative. "Ten Steps to Optimal MotherBaby Maternity Services." http://www.imbci.org/ShowPage.asp?id=209.

Ip, Stanley, Mei Chung, Gowri Raman, Priscilla Chew, Nombulelo Magula, Deirdre DeVine, Thomas Trikalinos, and Joseph Lau. *Breastfeeding and Maternal and Infant*

Health Outcomes in Developed Countries. Evidence Report/Technology Assessment No. 153. AHRQ Publication No. 07-E007. Rockville, MD: Agency for Healthcare Research and Quality, 2007. http://www.ahrq.gov/clinic/tp/brfouttp.htm.

Irons, D. W., P. Sriskandbalan, and C. H. Bullough. "A Simple Alternative to Parenteral Oxytocics for the Third Stage of Labor." *International Journal of Gynecology and Obstetrics* 46, no. 1 (July 1994): 15–18.

Jabs, Jennifer, and Carol M. Devine. "Time Scarcity and Food Choices: An Overview." *Appetite* 47 (2006): 196–204.

Jacknowitz, Alison. "The Role of Workplace Characteristics in Breastfeeding Practices." *Women and Health* 47, no. 2 (2008): 87–111.

Jacknowitz, Alison, Daniel Novillo, and Laura Tiehen. "Special Supplemental Nutrition Program for Women, Infants, and Children and Infant Feeding Practices." *Pediatrics* 119, no. 2 (2007): 281–289.

Jacobs, Jerry A., and Kathleen Gerson. *The Time Divide: Work, Family, and Gender Inequality*. Cambridge: Harvard University Press, 2004.

Jhally, Sut. "Imaged-Based Culture: Advertising and Popular Culture." In *Gender, Race, and Class in Media: A Text-Reader*, 2nd ed., edited by Gail Dines and Jean M. Humez, 249–257. Thousand Oaks, CA: Sage, 2003.

Johnson, Sally, Iain Williamson, Steven Lyttle, and Dawn Leeming. "Expressing Yourself: A Feminist Analysis of Talk around Expressing Breast Milk." *Social Science and Medicine* 69, no. 6 (2009): 900–907.

Johnston, Deirdre D., and Debra H. Swanson. "Cognitive Acrobatics in the Construction of Worker-Mother Identity." *Sex Roles: A Journal of Research* 57, nos. 5–6 (2007): 447–459.

Johnston, Marina L., and Noreen Esposito. "Barriers and Facilitators for Breastfeeding among Working Women in the United States." *Journal of Obstetric, Gynecologic and Neonatal Nursing* 36 (2007): 9–20.

Johnston-Robledo, Ingrid, Melissa Ball, Kimberly Lauta, and Ann Zekoll. "To Bleed or Not to Bleed: Young Women's Attitudes toward Menstrual Suppression." *Women and Health* 38, no. 3 (2003): 59–75.

Jonas, W., E. Nissen, A.-B. Ransjö-Arvidson, I. Wiklund, P. Henriksson, and K. Uvnä-Moberg. "Short- and Long-Term Decrease of Blood Pressure in Women during Breastfeeding." *Breastfeeding Medicine* 3, no. 2 (2008): 103–109.

Jones, Camara P. "Invited Commentary: 'Race,' Racism, and the Practice of Epidemiology." *American Journal of Epidemiology* 154, no. 4 (2001): 299–304, 305–306.

———. "Levels of Racism: A Theoretic Framework and a Gardener's Tale." *American Journal of Public Health* 90, no. 8 (2000): 1212–1215.

———. "The Moral Problem of Health Disparities." *American Journal of Public Health* 100, no. 1 (2010): s47–s51.

Jones, Gareth, Richard W. Steketee, Robert E. Black, Zulfiqar A. Bhutta, Saul S. Morris, and the Bellagio Child Survival Study Group. "How Many Child Deaths Can We Prevent This Year?" *Lancet* 362, no. 9377 (2003): 65–71.

Jordan, Amy B. "Social Class, Temporal Orientation, and Mass Media Use within the Family System." *Critical Studies in Mass Communication* 9, no. 4 (1992): 374–386.

Jordan, Brigitte. *Birth in Four Cultures: A Cross-Cultural Study of Child Birth in Yucatan, Holland, Sweden and the United States*. Shelborne, VT: Eden Press, 1978.

Jordan, Miriam. "Nestlé Markets Baby Formula to Hispanic Mothers in U.S." *Wall Street Journal*, March 4, 2004, sec. B.

Jordan, Pamela L., and Virginia R. Wall. "Breastfeeding and Fathers: Illuminating the Darker Side." *Birth* 17, no. 4 (1990): 210–213.

Kahn, Robbie Pfeufer. "Lessons of the Milk." In *Bearing Meaning: The Language of Birth*, 361–392. Champaign: University of Illinois Press, 1995.

Kaminis, Markos. "A Growing Boost for Baby Formula." *BusinessWeek*, January 11, 2005. http://www.businessweek.com/investor/content/jan2005/pi20050111_1011_pi008.htm.

Kang, Cindy. "Mothers Rally to Back Breast-Feeding Rights." *Washington Post*, November 22, 2006, D1.

Kantor, Jodi. "On the Job, Nursing Mothers Are Finding a 2-Class System." *New York Times*, September 1, 2006. http://www.nytimes.com.

Karlsen, Morten O., and Carin Pettersson. "Milk Record: Woman Paid for a Car with Breast Milk." *Nettavisen*, March 31, 2004. http://pub.tv2.no/nettavisen/english/article208126.ece.

Katz-Rothman, Barbara. *In Labor: Women and Power in the Birthplace*. New York: W. W. Norton & Co., 1982.

Kay, Margarita Artschwager. *Anthropology of Human Birth*. Philadelphia: Davis, 1982.

Kedrowski, Karen M., and Michael E. Lipscomb. *Breastfeeding Rights in the United States*. Westport, CT: Praeger, 2008.

Kegel, Arnold H. "Milk." *Chicago's Health* 21 (1927): 299–300.

Kelleher, Christa M. "The Physical Challenges of Early Breastfeeding." *Social Science and Medicine* 63, no. 10 (2006): 2727–2738.

Kendall-Tackett, Kathleen. "Breastfeeding and the Sexual Abuse Survivor." *Journal of Human Lactation* 14 (1998): 125–130.

Kenny, James A. "Sexuality of Pregnant and Breastfeeding Women." *Archives of Sexual Behaviour* 2, no. 3 (1973): 215–229.

Kent, George. "The High Price of Infant Formula in the United States." *Agrofood* 17, no. 5 (2006): 21–23.

———. "WIC's Promotion of Infant Formula in the United States." *International Breastfeeding Journal* 1 (2006). http://www.internationalbreastfeedingjournal.com/content/1/1/8.

Khatib-Chahibi, Jane. "Milk Kinship in Shi'ite Islamic Iran." In *The Anthropology of Breastfeeding*, edited by Vanessa Maher, 109–132. Oxford: Berg, 1992.

Kitzinger, Shelia. *Ourselves as Mothers: The Universal Experience of Motherhood*. Reading, MA: Addison-Wesley, 1995.

Klarose. "Question: How Can I Come to Terms with My Guilty Feelings about Quitting Breastfeeding?" *Mom Answers*. Babycenter. January 1, 2007, http://www.babycenter.com/400_how-can-i-come-to-terms-with-my-guilty-feelings-about-quitti_500346_1000.bc.

Klaus, Marshall H., Richard Jerauld, Nancy C. Kreger, Willie McAlpine, Meredith Steffa, and John H. Kennell. "Maternal Attachment: Importance of the First Postpartum Days." *New England Journal of Medicine* 286 (1972): 460–463.

Kleinman, Arthur. "On Caregiving." *Harvard Magazine* 29 (2010): 25–29. http://www.harvardmagazine.com/2010/07/on-caregiving.

Kleinman, Arthur, and Peter Benson. "Anthropology in the Clinic: The Problem of Cultural Competency and How to Fix It." *PloS Medicine* 3, no. 10 (2006): 673–676. http://www.plosmedicine.org.

Klingelhafer, Susan Kathleen. "Sexual Abuse and Breastfeeding." *Journal of Human Lactation* 23, no. 2 (2007): 194–197.

Klofas, John. "Community Structure, Violence and Its Prevention." Public Health Grand Rounds, Department of Community and Preventive Medicine, University of

Rochester, Winter/Spring 2009. http://www.urmc.rochester.edu/cpm/departmental-seminars/public-health-grand-rounds.cfm.

Knaak, Stephanie. "Contextualizing Risk, Constructing Choice: Breastfeeding and Good Mothering in Risk Society." *Health, Risk and Society* 12, no. 4 (2010): 345–355.

Knipe, William. H. W. "Twilight Sleep: Its Future and Relation to the General Practitioner." *American Medicine* 21 (1915): 29–32.

Kogan, Michael D., Milton Kotelchuck, Gregg R. Alexander, and Wayne E. Johnson. "Racial Disparities in Reported Prenatal Care Advice from Health Care Providers." *American Journal of Public Health* 84, no. 1 (1994): 82–88.

Koh, Howard K., Sarah C. Oppenheimer, Sarah B. Massin-Short, Karen M. Emmons, Alan C. Geller, and K. Viswanath. "Translating Research Evidence into Practice to Reduce Health Disparities: A Social Determinants Approach." *American Journal of Public Health* 100, no. 1 (2010): s72–s80.

Kotler, Philip, and Gerald Zaltman. "An Approach to Planned Social Change." *Journal of Marketing* 35 (1971): 3–12.

Krantz-Kent, Rachel. "Measuring Time Spent in Unpaid Household Work: Results from the American Time Use Survey." *Monthly Labor Review* 132, no. 7 (July 2009): 46–59.

Krieger, Nancy. "Does Racism Harm Health? Did Child Abuse Exist before 1962? On Explicit Questions, Critical Science, and Current Controversies: An Ecosocial Perspective." *American Journal of Public Health* 93, no. 2 (2003): 194–199.

Kukla, Rebecca. "Ethics and Ideology in Breastfeeding Advocacy Campaigns." *Hypatia* 21, no. 1 (2006): 157–180.

———. *Mass Hysteria: Medicine, Culture, and Mothers' Bodies*. Lanham, MD: Rowman & Littlefield, 2005.

Kunz, Thomas H., and David J. Hosken. "Male Lactation: Why, Why Not and Is It Care?" *Trends in Ecology and Evolution* 24, no. 2 (2008): 80–85.

Kuznets, Simon. "National Income, 1929–1932." 73rd Cong., 2d sess., S. Doc. 124, 1934. http://library.bea/gov/u?/SOD,888.

Labbok, Miriam H. "Breastfeeding: A Woman's Reproductive Right." *International Journal of Gynecology and Obstetrics* 94 (2006): 277–286.

———. "Transdisciplinary Breastfeeding Support: Creating Program and Policy Synergy across the Reproductive Continuum." *International Breastfeeding Journal* 3 (2008). http://www.internationalbreastfeedingjournal.com/content/3/1/16.

Labbok, Miriam H., Alfredo Perez, Veronica Valdes, Francisco Sevilla, Karen Wade, Virginia Hight Laukaran, Kristin A. Cooney, Shirley Coly, Clifford Sanders, and John T. Queenan. "The Lactational Amenorrhea Method (LAM): A Postpartum Introductory Family Planning Method with Policy and Program Implications." *Advances in Contraception* 10 (1994): 93–109.

Labbok, Miriam H., Paige Hall Smith, and Emily C. Taylor. "Breastfeeding and Feminism: A Focus on Reproductive Health, Rights and Justice." *International Breastfeeding Journal* 3 (2008). http://www.internationalbreastfeedingjournal.com/content/3/1/8.

Labbok, Miriam, and Mary Rose Tully. Interview by Linda Fentiman, August 29, 2008. Chapel Hill, NC.

Labiner-Wolfe, Judith, Sara B. Fein, Katherine R. Shealy, and Cunlin Wang. "Prevalence of Breast Milk Expression and Associated Factors." *Pediatrics* 122, no. 2 (2008): S63–S68.

Lack, Evonne. "Top 7 Mommy Guilt Trips—And How to Handle Them." Babycenter. http://www.babycenter.com/0_top-7-mommy-guilt-trips-and-how-to-handle-them_3654967.bc.

Ladd-Taylor, Molly, and Lauri Umansky. "Introduction." In *"Bad" Mothers: The Politics of Blame in Twentieth-Century America,* edited by Molly Ladd-Taylor and Lauri Umansky, 1–28. New York: New York University Press, 1998.

La Leche League International. *The Womanly Art of Breastfeeding.* 7th ed. London: Plume, Penguin Books, 2004.

Landes, Elizabeth M., and Richard A. Posner. "The Economics of the Baby Shortage." *Journal of Legal Studies* 7 (1978): 323–348.

Lane, Sandra D. *Why Are Our Babies Dying? Pregnancy, Birth and Death in America.* Boulder, CO: Paradigm Publishers, 2008.

Lasswell, Harold D. "The Structure and Function of Communication in Society." In *The Communication of Ideas,* edited by Lyman Bryson, 37–51. New York: Harper, 1948.

Lauwers, Judith, and Anna Swisher. *Counseling the Nursing Mother: A Lactation Consultant's Guide.* Boston: Jones & Bartlett, 2005.

LaVeist, Thomas, A. *Minority Populations and Health: An Introduction to Health Disparities in the U.S.* San Francisco: Jossey-Bass, 2005.

Law, Jules. "The Politics of Breastfeeding: Assessing Risk, Dividing Labor." *Signs: Journal of Women in Culture and Society* 25, no. 2 (2000): 407–450.

Lawrence, Ruth A., and Robert M. Lawrence. *Breastfeeding: A Guide for the Medical Profession.* 6th ed. Philadelphia: Elsevier Mosby, 2005.

Leavitt, Judith Walzer. *Brought to Bed: Childbearing in America, 1950–1950.* New York: Oxford University Press, 1986.

Lee, Ellie J. "Infant Feeding in Risk Society." *Health, Risk and Society* 9, no. 3 (2007): 295–309.

———. "Living with Risk in the Age of 'Intensive Motherhood': Maternal Identity and Infant Feeding." *Health, Risk and Society* 10, no. 5 (2008): 467–477.

Lee, Helen J., Irma T. Elo, Kelly F. McCollum, and Jennifer F. Culhane. "Racial/Ethnic Differences in Breastfeeding Initiation and Duration among Low-Income Inner-City Mothers." *Social Science Quarterly* 90, no. 5 (2009): 1251–1271.

Lee, Katherine. "Nursing? Eat Organic." *Working Mother,* December/January 2008, 78.

Lee, Shirley. "Health and Sickness: The Meaning of Menstruation and Premenstrual Syndrome in Women's Lives." *Sex Roles* 46, nos. 1–2 (2002): 25–35.

Lee-St. John, Jeninne. "Milk Maids." *Time,* April 19, 2007.

Lefebvre, R. Craig, and June A. Flora. "Social Marketing and Public Health Intervention." *Health Education Quarterly* 15, no. 3 (1988): 300–301.

Lengermann, Patricia M., and Jill Neibrugge-Brantley. "Contemporary Feminist Theory." In *Sociology Theory,* edited by George Ritzer, 307–355. Boston: McGraw Hill, 2000.

Lens, Vicki. "Reading between the Lines: Analyzing the Supreme Court's Views on Gender Discrimination in Employment, 1971–1982." *Social Service Review* 77 (2003): 25–50.

Lepore, Jill. "Baby Food: If Breast Is Best, Why Are Women Bottling Their Milk?" *New Yorker,* January 19, 2009. http://www.newyorker.com/reporting/2009/01/19/090119fa_fact_lepore.

Levenstein, Harvey. "'Best for Babies' or 'Preventable Infanticide'? The Controversy over Artificial Feeding of Infants in America, 1880–1920." *Journal of American History* 70 (1983): 75–94.

Lewallen, Lynne P. "Healthy Behaviors and Sources of Health Information among Low-Income Pregnant Women." *Public Health Nursing* 21, no. 3 (2004): 200–206.

Lewis, Belinda, and Damien Ridge. "Mothers Reframing Physical Activity: Family Oriented Politicism, Transgression, and Contested Expertise in Australia." *Social Science and Medicine* 60 (2005): 2295–2306.

Li, Ruowei, Fred Fridinger, and Lawrence Grummer-Strawn. "Public Perceptions on Breastfeeding Constraints." *Journal of Human Lactation* 18, no. 3 (2002): 227–235.

Li, Ruowei, Jason Hsia, Fred Fridinger, Abeda Hussain, Sandra Benton-Davis, and Laurence Grummer-Strawn. "Public Beliefs about Breastfeeding Policies in Various Settings." *Journal of the American Dietetic Association* 104 (2004): 1162–1168.

Libbus, M. Kay, and Linda F. C. Bullock. "Breastfeeding and Employment: An Assessment of Employer Attitudes." *Journal of Human Lactation* 18, no. 3 (2002): 247–251.

Liechty, Janet M., and Elaine A. Anderson. "Flexible Workplace Policies: Lessons from the Federal Alternative Work Schedules Act." *Family Relations* 56 (2007): 304–317.

Limbert, Wendy M., and Heather E. Bullock. "'Playing the Fool': A Critical Analysis of U.S. Welfare Policy." *Feminism and Psychology* 15, no. 3 (2005): 253–274.

Lindberg, Laura Duberstein. "Trends in the Relationship between Breastfeeding and Maternal Employment in the United States." *Social Biology* 43, no. 3–4 (1996): 191–202.

———. "Women's Decisions about Breastfeeding and Maternal Employment." *Journal of Marriage and the Family* 58, no. 1 (1996): 239–251.

Littman, Heidi, Sharon V. Medendorp, and Johanna Goldfarb J. "The Decision to Breastfeed: The Importance of Fathers' Approval." *Clinical Pediatrics* 33 (1994): 214–219.

Liu, Meina, and Patrice M. Buzzanell. "Negotiating Maternity Leave Expectations: Perceived Tensions between Ethics of Justice and Care." *Journal of Business Communication* 41, no. 4 (2004): 323–349.

Lloyd, Carol. "Modern-Day Wet Nursing." *Salon*, April 26, 2007. http://www.salon.com/mwt/broadsheet/2007/04/26/nursing/index.html.

Lock, Margaret. "Situating Women in the Politics of Health." In *The Politics of Women's Health: Exploring Agency and Autonomy*, edited by Susan Sherwin, 48–63. Philadelphia: Temple University Press, 1998.

Locke, Abigail. "'Natural versus Taught': Competing Discourses in Antenatal Breastfeeding Workshops." *Journal of Health Psychology* 14, no. 3 (2009): 435–446.

Locke, Jill. "Shame and the Future of Feminism." *Hypatia* 22, no. 4 (2007): 146–162.

Longhurst, Robyn. "Pregnant Bodies, Public Scrutiny." In *Embodied Geographies*, edited by Elizabeth K. Teather, 78–90. New York: Routledge, 1999.

Lopez, Iris. "An Ethnography of the Medicalization of Puerto Rican Women's Reproduction." In *Pragmatic Women and Body Politics*, edited by Margaret Lock and Patricia Kaufert, 240–259. Cambridge: Cambridge University Press, 1998.

Lorber, Judith. *Paradoxes of Gender*. New Haven, CT: Yale University Press, 1994.

Lounsbury, David W., and Shannon G. Mitchell. "Introduction to Special Issue on Social Ecological Approaches to Community Health Research and Action." *American Journal of Community Psychology* 44 (2009): 213–220.

Lu, Michael C., Linda O. Lange, Wendy Slusser, Jean Hamilton, and Neal Halfon. "Provider Encouragement of Breastfeeding: Evidence from a National Survey." *Obstetrics and Gynecology* 97 (2001): 290–295.

Lu, Michael C., Julia Prentice, Stella M. Yu, Moir Inkelas, Linda O. Lange, and Neal Halfon. "Childbirth Education Classes: Sociodemographic Disparities in Attendance and the Association of Attendance with Breastfeeding Initiation." *Maternal and Child Health Journal* 7, no. 2 (2003): 87–93.

Lupton, Deborah. "Consumerism, Commodity Culture and Health Promotion." *Health Promotion International* 9, no. 2 (1994): 111–118.

Mac1444. "Question: How Can I Come to Terms with My Guilty Feelings about Quitting Breastfeeding?" *Mom Answers*. Babycenter. April 2, 2007. http://www.babycenter.com/400_how-can-i-come-to-terms-with-my-guilty-feelings-about-quitti_500346_1000.bc.

MacDonald, Margaret. *At Work in the Field of Birth: Midwifery Narratives of Nature, Tradition, and Home.* Nashville: Vanderbilt University Press, 2007.

MacKinnon, Catharine A. *Feminism Unmodified: Discourses on Life and Law.* Cambridge, MA: Harvard University Press, 1987.

Magazine Publishers of America. "10-Year Magazine Readership Trend, 1997–2006." *Magazine Publishers of America.* http://www.magazine.org/.

Maher, Bill. "Bill Maher on Breastfeeding." *YouTube.com.* http://www.youtube.com/.

Maher, Vanessa. "Breast-Feeding in Cross-Cultural Perspective: Paradoxes and Proposals." In *The Anthropology of Breast-Feeding: Natural Law or Social Construct,* edited by Vanessa Maher, 1–36. Providence, RI: Berg Publishers, 1992.

Mahon-Daly, Patricia, and Gavin Andrews. "Liminality and Breastfeeding: Women Negotiating Space and Two Bodies." *Health and Place* 8 (2002): 61–76.

MamaBear. "Thinking of Donating Your Breastmilk? Read This First." *International Breastfeeding Symbol Blog.* September 2, 2007. http://www.breastfeedingsymbol.org/2007/09/02/thinking-of-donating-your-breastmilk-read-this-first.

Manion, Jennifer C. "Girls Blush, Sometimes: Gender, Moral Agency, and the Problem of Shame." *Hypatia* 18, no. 3 (2003): 21–41.

———. "The Moral Relevance of Shame." *American Philosophical Quarterly* 39, no. 1 (2002): 73–90.

Marmet, Chele, and Ellen Shell. "The New Lactation Professional: The Lactation Institute Training Programme." In *Programmes to Promote Breastfeeding,* edited by Derrick B. Jelliffe and E. F. Patrice Jelliffe, 323–325. Oxford: Oxford University Press, 1988.

Marshall, Joyce. L., Mary Godfrey, and Mary J. Renfrew. "Being a 'Good Mother': Managing Breastfeeding and Merging Identities." *Social Science and Medicine* 65, no. 10 (2007): 2147–2159.

Marshall, Joyce L., Mary J. Renfrew, and Mary Godfrey. "Using Evidence in Practice: What Do Health Professionals Really Do? A Study of Care and Support for Breast-feeding Women in Primary Care." In "Women's Health and Maternity Care," special issue, *Clinical Effectiveness in Nursing* 9, Supp. 2 (2006): e181–e190.

Martin, Emily. *The Woman in the Body: A Cultural Analysis of Reproduction.* Boston: Beacon Press, 1987.

Martin, Graham, Helen A. Bergen, Angela S. Richardson, Leigh Roeger, and Stephen Allison. "Sexual Abuse and Suicidality: Gender Differences in a Large Community Sample of Adolescents." *Child Abuse and Neglect* 28, no. 5 (2004): 491–503.

Martines Jose, Vinod K. Paul, Zulfiqar A. Bhutta, Marjorie Koblinsky, Agnes Soucat, Neff Walker, Rajiv Bahl, Helga Fogstad, and Anthony Costello. "Neonatal Survival: A Call for Action." *Lancet* 365, no. 9465 (2005): 1189–1197.

Masters, William H., and Virginia E. Johnson. *Human Sexual Response.* Boston: Little & Brown, 1966.

"Maternal and Child Health Pyramid of Health Services." Reprinted from *Understanding Title V of the Social Security Act.* Washington, DC: U.S. Department of Health and Human Services, Maternal and Child Health Bureau, 2008. http://www.amchp.org/AboutTitleV/Documents/MCH_Pyramid_Purple.pdf.

"Maternity Department Shows a Great Increase." *Presbyterian Hospital of the City of Chicago Bulletin* 35 (1943).

McBurney, Lesley. "Guilty Secrets." Australian Breastfeeding Association, 1999. http://www.breastfeeding.asn.au/bfinfo/guilty.html. Reprinted from *Essence* 35, no. 4 (1999).

McCaughey, Martha. "Got Milk? Breastfeeding as an 'Incurably Informed' Feminist STS Scholar." *Science as Culture* 19, no. 1 (2010): 57–78.

McClain, Valerie. "Banked Donor Human Milk, Human Rights, and Patents." *International Breastfeeding Journal* 1 (2006). http://www.internationalbreastfeedingjournal .com/content/1/1/26/comments.

McCormick, James. "Health Scares Are Bad for Your Health." In *Pleasure and the Quality of Life*, edited by David W. Warburton and Neil Sherwood, 189–198. New York: Wiley, 1996.

McGregor, Deborah Kuhn. *From Midwives to Medicine: The Birth of American Gynecology*. New Brunswick: Rutgers University Press, 1998.

McKee, Alan. "Looking for Fun in Cultural Sciences." *Cultural Science* 1, no. 2 (2008): 1–9.

McKenzie, Pamela L. "A Model of Information Practices in Accounts of Everyday-Life Information Seeking." *Journal of Documentation* 59, no. 1 (2003): 19–40.

McLaughlin, Joan E., Nancy R. Burstein, Fumiyo Tao, and Mary Kay Fox. *Breastfeeding Intervention Design Study*. Special Nutrition Programs Report Number WIC-04-BFDSN. Alexandria, VA: U.S. Department of Agriculture, Food and Nutrition Service, 2004. http://www.fns.usda.gov/ora/menu/published/wic/FILES/Breastfeeding Study.pdf.

McLean, Dan. "Breast-feeding Mom Sues Delta." *BurlingtonFreePress.com*, October 8, 2009. http://www.burlingtonfreepress.com/article/20091008/NEWS02/91007028/ Breast-feeding-mom-sues-Delta.

McLeod, Carolyn. *Self-Trust and Reproductive Autonomy*. Cambridge, MA: MIT Press, 2002.

McLeroy, Kenneth R., Daniel Bibeau, Allan Steckler, and Karen Glanz. "An Ecological Perspective on Health Promotion Programs." *Health Education Quarterly* 15, no. 4 (1988): 351–377.

McNiel, Melinda E., Miriam H. Labbok, and Sheryl W. Abrahams, "What Are the Risks Associated with Formula Feeding? A Re-Analysis and Review." *Birth* 37, no. 1 (2010): 50–58.

Meckel, Richard A. *Save the Babies: American Public Health Reform and the Prevention of Infant Mortality, 1850–1929*. Baltimore: Johns Hopkins University Press, 1990.

Meier, Paula P. "Breastfeeding in the Special Care Nursery: Prematures and Infants with Medical Problems." *Pediatric Clinics of North America* 48, no. 2 (2001): 425–442.

Mercer, Ramona T. "Becoming a Mother versus Maternal Role Attainment." *Journal of Nursing Scholarship* 36, no. 3 (2004): 226–232.

Merewood, Anne. "Race, Ethnicity, and Breastfeeding." *Pediatrics* 118, no.4 (October 1, 2006): 1742–1743.

Merewood, Anne, and Barbara L. Philipp. "Becoming Baby-Friendly: Overcoming the Issue of Accepting Free Formula." *Journal of Human Lactation* 16 (2000): 279–282.

Meyers, Diana Tietjens. "The Rush to Motherhood: Pronatalist Discourse and Women's Autonomy." *Signs* 26, no. 3 (2001): 735–773.

Mezzacappa, Elizabeth Sibolboro, Robert M. Kelsey, Edward S. Katkin. "Breast Feeding, Bottle Feeding, and Maternal Autonomic Responses to Stress." *Journal of Psychosomatic Research* 58, no. 4 (2005): 351–365.

Michie, Helena, and Naomi R. Cahn. *Confinements: Fertility and Infertility in Contemporary Culture*. New Brunswick, NJ: Rutgers University Press, 1997.

"Milk Bank Mothers Help Children throughout the World." *Capital Health News*, January 22, 2007. http://www.capitalhealth.org/news.cfm?action=detail&ref=24.

Miller, Julie. "To Stop the Slaughter of the Babies: Nathan Straus and the Drive for Pasteurized Milk, 1893–1920." *New York History* 74 (1993): 159–184.

Milligan, Renee A., Linda C. Pugh, Yvonne L. Bronner, Diane L. Spatz, and Linda P. Brown. "Breastfeeding Duration among Low Income Women." *Journal of Midwifery and Women's Health* 45, no. 3 (2000): 246–252.

Minkler, Meredith. "Linking Science and Policy through Community-Based Participatory Research to Study and Address Health Disparities." *American Journal of Public Health* 100, S1 (2010): s81–s87.

Mitchinson, Wendy. *Giving Birth in Canada, 1900–1950*. Toronto: University of Toronto Press, 2002.

Mittell, Jason. *Television and American Culture*. New York: Oxford University Press, 2010.

Mohrbacher, Nancy. "How Much Milk Should I Expect." *Breast Pumping*. Ameda. http://www.ameda.com/breast-pumping/how-much-milk-should-i-expect.

Mojab, Cynthia Good. "The Real Breastfeeding Issue Goes Far beyond Mere Guilt." *Oregonian*, July 25, 2002. http://home.comcast.net/%7Eammawell/realbreastfeeding issue.html.

Montalto, Simon Attard, Helen Borg, Mary Buttigieg-Said, and Edward J. Clemmer. "Incorrect Advice: The Most Significant Negative Determinant of Breastfeeding in Malta." *Midwifery* 26, no. 1 (2010): e6–e13.

Montgomery, Debbie L., and Patricia L. Splett. "Economic Benefit of Breastfeeding Infants Enrolled in WIC." *Journal of the American Dietetic Association* 97 (1997): 379–385.

Moriarty, Sandra E. "A Content Analysis of Visuals Used in Print Media Advertisements." *Journalism Quarterly* 64, no. 2–3 (1987): 550–554.

Morse, Janice M., and Joan L. Bottorff. "The Emotional Experience of Breast Expression." In *Qualitative Health Research*, edited by Janice M. Morse, 319–332. Newbury Park, CA: Sage, 1992.

Morsy, Soheir A. "Deadly Reproduction among Egyptian Women: Maternal Mortality and the Medicalization of Population Control." In *Conceiving the New World Order: The Global Politics of Reproduction*, edited by Faye Ginsburg and Rayna Rapp, 162–176. Berkeley: University of California Press, 1995.

Moskin, Julia. "For an All-Organic Formula, Baby, That's Sweet." *New York Times*, May 19, 2008, sec. A.

Mulford, Chris. "Swimming Upstream: Breastfeeding Care in a Nonbreastfeeding Culture." *Journal of Obstetric, Gynecologic, and Neonatal Nursing* 24, no. 5 (1995): 464–474.

Mulvihill, Kim. "Breast Milk as Cancer Treatment?" *Health Watch*. CBS 5. http://cbs5.com/health/Health.Dr.Kim.2.455691.html.

Muñoz, Sara Schaefer. "Mothers Who Share Breast Milk." *Wall Street Journal*, January 4, 2005, sec. D.

Murphy, Elizabeth. "Expertise and Forms of Knowledge in the Government of Families." *Sociological Review* 51, no. 4 (2003): 433–462.

———. "Risk, Responsibility, and Rhetoric in Infant Feeding." *Journal of Contemporary Ethnography* 29, no. 3 (2000): 291–325.

Myers, Phillip N., and Frank A. Biocca. "The Elastic Body Image: The Effects of Television Advertising and Programming on Body Image Distortions in Young Women." *Journal of Communications* 42, no. 3 (1992): 108–133.

Nakar, Sasson, Oded Peretz, Robert Hoffman, Zachi Grossmn, Boris Kaplan, and Shlomo Vinker. "Attitudes and Knowledge on Breastfeeding among Paediatricians, Family Physicians, and Gynaecologists in Israel." *Acta Paediatrica* 96 (2007): 848–851.

Naples, Nancy A. "Deconstructing and Locating Survivor Discourse: Dynamics of Narrative, Empowerment, and Resistance for Survivors of Childhood Sexual Abuse." *Journal of Women in Culture and Society* 28, no. 4 (2003): 1151–1185.

Nathoo, Tasnim, and Aleck Ostry. *The One Best Way: Breastfeeding History, Politics and Policy in Canada*. Waterloo, Canada: Wilfred Laurier University Press, 2009.

National Conference of State Legislatures. "Breastfeeding Laws." 2010. http://www
.ncsl.org/IssuesResearch/Health/BreastfeedingLaws/tabid/14389/Default.aspx.

National Health and Medical Research Council Dietary Guidelines for Children and Adolescents in Australia Incorporating the Infant Feeding Guidelines for Health Workers.
2003. http://www.nhmrc.gov.au/_files_nhmrc/file/publications/synopses/n34.pdf.

National Institutes of Health, Panel on Treatment of HIV-Infected Pregnant Women and
Prevention of Perinatal Transmission. *Recommendations for Use of Antiretroviral
Drugs in Pregnant HIV-1-Infedected Women for Maternal Health and Interventions to
Reduce Perinatal HIV Transmission in the United States*. May 24, 2010. http://
aidsinfo.nih.gov/ContentFiles/PerinatalGL.pdf.

Nattinger, Ann B., Raymond G. Hoffmann, Alicia Howell-Pelz, and James S. Goodwin.
"Effect of Nancy Reagan's Mastectomy on Choice of Surgery for Breast Cancer by U.S.
Women." *Journal of the American Medical Association* 279, no. 10 (1998): 762–767.

Negishi, H., Tatsuro Kishida, Hideto Yamada, E. Hirayama, Masato Mikuni, and
Seiichiro Fujimoto. "Changes in Uterine Size after Vaginal Delivery and Cesarean
Section Determined by Vaginal Sonography in the Puerperium." *Archives of Gyne-
cology and Obstetrics* 263, nos. 1–2 (1999): 13–16.

Nelson, Antonia M. "Transition to Motherhood." *Journal of Obstetric, Gynecologic and
Neonatal Nursing* 32 (2003): 465–477.

Newell, Franklin S. "The Effect of Overcivilization on Maternity." *American Journal of
the Medical Sciences* 136 (1908): 532–541.

Newman, Jack. *Breastfeeding and Guilt*. 2000. http://www.kellymom.com/newman/
bf_and_guilt_01–00.html.

Nisbett, Robert E. *The Geography of Thought*. New York: Free Press, 2003.

Noll, Jennie G., Penelope K. Trickett, and Frank Putnam. "A Prospective Investigation of
the Impact of Childhood Sexual Abuse on the Development of Sexuality." *Journal of
Consulting and Clinical Psychology* 71 (2003): 575–586.

Noll, Jennie G., Penelope K. Trickett, Elizabeth J. Susman, and Frank W. Putnam. "Sleep
Disturbances and Childhood Sexual Abuse." *Journal of Pediatric Psychology* 31, no. 5
(2006): 469–480.

Noor, Rushdan. "Breast Milk: Benefits and Comparison with Formula Milk." *Guide for
Women's Heath*. September 24, 2008. http://www.guide4womenshealth.com/2008/
09/breast-milk-benefits-and-comparison.html.

Nuru-Jeter, Amani, Tyan P. Dominguez, Wizdom P. Hammond, Janix Leu, Marilyn Skaff,
Susan Egerter, Camara P. Jones, and Paula Braveman. "'It's the Skin You're In':
African-American Women Talk about Their Experiences of Racism. An Exploratory
Study to Develop Measures of Racism for Birth Outcome Studies." *Maternal and Child
Health Journal* 13, no. 1 (2009): 29–39.

O'Brien, Ruth. "Other Voices at the Workplace: Gender, Disability, and an Alternative Ethic
of Care." *Signs: Journal of Women in Culture and Society* 30, no. 2 (2005): 1529–1552.

Oberman, Michelle. "When the Truth Is Not Enough: Tissue Donation, Altruism, and the
Market." *DePaul Law Review* 55, no. 3 (2006): 903–942.

Ockene, Judith K., Elizabeth A. Edgerton, Steven M. Teutsch, Lucy N. Marion, Therese
Miller, Janice L. Genevro, Carol J. Loveland-Cherry, Jonathan E. Fielding, and Peter A.
Briss. "Integrating Evidence-Based Clinical and Community Strategies to Improve
Health." *American Journal of Preventative Medicine* 32, no. 3 (2007): 244–252.

O'Connor, Barbara, and Elisabeth Klaus. "Pleasure and Meaningful Discourse: An
Overview of Research Issues." *International Journal of Cultural Studies* 3, no. 3
(2000): 369–387.

Ohene, Sally-Ann, Linda Halcon, Marjorie Ireland, Peter Carr, and Clea McNeely. "Sexual Abuse History, Risk Behavior, and Sexually Transmitted Diseases: The Impact of Age at Abuse." *Journal of the American Sexually Transmitted Disease Association* 32, no. 6 (2004): 358–363.

Oliveira, Victor. "Cost of Infant Formula for the WIC Program Rising." *Amber Waves*, November 2006. http://www.ers.usda.gov/AmberWaves/November06/Findings/Cost.htm.

Oliveira, Victor, Elizabeth Frazao, and David Smallwood. *Rising Infant Formula Costs to the WIC Program: Recent Trends in Rebates and Wholesale Prices.* Economic Research Report 93. Washington, DC: U.S. Department of Agriculture, 2010.

Oliviera, Victor, Mark Prell, David Smallwood, and Elizabeth Frazao. *WIC and the Retail Price of Infant Formula.* Food Assistance and Nutrition Research Report 1. Washington, DC: U.S. Department of Agriculture, 2005. http://www.ers.usda.gov/publications/fanrr39-1/.

Ong, Aihwa. *Neoliberalism as Exception: Mutations in Citizenship and Sovereignty.* Durham, NC: Duke University Press, 2006.

Oppenheimer, Gerald M. "Paradigm Lost: Race, Ethnicity, and the Search for a New Population Taxonomy." *American Journal of Public Health* 91, no. 7 (2001): 1049–1055.

Oppong, Christine. "A Synopsis of Seven Roles and Status of Women: An Outline of a Conceptual and Methodological Approach and a Framework for Collection and Analysis of Qualitative and Quantitative Data Relevant to Women's Productive and Reproductive Activities and Demographic Change." Paper presented at expert meeting of the United Nations Educational, Scientific and Cultural Organisation, Paris, November 25–28, 1980.

Oppong, Christine, and Katherine Abu. *Handbook for Data Collection and Analysis of the Seven Roles and Status of Women.* Population and Labour Policies Program, World Employment Program Research Working Paper No. 106, 1985.

Orbach, Susie. *Bodies.* New York: Picador, 2009.

Orent, Wendy. "A Formula to Put Babies at Risk: The Bush Administration Squelched Ads that Promoted the Benefits of Breast-Feeding." *Los Angeles Times*, September 30, 2007. http://articles.latimes.com/2007/sep/30/opinion/op-orent30.

Ortiz, Joan, Kathryn McGilligan, and Patricia Kelly. "Duration of Milk Expression among Working Mothers Enrolled in an Employer-Sponsored Lactation Program." *Pediatric Nursing* 30 (2004): 111–119.

Ortner, Sherry B. "Gender Hegemonies." In *Making Gender: The Politics and Erotics of Culture,* by Sherry B. Ortner, 139–172. Boston: Beacon Press, 1996.

Oshaug Arne, and Grete Botten. "Human Milk in Food Supply Statistics." *Food Policy* 19, no. 5 (1994): 479–482.

Ott, Brian. "(Re)locating Pleasure in Media Studies: Toward an Erotics of Reading." *Communication and Critical/Cultural Studies* 1, no. 2 (2004): 194–212.

Page, David C. "Breastfeeding in Early Functional Jaw Orthopaedics (An Introduction)." *Functional Orthodontist* 18, no 3 (2001): 24–27.

Pain, Rachel, Cathy Bailey, and Graham Mowl. 2001. "Infant Feeding in North East England: Contested Spaces of Reproduction." *Area* 33, no. 3 (2001): 261–272.

Palmer, Gabrielle. *The Politics of Breastfeeding: When Breasts Are Bad for Business.* 3rd ed. London: Pinter and Martin, 2009.

Palmer, Gabrielle, and Saskia Kemp. "Breastfeeding Promotion and the Role of the Professional Midwife." In *Baby Friendly/Mother Friendly: Perspectives in International Midwifery,* edited by Susan F. Murray, 1–18. London: Mosby, 1996.

Park, Alice. "Why the U.S. Gets a D on Preterm Birth Rates." *Time*, November 17, 2009. http://www.time.com/time/health/article/0,8599,1940140,00html.

Parker, Rozsika. *Torn in Two: The Experience of Maternal Ambivalence*. London: Virago Press, 1995.

Parkes, Peter. "Alternative Social Structures and Foster Relations in the Hindu Kush: Milk Kinship Allegiance in Former Mountain Kingdoms of Northern Pakistan." *Comparative Studies in Society and History* 43, no. 1 (2001): 4–36.

Pascale, Celine-Marie. *Cartographies of Knowledge: Exploring Qualitative Epistemologies*. Los Angeles: Sage Publications, 2010.

Patient Protection and Affordable Health Care Act. Pub. L. 118-148, s.4207 (2010).

Patton, Carla, Margaret Beaman, Norma Csar, and Charlotte Lewinski. "Nurses' Attitudes and Behaviors that Promote Breastfeeding." *Journal of Human Lactation* 12, no. 2 (1996): 111–115.

Payne, Cynthia. "Japanese Culture and Breastfeeding." *New Beginnings* 20, no. 5 (2003): 181.

Pearce, Tralee. "Breast Friend." *Toronto Globe and Mail*, May 1, 2007, sec. L.

PEI Advisory Council on the Status of Women. "Women and Unpaid Work—Milestones in Canada." http://www.gov.pe.ca/photos/original/acsw_paid_full.pdf.

Perry-Jenkins, Maureen. "Work in the Working Class: Challenges Facing Families." In *Work, Family, Health and Well-being*, edited by Suzanne M. Bianchi, Lynne M. Casper, and Rosalind B. King, 453–472. New York: Routledge, 2003.

Phares, Tanya M., Brian Morrow, Amy Lansky, Wanda D. Barfield, Cheryl B. Prince, Kristen S. Marchi, Paula A. Braveman, Letitia M. Williams, and Brooke Kinniburg. "Surveillance for Disparities in Maternal Health Related Behaviors—Selected States, Pregnancy Risk Assessment Monitoring System (PRAMS), 2000–2001." *Morbidity and Mortality Weekly Report* 53, no. 4 (2004): 1–13.

PhD in Parenting. "Sabotage." Weblog, 2009. http://www.phdinparenting.com/2009/05/04/Sabotage.

Pheifer, Pat. "Breast-feeding Mother Says Maplewood Restaurant Told Her to Cover Up." *Star Tribune*, April 7, 2010. http://www.startribune.com/.

Philipp, Barbara L., Anne Merewood, Lisa W. Miller, Neetu Chawla, Melissa M. Murphy-Smith, Jenifer S. Gomes, Sabrina Cimo, and John T. Cook. "Baby-Friendly Hospital Initiative Improves Breastfeeding Initiation Rates in a US Hospital Setting." *Pediatrics* 108 (2001): 677–680.

Philpott, Anne, Wendy Knerr, and Vicky Boydell. "Pleasure and Prevention: When Good Sex Is Safer Sex." *Reproductive Health Matters* 14, no. 28 (2006): 23–31.

Pinkston, Ashley Nicole. "Being Cyborg, Teaching Writing: Figuring a Feminist Practice in the Computer Composition Classroom." Master's thesis, North Carolina State University, 2004. http://www.lib.ncsu.edu/theses/available/etd-11232004-171817/unrestricted/etd.pdf.

Pollak, Michael. "A Mother's Memory." *New York Times*, May 14, 2006, 14.

Poncher, H. G. "Relation to Supplementary Feeding in the Newborn." *Illinois Medical Journal* 70 (1936): 258–261.

Porter, Donna V. "Breast-Feeding: Impact on Health, Employment and Society." Congressional Research Service. Report for Congress, RL32002, July 18, 2003. http://maloney.house.gov/documents/olddocs/breastfeeding/CRS_Report_on_Benefits_of_Breastfeeding.pdf.

Potter, Beth, Judy Sheeshka, and Ruta Valaitis. "Content Analysis of Infant Feeding Messages in a Canadian Women's Magazine, 1945 to 1995." *Journal of Nutrition Education* 32 (2000): 196–203.

Prentice, Julia C., Michael C. Lu, Linda Lange, and Neal Halfon. "The Association between Reported Childhood Sexual Abuse and Breastfeeding Initiation." *Journal of Human Lactation* 18, no. 3 (2002): 219–226.

Prentiss, D. W. "A Report of Five Hundred Consecutive Cases of Labor in Private Practice, in the District of Columbia, between the Years 1864 and 1888." *American Journal of Obstetrics and Diseases of Women and Children* 21 (1888): 956–970.

Pridham, Karen F. "Transition to Being the Mother of a New Infant in the First Three Months: Maternal Problem Solving and Self-Appraisals." *Journal of Advanced Nursing* 17, no. 2 (1992): 204–216.

Profitt, Norma Jean. *Women Survivors, Psychological Trauma, and the Politics of Resistance.* Binghamton, NY: Haworth Press, 2000.

Prolacta Bioscience, Inc. "Prolacta Bioscience Closes on Over $5 Million in Private Funding." News release, May 23, 2007. http://www.prolacta.com/pressreleases.php.

———. "Prolacta Bioscience Closes on Over $5 Million in Private Funding." News release, October 4, 2006. http://www.prolacta.com/pressreleases.php.

———. "Research and Development." *Prolacta Bioscience: Advancing the Science of Human Milk.* http://www.prolacta.com/research.php.

———. "Standardized Human Milk Formulations." *Prolacta Bioscience: Advancing the Science of Human Milk.* http://www.prolacta.com/humanmilk.php.

Pugin, Edda, Verónica Valdés, Miriam H. Labbok, Alfredo Pérez, and Ricardo Aravena. "Does Parental Breastfeeding Skills Group Education Increase the Effectiveness of a Comprehensive Breastfeeding Promotion Program?" *Journal of Human Lactation* 12, no. 1 (March 1996). 15–19.

Quandt, Sara A. "Patterns of Variation in Breast-Feeding Behaviors." *Social Science and Medicine* 23, no. 5 (1986): 445–453.

Racine, Elizabeth, Kevin Frick, Joanne F. Guthrie, and Donna Strobino. "Individual Net-Benefit Maximization: A Model for Understanding Breastfeeding Cessation among Low-Income Women." *Maternal Child Health* 13 (2009): 241–249.

Radey, Melissa, and Karin L. Brewster. "The Influence of Race/Ethnicity on Disadvantaged Mothers Child Care Arrangements." *Early Childhood Research Quarterly* 22, no. 3 (2007): 279–293.

Radin, Margaret. "Contested Commodities." In *Rethinking Commodification: Cases and Readings in Law and Culture,* edited by Martha M. Ertman and Joan C. Williams, 81–95. New York: New York University, 2005.

Ragin, Charles. *Fuzzy-Set Social Science.* Chicago: University of Chicago Press, 2000.

Raisler, Jeanne. "Against the Odds: Breastfeeding Experiences of Low Income Mothers." *Journal of Midwifery and Women's Health* 45, no. 3 (2000): 253–263.

Raisler, Jeanne, Cheryl Alexander, and Patricia O'Campo. "Breastfeeding and Infant Illness: A Dose-Response Relationship?" *American Journal of Public Health* 89 (1999): 25–30.

Raj, Roop. "Nursing Mom: Target Called the Cops." *MyFoxDetroit.com*, November 30, 2009. http://www.myfoxdetroit.com/dpp/news/breast-feeding-incident-at-local-target.

Randall, Clyde L. *Developments in the Certification of Obstetricians and Gynecologists in the United States, 1930–1980: The American Board of Obstetrics and Gynecology.* Washington, DC: American Board of Obstetrics and Gynecology, 1989.

Rapp, Rayna. "Moral Pioneers: Women, Men, and Fetuses on a Frontier of Reproductive Technology." In *Gender at the Crossroads of Knowledge: Feminist Anthropology in the Postmodern Era,* edited by Micaela di Leonardo, 383–395. Berkeley: University of California Press, 1991.

Razavi, Shahra. "The Political and Social Economy of Care in a Development Context: Conceptual Issues, Research Questions and Policy Options." Gender and Development Programme Paper Number 3. Geneva: United Nations Research Institute for Social Development, 2007. http://www.unrisd.org/80256B3C005BCCF9/(http AuxPages)/2DBE6A93350A7783C12573240036D5A0/$file/Razavi-paper.pdf.

Regales, Jackie. "Nursing at Starbucks: An Interview with Lorig Charkoudian." *hipmama.com*. http://hipmama.com/node/8598.

Rempel, Lynn A., and John K. Rempel. "Partner Influence on Health Behavior Decision Making: Increasing Breastfeeding Duration." *Journal of Social and Personal Relationships* 21, no. 1 (2004): 92–111.

Renfrew, Mary J., Mike W. Woolridge, and Helen Ross McGill. *Enabling Women to Breastfeed: A Review of Practices Which Promote or Inhibit Breastfeeding—With Evidence-Based Guidance for Practice*. London: Stationery Office, 2000.

Reskin, Barbara F. "Occupational Segregation by Race and Ethnicity among Women Workers." In *Latinas and African American Women at Work*, edited by Irene Browne, 183–204. New York: Russell Sage Foundation, 1999.

Reyes, Sonia. "Organic Baby Formula Segment Growing Fast: Wal-Mart, Similac, Hain Celestial Ga-Ga over 'Yoga Mommies.'" *BrandWeek*, October 2, 2006.

Riad, Sally. "Under the Desk: On Becoming a Mother in the Workplace." *Culture and Organization* 15, no. 4 (2007): 475–512.

Rideout, Victoria. "Television as a Health Educator: A Case Study of *Grey's Anatomy*." *A Kaiser Family Foundation Report*. September 16, 2008. http://www.kff.org/ent-media/upload/7803.pdf.

Rion, Hanna. *The Truth about Twilight Sleep*. New York: McBride, Nast & Co., 1915.

Riordan, Jan. "Breastfeeding Education." In *Breastfeeding and Human Lactation*, 4th ed., edited by Jan Riordan and Karen Wambach, 689–712. Boston, MA: Jones & Bartlett, 2010.
———. *Breastfeeding and Human Lactation*. 3rd ed. Boston: Jones & Bartlett, 2005.

Riordan, Jan, and Kathleen Auerbach. *Breastfeeding and Human Lactation*. Boston: Jones & Bartlett, 1993.
———. "Lactation Consultant Certification Candidates: The Influence of Background Characteristics on Test Scores." *Birth* 14, no. 4 (1987): 196–198.

Riordan, Jan, and Karen Wambach, eds. *Breastfeeding and Human Lactation*. 4th ed. Boston: Jones & Bartlett, 2010.

Riordan, Janice M., and Emily T. Rapp. "Pleasure and Purpose: The Sensuousness of Breastfeeding." *Journal of Obstetric and Gynecological Nursing* 9, no. 2 (1980): 109–112.

Rippeyoung, Phyllis L. F. "Feeding the State: Breastfeeding and Women's Well-Being in Context." *Journal of the Association for Research on Mothering* 11, no. 1 (2009): 36–48.

Riss, Suzanne, Teresa Palagano, and Angela Ebron, eds. "Fifty Best Law Firms for Women." *Working Mother*, August–September 2007, 67–91.

Roberts, Dorothy E. "The Social and Moral Cost of Mass Incarceration in African American Communities." *Stanford Law Review* 56 (2004): 1271–1305.
———. "Spiritual and Menial Housework." *Yale Journal of Law and Feminism* 9 (1997): 51–80.

Rodgers, Mary F., and Susan E. Chase. "Mothers, Sexuality, and Eros." In *Mothers and Children Feminist Analyses and Personal Narratives*, edited by Susan E. Chase and Mary F. Rodgers, 115–134. New Brunswick: Rutgers University Press, 2001.

Roe, Brian, Leslie A. Whittington, Sara Beck Fein, and Mario F. Teisl. "Is There Competition between Breastfeeding and Maternal Employment?" *Demography* 36 (1999): 157–171.

Rojjanasrirat, Wilaiporn. "Working Women's Breastfeeding Experiences." *MCN: The American Journal of Maternal Child Nursing* 29, no. 4 (2004): 222–227.

Rosenberg, Kenneth D., Carissa A. Eastham, Laurin J. Kasehagen, and Alfredo P. Sandoval. "Marketing Infant Formula through Hospitals: The Impact of Commercial Hospital Discharge Packs on Breastfeeding." *American Journal of Public Health* 98, no. 2 (2008): 290–295.

Rosin, Hanna. "The Case Against Breast-Feeding." *Atlantic Online*, April, 2009. http://www.theatlantic.com/doc/200904/case-against-breastfeeding.

Rotch, Thomas Morgan. *Pediatrics: The Hygienic and Medical Treatment of Children.* Philadelphia: J. B. Lippincott Co., 1896.

———. "The Value of Milk Laboratories for the Advancement of Our Knowledge of Artificial Feeding." *Archives of Pediatrics* 10 (1893): 97–111.

Rubio, Mercedes, and David R. Williams. "The Social Dimension of Race." In *Race and Research*, edited by Bettina Beech and Maurine Goodman, 1–26. Washington, DC: American Public Health Association, 2004.

Ruccadog. "I Stopped Breastfeeding My Baby Today." *July 2009 Birth Club.* Babycenter Community. July 11, 2009. community.babycenter.com/post/a11831855/i_stopped_breastfeeding_my_baby_today.

Russett, Cynthia Eagle. *Sexual Science: The Victorian Construction of Womanhood.* Cambridge, MA: Harvard University Press, 1989.

Ryan, Alan S., and Wenjun Zhou. "Lower Breastfeeding Rates Persist among the Special Supplemental Nutrition Program for Women, Infants, and Children Participants, 1978–2003." *Pediatrics* 117, no. 4 (2006): 1136–1146.

Ryan, Alan S., Wenjun Zhou, and Mary Beth Arensberg. "The Effect of Employment Status on Breastfeeding in the United States." *Women's Health Issues* 16 (2006): 243–251.

Ryan, Kath, Paul Bissell, and Jo Alexander. "Moral Work in Women's Narratives of Breastfeeding." *Social Science and Medicine* 70, no. 6 (2010): 951–958.

Ryser, Faun G. "Breastfeeding Attitudes, Intention, and Initiation in Low-Income Women: The Effect of the Best Start Program." *Journal of Human Lactation* 20, no. 3 (2004): 300–305.

Saha, Prantik. "Breastfeeding and Sexuality: Professional Advice Literature from the 1970s to the Present." *Health Education and Behaviour* 29, no. 1 (2002): 61–72.

Saini, A. N. "U.S. Television Product Placements Declined by 15% in the First Half of 2008." *Journal of Promotion Management* 14 (2008): 77–83.

Salmon, Marylynn. "The Cultural Significance of Breastfeeding and Infant Care in Early Modern England and America." *Journal of Social History* 18 (1994): 247–269.

Samuels, Gina M., and Fariyal Ross-Sheriff. "Identity, Oppression, and Power: Feminisms and Intersectionality Theory." *Journal of Women and Social Work* 23 (2008): 5–9.

Sandel, Michael J. "What Money Can't Buy: The Moral Limits of Markets." In *Rethinking Commodification: Cases and Readings in Law and Culture*, edited by Martha M. Ertman and Joan C. Williams, 122–127. New York: New York University, 2005.

San Jose Mercury News. "Protests Mount over Facebook Ban on Breast-Feeding Photos." December 27, 2008. http://www.mercurynews.com/.

Scanlon, Karen S., Laurence Grummer-Strawn, Rowena Li, J. Chen, N. Molinari, and C. G. Perrine. "Racial and Ethnic Differences in Breastfeeding Initiation and Duration, by State—National Immunization Survey, United States, 2004–2008." *Morbidity and Mortality Weekly Report* 59, no. 11 (2010): 327–334.

Schanler, Richard J., Karen G. O'Connor, and Ruth A. Lawrence. "Pediatricians' Practices and Attitudes Regarding Breastfeeding Promotion." *Pediatrics* 103, no. 3 (1999): e35.

Scheper-Hughes, Nancy. *Death without Weeping: The Violence of Everyday Life in Brazil.* Berkeley: University of California Press, 1992.

Schmied, Virginia, and Lesley Barclay. "Connection and Pleasure, Disruption and Distress: Women's Experience of Breastfeeding." *Journal of Human Lactation* 15, no. 4 (1999): 325–334.

Schmied, Virginia, and Deborah Lupton. "Blurring the Boundaries: Breastfeeding and Maternal Subjectivity." *Sociology of Health and Illness* 23, no. 2 (2001): 234–250.

Schmidt, Johanna. "Gendering in Infant Feeding Discourses: The Good Mother and the Absent Father." *New Zealand Sociology* 23, no. 2 (2008): 61–74.

Schneider, Anne L., and Helen M. Ingram. *Policy Design for Democracy.* Lawrence: University of Kansas Press, 1997.

Schultz, Amy, Edith Parker, Barbara Israel, and Tomkio Fisher. "Social Context, Stressors and Disparities in Women's Health." *Journal of the American Medical Women's Association* 56 (2001): 143–149.

Scott, Jane A., and Tricia Mostyn. "Women's Experiences of Breastfeeding in a Bottle-Feeding Culture." *Journal of Human Lactation* 19, no. 3 (2003): 270–277.

Seavey, Heather. "Mother Exposed for Breastfeeding." *WCSH6.com.* August 20, 2009. http://www.wcsh6.com/news/health/story.aspx?storyid=108332.

Sedlak, Andrea J., Jane Mettenburg, Monica Basena, Karla McPherson, Angela Greene and Spencer Li. *Fourth National Incidence Study of Child Abuse and Neglect (NIS–4): Report to Congress.* Washington, DC: U.S. Department of Health and Human Services, Administration for Children and Families, 2010.

"Service Extended by Milk Bureau." *New York Times*, March 10, 1935, sec N.

Shaw, Rhonda. "The Virtues of Cross-Nursing and the 'Yuk Factor.'" *Australian Feminist Studies* 19, no. 45 (2004): 287–299.

Shealy, Katherine R., Rouwei Li, Sandra Benton-Davis, and Lawrence M. Grummer-Strawn. *The CDC Guide to Breastfeeding Interventions.* Atlanta: Centers for Disease Control and Prevention, 2005.

Sheehan, Athena, Virginia Schmied, and Margaret Cooke. "Australian Women's Stories of Their Baby-Feeding Decisions in Pregnancy." *Midwifery* 19 (2003): 259–266.

Sheeshka, Judy, Beth Potter, Emilie Norrie, Ruta Valaitis, Gerald Adams, and Leon Kuczynski. "Women's Experiences Breastfeeding in Public Places." *Journal of Human Lactation* 17, no. 1 (2001): 31–38.

Shildrick, Margrit. *Leaky Bodies and Boundaries: Feminism, Post-Modernism and (Bio) Ethics.* New York: Routledge, 1997.

Sibeko, Lindiwe, Anna Coutsoudis, S'phindile Nzuza, and Katherine Gray-Donald. "Mothers' Infant Feeding Experiences: Constraints and Supports for Optimal Feeding in an HIV-Impacted Urban Community in South Africa." *Public Health Nutrition* 12, no. 11 (2009): 1983–1990.

Sibeko, Lindiwe, Mohammed Ali Dhansay, Karen E. Charlton, Timothy Johns, and Katherine Gray-Donald. "Beliefs, Attitudes, and Practices of Breastfeeding Mothers from a Periurban Community in South Africa." *Journal of Human Lactation* 21, no. 1 (2005): 31–38.

Siegel, Matt. "Formula for Disaster." *American Lawyer* 16, no. 1 (1994): 63.

Sievert, Lynnette Leidy. "The Medicalization of Female Fertility: Points of Significance for the Study of Menopause." *Collegium Antropologicum* 27, no. 1 (2003): 67–78.

Silbaugh, Katharine A. "Commodification and Women's Household Labor." In *Rethinking Commodification: Cases and Readings in Law and Culture*, edited by Martha M. Ertman and Joan C. Williams, 297–302. New York: New York University, 2005.

Simkin, Penny. *When Survivors Give Birth: Understanding and Healing the Effects of Early Sexual Abuse on Childbearing Women*. Seattle: Classic Day, 2004.

Singh, Gopal K., Michael D. Kogan, and Deborah L. Dee. "Nativity/Immigrant Status, Race/Ethnicity, and Socioeconomic Determinants of Breastfeeding Initiation and Duration in the United States, 2003." *Pediatrics* 119, supplement 1 (2007): 538–546.

Slater, Shelly. "Breast Milk Used to Treat Cancer Patients." News story. WFAA Channel 8, Dallas. February 16, 2008. http://www.wfaa.com/sharedcontent/dws/news/local-news/tv/stories/wfaa080215_lj_breastmilk.c618de8d.html.

Slaw, Robin. "1999 LLLI Conference Sessions: Promoting Breastfeeding or Promoting Guilt?" *New Beginnings* 16, no. 5 (1999): 171. http://www.llli.org/NB/NBSepOct99 p171.html.

Sloan, Seaneen, Helga Sneddon, Moira Stewart, and Dorota Iwaniec. "Breast Is Best? Reasons Why Mothers Decide to Breastfeed or Bottlefeed Their Babies and Factors Influencing the Duration of Breastfeeding." *Child Care in Practice* 12 (2006): 283–297.

Sloan Work and Family Research Network. "Glossary." *References and Research*. wfnetwork.bc.edu/glossary_entry.php?term=Carework,%20Definition(s)%20of&area=All.

———. "Questions and Answers about Child Care: A Sloan Work and Family Research Network Fact Sheet." July 2008. http://wfnetwork.bc.edu/pdfs/childcare.pdf.

Smale, Mary. "The Stigmatisation of Breastfeeding." In *Stigma and Social Exclusion in Healthcare*, edited by Tom Mason, Caroline Carlisle, Caroline Watkins, and Elizabeth Whitehead, 234–245. New York: Routledge, 2001.

Smedley, Brian D., Adrienne Y. Stith, and Alan R. Nelson, eds. *Unequal Treatment: Confronting Racial and Ethnic Disparities in Health Care*. National Institute of Medicine. Washington, DC: National Academies Press, 2003.

Smith, Julie. "Mothers' Milk and Markets." *Australian Feminist Studies* 19, no. 45 (2004): 369–379.

Smith, Julie P., and Lindy H. Ingraham. "Mother's Milk and Measures of Economic Output." *Feminist Economics* 11, no. 1 (2005): 41–62.

Smith, Linda T. *Decolonizing Methodologies: Research and Indigenous Peoples*. New York: Zed Books, 1999.

Smith, Paige, Miriam Labbok, Susan Cupito, Ea Nwokah, and Sheryl Coley. "Choosing Feeding: Enhancing Breastfeeding Education for Teen Mothers." Presentation, American Public Health Association Annual Conference, Denver, November 2010.

Smyth, Lisa. "Gendered Spaces and Intimate Citizenship: The Case of Breastfeeding." *European Journal of Women's Studies* 15, no. 2 (2008): 83–99.

———. "Intimate Citizenship and the Right to Care: The Case of Breastfeeding." In *Intimate Citizenship: Gender, Sexualities, Politics*, edited by Elzbieta H. Olesky, 118–132. New York: Routledge, 2009.

Soumerai, Stephen B., Dennis Ross-Degnan, and Jessica S. Kahn. "The Effects of Professional and Media Warnings About the Association between Aspirin Use in Children and Reye's Syndrome." In *Public Health Communication: Evidence for Behavior Change*, edited by Robert Hornik, 265–288. Mahwah, NJ: Lawrence Erlbaum Associates, 2002.

Sparks, P. Johnelle. "Rural-Urban Differences in Breastfeeding Initiation in the United States." *Journal of Human Lactation* 26, no. 2 (2010): 118–129.

Spataro, Josie, Philip M. Burgess, David L. Wells, and Simon A. Moss. "Impact of Child Sexual Abuse on Mental Health: Prospective Study in Males and Females." *British Journal of Psychiatry* 184 (2004): 416–421.

Spitzer, Denise L. "In Visible Bodies: Minority Women, Nurses, Time and the New Economy of Care." *Medical Anthropology Quarterly* 18, no. 4 (2004): 490–508.

Stander, H. J. "Undergraduate and Graduate Instruction in Obstetrics and Gynecology." *American Journal of Obstetrics and Gynecology* 51 (1946): 771–779.

Stanway, Penny. *Breast Is Best*. London: Pan Macmillan, 2005.

Starr, Paul. *The Social Transformation of American Medicine: The Rise of a Sovereign Profession and the Making of a Vast Industry*. New York: Basic Books, 1982.

Stearns, Cindy A. "Breastfeeding and the Good Maternal Body." *Gender and Society* 13, no. 3 (1999): 308–325.

Steffensmeier, Renee Hoffman. "A Role Model of the Transition to Parenthood." *Journal of Marriage and Family* 44, no. 2 (1982): 31–34.

Steingraber, Sandra. "The Benefits of Breast Milk Outweigh Any Risks." *Healthy Child Healthy World Blog*. August 1, 2010. http://healthychild.org/blog/comments/the_benefits_of_breast_milk_outweigh_any_risks/.

Stern, Linda. "Breast-Feeding Supplies Deductible, U.S. IRS Rules." Reuters. February 10, 2011. http://blogs.reuters.com/linda-stern/.

Stevens, Rosemary. *American Medicine and the Public Interest*. New Haven, CT: Yale University Press, 1971.

Stiglitz, Joseph E., Amartya Sen, and Jean-Paul Fitoussi. "Report by the Commission on the Measurement of Economic Performance and Social Progress." September 14, 2009. http://www.stiglitz-sen-fitoussi.fr/en/index.htm.

Stobbe, Mike. "AP Impact: More U.S. Babies Born, Fertility Rate Up, Defying Low-Birth Trend in Europe." *San Diego Union Tribune*, January 15, 2007. http://www.signonsandiego.com/news/nation/20080115-2055-babyboomlet.html.

Stone, Deborah. *Policy Paradox: The Art of Political Decision Making*. Rev. ed. New York: Norton, 1997.

Sullivan, Gerald. "Of External Habits and Maternal Attitudes: Margaret Mead, Gestalt Psychology, and the Reproduction of Character." *Pacific Studies* 32, nos. 2–3 (2009): 222–250.

Sullivan, Sandra. "A Historically Controlled Cohort Study of a Novel Breast-Milk Based Human Milk Fortifier in Pre-Term Infants: Effects of Growth, Respiratory Status, and ROP." Poster, the American Academy of Pediatrics National Conference and Exhibition, Boston, October 10, 2008.

Sundstrom, Kathy. "Breast Milk Used in Cancer Fight." *Peaceful Parenting Blog*. 2009. http://drmomma.blogspot.com/2009/08/breast-milk-used-in-cancer-fight.html.

Sutherland, Katherine. "Of Milk and Miracles: Nursing, the Life Drive, and Subjectivity." *Frontiers* 20, no. 2 (1999): 1–20.

Sweet, Linda. "Breastfeeding a Preterm Infant and the Objectification of Breast Milk." *Breastfeeding Review* 14 (2006): 5–13.

Taylor, Emily C. *Constraints to Exclusive Breastfeeding: Findings and Recommendations*. Poster, American Public Health Association Annual Meeting, Philadelphia, November 2011. http://apha.confex.com/apha/137am/recordingredirect.cgi/32972.

Teather, Elizabeth K., ed. *Embodied Geographies: Spaces, Bodies, and Rites of Passage*. New York: Routledge, 1999.

Teghtsoonian, Katherine. "Promises, Promises: 'Choices for Women' in Canadian and American Child Care Policy Debates." *Feminist Studies* 22, no. 1 (1996): 119–147.

Thomas, Sari, and Brian P. Callahan. "Allocating Happiness: TV Families and Social Class." *Journal of Communication* 32, no. 3 (1982): 184–190.

Thulier, Diane, and Judith Mercer. "Variables Associated with Breastfeeding Duration." *Journal of Obstetric, Gynecologic and Neonatal Nursing* 38 (2009): 259–268.

Tierney, John. "Message in What We Buy, But Nobody's Listening." *New York Times*, May 19, 2009, sec. D.

Today Food. "Chef Dishes up Breast-Milk Cheese." March 9, 2010. today.msnbc.msn .com/id/35778477/ns/today-today_food_and_wine/.

Toledo, Elizabeth, and Jan Erickson. "NOW Demands Greater Acceptance and Access for Breastfeeding Mothers." *National NOW Times*, Summer 1998. http://www.now.org/ nnt/05–98/breastfd.html.

Tomaselli, Keyan G., Lauren Dyll, and Michael Francis. "Self and Other: Auto-Reflexive and Indigenous Ethnography." In *Handbook of Critical and Indigenous Methodologies*, compiled by Norman K. Denzin, Yvonna S. Lincoln, and Linda Tuhiwai Smith, 347–372. Los Angeles: Sage, 2008.

Torres, Jennifer. "Pumps and Scales: The Medicalization of Breastfeeding and the Ideology of Insufficient Milk." American Sociological Association Annual Meeting, San Francisco, August 8, 2009.

Tow, Abraham. "The Rationale of Breast Feeding: A Modern Concept." *Hygeia* 12 (1934): 406–408.

Traina, Christina. "Maternal Experience and the Boundaries of Christian Sexual Ethics." *Signs: Journal of Women in Culture and Society* 25, no. 2 (2000): 369–405.

Triolo, Nancy. "Fascist Unionization and the Professionalization of Midwives in Italy: A Sicilian Case Study." *Medical Anthropology Quarterly* 8, no. 3 (1994): 259–281.

Tucker, Beatrice E., and Harry B. Benaron. "Maternal Mortality of the Chicago Maternity Center." *American Journal of Public Health* 27 (1937): 33–36.

Tünte, Markus. "Man's Work in a Female World? Gender Paradoxes of Male Childcare Workers." *Gender Forum* 17 (2007). http://www.genderforum.org/no_cache/issues/ working-out-gender/a-mans-work-in-a-female-world/.

Turner, Heather A. "The Significance of Employment for Chronic Stress and Psychological Distress among Rural Single Moms." *American Journal of Community Psychology* 40 (2007): 181–193.

UK Department of Health. *Maternal and Infant Nutrition*. 2010. http://www.dh.gov .uk/en/Healthcare/Children/Maternity/Maternalandinfantnutrition/index.htm.

UN Research Institute for Social Development. "Political and Social Economy of Care." 2009. http://www.unrisd.org/80256B3C005BB128/(httpProjects)/37BD128E275F1F8 BC1257296003210EC?OpenDocument.

U.S. Breastfeeding Committee. "USBC Applauds Workplace Breastfeeding Support Provision in Health Care Reform." News release, April 1, 2010. http://www.usbreast feeding.org/NewsInformation/NewsRoom/201004WorkplaceBreastfeedingSupport Provision/tabid/177/Default.aspx.

U.S. Department of Agriculture, Food and Nutrition Service. "WIC at a Glance." *About WIC*. 2011. http://www.fns.usda.gov/wic/aboutwic/wicataglance.htm.

U.S. Department of Health and Human Services. "News Release," January 20, 2011. http://www.hhs.gov/news/press/2011pres/01/20110120a.html.

———. *The Surgeon General's Call to Action to Support Breastfeeding*. Washington, DC: U.S. Department of Health and Human Services, Office of the Surgeon General, 2011.

———. "A Systematic Approach to Health Improvement." In *Healthy People 2010*, 2nd ed., 1:6. Washington, DC: Government Printing Office, 2000.

U.S. Department of Health and Human Services, Centers for Disease Control and Prevention. "Adverse Childhood Experiences (ACE) Study: Prevalence of Individual Adverse Childhood Experiences: Data and Statistics." 2010. http://www.cdc.gov/nccdphp/ace/prevalence.htm.

———. "Breastfeeding among U.S. Children Born 1999–2006, CDC National Immunization Survey." 2010. http://www.cdc.gov/breastfeeding/data/NIS_data/index.htm.

———. "A Framework for Assessing the Effectiveness of Disease and Injury Prevention." *Morbidity and Mortality Weekly Reports* 41 (March 27, 1992): 1

———. *Healthy People 2010.* 2nd ed. Washington, DC: Government Printing Office, 2000. http://www.healthypeople.gov/Document/tableofcontents.htm.

———. *Healthy People 2020 Summary of Objectives: Maternal, Infant, and Child Health.* 2011. http://healthypeople.gov/2020/topicsobjectives2020/pdfs/MaternalChild Health.pdf.

U.S. Department of Health and Human Services, National Institute of Mental Health. *Television and Behavior: Ten Years of Scientific Progress and Implications for the Eighties* (DHHS Publication No. ADM 82-11985). Washington, DC: U.S. Government Printing Office, 1982.

U.S. Department of Health and Human Services, Office on Women's Health. *Breastfeeding: HHS Blueprint for Action on Breastfeeding.* 2000. http://www.womenshealth.gov/archive/breastfeeding/programs/blueprints/bluprntbk2.pdf.

———. "The Business Case for Breastfeeding Steps for Creating a Breastfeeding Friendly Worksite." *Women's health.gov.* 2010. http://www.womenshealth.gov/breastfeeding/government-programs/business-case-for-breastfeeding/index.cfm.

———. "'Log Rolling' Spot Transcript." 2010. http://www.womenshealth.gov/breastfeeding/government-programs/national-breastfeeding-campaign/adcouncil/transcript_logroll.cfm.

———. "National Breastfeeding Campaign." 2010. http://www.womenshealth.gov/breastfeeding/government-programs/national-breastfeeding-campaign.

U.S. Department of Labor, Bureau of Labor Statistics. "Labor Force Participation of Mothers with Infants in 2008." *TED: The Editor's Desk*, May 29, 2009, http://www.bls.gov/opub/ted/2009/may/wk4/art04.htm.

U.S. Department of Labor, Bureau of Labor Statistics. "Labor Force Characteristics by Race and Ethnicity, 2008." Report Number 1020, November 2009, http://www.bls.gov/cps/cpsrace2008.pdf.

U.S. Government Accountability Office. *Breastfeeding: Some Strategies Used to Market Infant Formula May Discourage Breastfeeding; State Contracts Should Better Protect Against Misuse of WIC Name.* Report to Congressional Addressees. Washington, DC: U.S. Government Accountability Office, 2006.

Van Esterik, Penny. *Beyond the Breast-Bottle Controversy.* New Brunswick, NJ: Rutgers University Press, 1989.

———. "Breastfeeding and Feminism." *International Journal of Gynecology and Obstetrics* 47, no. 1 (1994): s41–s54.

———. "Contemporary Trends in Infant Feeding Research." *Annual Review of Anthropology* 31 (2002): 257–278.

———. "Expressing Ourselves: Breast Pumps." *Journal of Human Lactation* 12, no. 4 (1996): 273–274.

———. "Thank You Breasts: Breastfeeding as a Global Feminist Issue." In *Ethnographic Feminisms*, edited by Sally Cole and Lynne Philips, 75–91. Ottawa: Carleton University Press, 1995.

Van Esterik, Penny, and Terry Elliot. "Infant Feeding Style in Urban Kenya." *Ecology of Food and Nutrition* 18, no. 3 (1986): 183–195.

Van Esterik, Penny, and Ted Greiner. "Breastfeeding and Women's Work: Constraints and Opportunities." Special Issue: Breastfeeding: Program, Policy, and Research Issues. *Studies in Family Planning* 12, no. 4 (1981): 184–197.

Van Gennep, Arnold. *The Rites of Passage.* Chicago: University of Chicago Press, 1960.

Van Hollen, Cecilia. *Birth on the Threshold: Childbirth and Modernity in South India.* Berkeley: University of California Press, 2003.

Vance, Melissa R. "Breastfeeding Legislation in the United States: A General Overview and Implications for Helping Mothers." *Leaven* 41, vol. 3 (2005): 51–54.

Vesely, Colleen. "Child Care and Development Fund: A Policy Analysis." *Journal of Sociology and Social Welfare* 36, no. 1 (2009): 39–59.

Vogel, Lise. "Debating Difference: Feminism, Pregnancy and the Workplace." *Feminist Studies* 16, no. 1 (1990): 9–32.

Waggoner, Miranda. "Emergence of a Gendered Profession: The Work of Lactation Consultants and New Expert Knowledge." American Sociological Association Annual Meeting, Boston, July 31, 2008.

Wagner, Marsden. *Born in the USA: How a Broken Maternity System Must Be Fixed to Put Women and Children First.* Berkeley: University of California Press, 2006.

Walker, Marsha. "Breast Pumps and Other Technologies." In *Breastfeeding and Human Lactation*, 4th ed., edited by Jan Riordan and Karen Wambach, 379–407. Sudbury, MA: Jones & Bartlett, 2010.

Wall, Glenda. "Moral Constructions of Mothers in Breastfeeding Discourse." *Gender and Society* 15, no. 4 (2001): 592–610.

Wallace, Louise M., Orla M. Dunn, Elizabeth M. Alder, Sally Inch, Robert K. Hills, and Susan M. Law. "Breastfeeding Best Start Randomized Controlled Trial of a Midwifery Intervention to Promote the Duration of Breastfeeding in Primiparous Mothers in England." *Midwifery* 22 (2006): 262–273.

Wallace, Louise M., and Joanna Kosmala-Anderson. "A Training Needs Survey of Doctors' Breastfeeding Support Skills in England." *Maternal and Child Nutrition* 2 (2006): 217–231.

Wambach, Karen, Suzanne Hetzel Campbell, Sara L. Gill, Joan E. Dodgson, Titilayo C. Abiona, and M. Jane Heining. "Clinical Lactation Practice: 20 Years of Evidence." *Journal of Human Lactation* 21, no. 3 (2005): 245–258.

Warburton, David M., and Neil Sherwood, eds. *Pleasure and the Quality of Life.* New York: Wiley, 1996.

Ward, Kate A., Judith E. Adams, M. Zulf Mughal. "Bone Status during Adolescence, Pregnancy, and Lactation." *Current Opinion in Obstetrics and Gynecology* 17, no. 4 (2005): 435–439.

Waring, Marilyn. *Counting for Nothing: What Men Value and What Women Are Worth.* Toronto: University of Toronto Press, 1988.

Warner, Dorothy, and J. Drew Procaccino. "Toward Wellness: Women Seeking Health Information." *Journal of the American Society for Information Science and Technology* 55, no. 8 (2004): 709–730.

Warner, W. Lloyd, and Paul S. Lunt. *The Social Life of a Modern Community.* New Haven, CT: Yale University Press, 1941.

Waserman, Manfred J. "Henry L. Coit and the Certified Milk Movement in the Development of Modern Pediatrics." *Bulletin of the History of Medicine* 46 (1972): 359–390.

Weichert. Carol, "Sexual Arousal from Breast-Feeding." *Medical Aspects of Human Sexuality* 11 (1977): 99.

Weimer, Douglas R. "Summary of State Breastfeeding Laws and Related Issues." Congressional Research Service. Report for Congress, RL31633. January 12, 2005. http://maloney.house.gov/documents/olddocs/breastfeeding/050505CRSReport.pdf.

Weinreich, Nedra Kline. "What Is Social Marketing?" *Weinreich Communications* (2010). http://www.social-marketing.com/Whatis.html.

Weisskopf, Susan (Contratto). "Maternal Sexuality and Asexual Motherhood." *Signs* 5, no. 4 (1980): 766–782.

Whit, Angela. "Breast Milk Cures Pink Eye (Conjunctivitis)." *Blisstree*, November 30, 2006. http://www.blisstree.com/breastfeeding123/breast-milk-cures-pink-eye-conjunctivitis.

Whit, Angela. "Should You Support the International Breast Milk Project?" *Blisstree*, June 4, 2007. http://www.blisstree.com/breastfeeding123/should-you-support-the-international-breast-milk-project.

Whitaker, Elizabeth Dixon. *Measuring Mamma's Milk: Fascism and the Medicalization of Maternity in Italy*. Ann Arbor: University of Michigan Press, 2000.

Whiteford, Linda, and Lois Gonzalez. "Stigma: The Hidden Burden of Infertility." *Social Science and Medicine* 40, no. 1 (1995): 27–36.

Whitehead, Dean. "In Pursuit of Pleasure: Health Education as a Means of Facilitating the 'Health Journey' of Young People." *Health Education* 105, no. 3 (2005): 213–227.

Wiessinger, Diane. "A Breastfeeding Teaching Tool Using Sandwich Analogy for Latch-On." *Journal of Human Lactation* 14 (1998): 51–56.

———. "Watch Your Language!" *Journal of Human Lactation* 12, no. 1 (1996): 1–4.

Wight, Nancy E. "The Guilt Issue." San Diego County Breastfeeding Coalition, n.d. http://66.63.136.173/articles/guilt.html.

Williams, David R., and Michelle Sternthal. "Understanding Racial-Ethnic Disparities in Health: Sociological Contributions." *Journal of Health and Social Behavior* 51 (2010): S15–27.

Williams, Joan. "A Reconstructive Feminism: Reconstructing the Relationship of Market Work and Family Work." *Northern Illinois University Law Review* 19 (1998): 89–108.

———. *Unbending Gender: Why Family and Work Conflict and What to Do about It*. New York: Oxford University Press, 2000.

Williams, Joan C., and Heather Boushey. *The Three Faces of Work-Family Conflict: The Poor, the Professionals, and the Missing Middle*. Center for American Progress and Work Life Law, 2010. http://www.worklifelaw.org/pubs/ThreeFacesofWorkFamilyConflict.pdf.

Williams, Wendy W. "Equality's Riddle: Pregnancy and the Equal Treatment/Special Treatment Debate." *NYU Review of Law and Social Change*. Reprinted in *Feminist Legal Theory Foundations*, edited by D. Kelly Weisberg, 128–155. Philadelphia: Temple University Press, 1993.

Wilson, Doreen, and Anne Colquhoun. "Influences in the Decision to Breastfeed: A Study of Pregnant Women and Their Feeding Intentions." *Nutrition and Food Science* 98, no. 4 (1998): 185–192.

Win, Nwet N., Colin W. Binns, Yun Zhao, Jane A. Scott, and Wendy H. Oddy. "Breastfeeding Duration in Mothers Who Express Breast Milk: A Cohort Study." *International Breastfeeding Journal* 1 (2006). http://www.internationalbreastfeedingjournal.com/content/1/1/28/comments.

Wing, Adrien Katherine, and Laura Weselmann. "Transcending Traditional Notions of Mothering: The Need for Critical Race Feminist Praxis." *Journal of Gender, Race, and Justice* 3 (1999): 257–263.

Winslow, Charles-Edward Amory. "The Untilled Fields of Public Health," *Science* 51 (1920): 23.

Winsten, Jay A. "Promoting Designated Drivers: The Harvard Alcohol Project." *American Journal of Preventive Medicine* 10, no. 3 (1994): 11–14.

Wolf, Jacqueline H. *Deliver Me from Pain: Anesthesia and Birth in America.* Baltimore: Johns Hopkins University Press, 2009.

———. *Don't Kill Your Baby: Public Health and the Decline of Breastfeeding in the Nineteenth and Twentieth Centuries.* Columbus: Ohio State University Press, 2001.

———. "Got Milk? Not in Public!" *International Breastfeeding Journal* 3, no. 11 (2008). http://www.international breastfeedingjournal.com/content/3/1/11.

———. *Is Breast Best? Taking on the Breastfeeding Experts and the New High Stakes of Motherhood.* New York: New York University Press, 2011.

———. "Is Breast Really Best? Risk and Total Motherhood in the National Breastfeeding Awareness Campaign." *Journal of Health Politics, Policy, and Law* 32, no. 4 (2007): 595–636.

Wolf, Joan B. "Low Breastfeeding Rates and Public Health in the United States." *American Journal of Public Health* 93, no. 12 (2003): 2000–2010.

———. "What Feminists Can Do for Breastfeeding and What Breastfeeding Can Do for Feminists." *Signs* 31, no. 2 (2006): 397–424.

Working Mother. "2007 Working Mother 100 Best Companies Hall of Fame." November 2007. 75–80.

World Health Organization. "Constitution of the World Health Organization." *Basic Documents.* 45th ed. Geneva: WHO Press, 2006. http://www.who.int/governance/eb/who_constitution_en.pdf.

———. "Definition of Health." Preamble to the Constitution of the World Health Organization as adopted by the International Health Conference, New York, June 19–22, 1946; signed on July 22, 1946, by the representatives of 61 States (Official Records of the World Health Organization, no. 2, p. 100) and entered into force on April 7, 1948.

———. *Evidence for the Ten Steps to Successful Breastfeeding.* Geneva: WHO Press, 1998.

———. "Infant and Young Child Feeding Data by Country." *WHO Global Data Bank on Infant and Young Child Feeding.* 2011. http://www.who.int/nutrition/databases/infantfeeding/countries/en/index.html.

———. *International Code of Marketing of Breast-Milk Substitutes.* Geneva: WHO Press, 1981.

World Health Organization and UNICEF. *Global Strategy for Infant and Young Child Feeding.* Geneva: WHO Press, 2003.

World Health Organization and UNICEF. *Innocenti Declaration on the Protection, Promotion and Support of Breastfeeding.* 1990. http://www.unicef.org/programme/breastfeeding/innocenti.htm.

———. "Protecting, Promoting and Supporting Breastfeeding. The Special Role of Maternity Services." Geneva: WHO Press, UNICEF, 1989.

Wright, Peter W. G. "Babyhood: The Social Construction of Infant Care as a Medical Problem in England in the Years around 1900." In *Biomedicine Examined*, edited by Margaret Lock and Deborah Gordon, 299–329. Dordrecht: Kluwer, 1988.

"Writer Doesn't Want to See Moms Nursing at Starbucks." *Starbucks Gossip: Monitoring America's Favorite Drug Dealer.* August 11, 2004. http://starbucksgossip.typepad .com/_/2004/08/writer_doesnt_w.html.

Young, Iris Marion. "Breasted Experience: The Look and the Feeling." In *On Female Body Experience: "Throwing Like a Girl" and Other Essays,* 75–96. New York: Oxford University Press, 2005.

Young, Kathryn T. "American Conceptions of Infant Development from 1995 to 1984: What the Experts Are Telling Parents." *Child Development* 61 (1990): 17–28.

YouTube. "Breast Is Best—The Graham Norton Show—Preview—BBC One." http://www.youtube.com/watch?v=1R1c8pn4KIc.

————. "U Tampon by Kotex, Produced by the Brandshop." March 2008. http://www .youtube.com/watch?v=mxkUE5TtOFQ.

Ziegler, Charles Edward. "How Can We Best Solve the Midwifery Problem." *American Journal of Public Health* 12 (1922): 409.

————. "The Teaching of Obstetrics." *American Journal of Obstetrics and Diseases of Women and Children* 73 (1916): 50–57.

Zita, Jacquelyn N. "The Premenstrual Syndrome: 'Dis-easing' the Female Cycle." In "Feminism and Science, Part 2," special issue, *Hypatia* 3, no. 1 (March 1988): 77–99.

Zola, Irving Kenneth. *Socio-Medical Inquiries: Recollections, Reflections, and Reconsiderations.* Philadelphia: Temple University Press, 1983.

Notes on Contributors

Nancy Chin, PhD, MPH, is an associate professor in the Department of Community and Preventive Medicine at the University of Rochester School of Medicine and an associate of the Susan B. Anthony Institute at the University of Rochester. An anthropologist by training, Professor Chin's work focuses on the intersection of gender, social class, culture, and health. She has conducted ethnographic fieldwork on gender and health in Ladakh, Antarctica, Tibet, and Rochester, New York.

Joan E. Dodgson, PhD, FAAN, is an associate professor at the College of Nursing and Health Innovation at Arizona State University. She is a perinatal and lactation clinical specialist and a breastfeeding researcher who has conducted federally funded studies related to historic changes in infant feeding behavior, as well as the effects of culture on infant feeding and perinatal health disparities over the past twenty years.

Ann Dozier, PhD, works in the School of Medicine and Dentistry at the University of Rochester. Her current research and fieldwork focus is program evaluation methods, including integration of qualitative and quantitative research methods, and maternal child health outcomes.

Sally Dowling, MA, MPH, has an academic and work background in nursing and public health. She is currently a faculty member of the Department of Nursing and Midwifery, University of the West of England, Bristol. She has worked for many years in the National Health Service (NHS) in a variety of roles, most recently in Public Health, and is a member of the faculty of Public Health of the Royal College of Physicians of London. Her research interests include experiences of breastfeeding, breastfeeding in public, and the use of online methods in qualitative research.

N. Danielle Duckett is finishing a PhD in sociology at the University of Kentucky in 2012. Her dissertation concerns the ways in which breastfeeding decisions affect the identity work performed by new mothers in Appalachia. Most of her previous research has been in the field of domestic violence, where her work has been published in *Violence and Victims*, *Homicide Studies*, and *Violence Against Women*. She teaches courses in sociology, as well as gender and women's studies, at several colleges and universities in the Bluegrass Region of Kentucky.

Aimee R. Eden is a doctoral candidate in the Department of Anthropology at the University of South Florida, where she is also working on her MPH in maternal-child health. She is engaged in breastfeeding-related work in her community and at the international level, serving on boards of directors of the International Board of Lactation Consultant Examiners (IBLCE) and the Kids Healthcare Foundation.

She holds a master's degree in international development from Ohio University and is a returned Peace Corps volunteer (Kazakhstan 2000–2002).

Linda C. Fentiman, JD, LLM, is the James D. Hopkins Professor at Pace University Law School in New York, specializing in health care law. She has also taught at the law schools of Columbia University, the University of Houston, Suffolk University, and the University of Warsaw in Poland, where she was a Fulbright Scholar. She has written extensively about bioethics, health care access and regulation, mental disability law, and criminal law, and is a Fellow of the New York Academy of Medicine. In 2010 she was a visiting scholar at the Center for Reproductive Rights in New York.

Katherine A. Foss, PhD, is an assistant professor, Department of Journalism, Middle Tennessee State University, where she serves as graduate faculty and Women's Studies faculty. Her research interests include media representations of breastfeeding, constructions of deafness and hearing loss in television, influence of historical context on fictional television programming, media constructions of health responsibility, and victimization and gender in contemporary television.

Fiona Giles, PhD, is a senior lecturer in the Department of Media and Communications at Sydney University. She is the author of *Fresh Milk: The Secret Life of Breasts* and "The Uses of Pleasure: Reconfiguring Lactation, Sexuality and Mothering," in *Theorising and Representing Maternal Realities.*

Danielle Groleau, PhD, is an associate professor at McGill University in the Faculty of Medicine, Division of Social and Transcultural Psychiatry, and is a member of the Family Medicine Department. She is also senior investigator at the Culture and Mental Health Unit, Lady Davis Medical Institute, Jewish General Hospital, Montreal. She serves on the editorial board of the journal *Transcultural Psychiatry* and has graduate training in Medical Anthropology, Public Health, and Transcultural Psychiatry. She has completed multiple research projects on breastfeeding among Vietnamese immigrants, low-income French Canadians, and mothers of low birth weight babies in Canada and Brazil.

Bernice L. Hausman, PhD, is professor of English at Virginia Tech and professor in the Department of Interprofessionalism at the Virginia Tech Carilion School of Medicine. She is author of *Changing Sex: Transsexualism, Technology, and the Idea of Gender; Mother's Milk: Breastfeeding Controversies in American Culture;* and *Viral Mothers: Breastfeeding in the Age of HIV/AIDS.* She has served as director of the Women's Studies program at Virginia Tech and currently coordinates the undergraduate minor in medicine and society. Her current research includes collaborative projects on vaccination controversies and the rhetoric of genetic testing.

Carol Grace Hurst, PhD, is a social work educator and a clinical social worker. She teaches for a private behavioral health care company corporate training division and as an adjunct instructor with Virginia Commonwealth University School of Social Work.

Sally Johnson, PhD, is a lecturer in psychology at the University of Bradford, United Kingdom. She has previously worked in psychology teaching and research posts at the University of Hull, University of Northampton, and Leeds Metropolitan University in the United Kingdom. Her research interests are in feminist and qualitative approaches to women's reproductive health, specifically bodily changes as a result of pregnancy, breastfeeding, and menstruation; the female body; and motherhood.

Miriam Labbok, MD, MPH, is professor of maternal and child health and director of the Carolina Global Breastfeeding Institute at the University of North Carolina at Chapel Hill. Previously, she served as senior advisor to Infant and Young Child Feeding and Care, UNICEF, and chief of Maternal Health and Nutrition, USAID, as well as faculty at Georgetown and Johns Hopkins. She has nearly three hundred chapters, books, refereed articles, abstracts, and monographs in print.

Dawn Leeming, PhD, is a senior lecturer in the Psychology and Counselling Division at Huddersfield University in the United Kingdom. She has previously worked elsewhere in the United Kingdom in academic posts within psychology and health and as a clinical psychologist within a community mental health team. Currently, she is researching women's experiences of breastfeeding, the management and repair of shame, and the impact of mental health stigma on users of mental health services.

Abigail Locke, PhD, is a principal lecturer in psychology at the University of Huddersfield, United Kingdom. Her current work focuses on the representation of parenting in health care and popular culture. She has studied the representations of infant feeding in antenatal classes, choice and risk in antenatal care, and constructions of the parenting role. She has a wider interest in discourse analysis and qualitative methodologies applied to health care, gender, emotion, and parenting, and has recently cofounded the Institute for Health Citizenship at the University of Huddersfield.

Amanda Marie Lubold is a graduate research assistant, Department of Sociology, University of Arizona. Previously she served as Mental Health Worker II at Children's Home of York, Tindall House Program, York, Pennsylvania.

Jennifer C. Lucas, PhD, is an assistant professor of politics at Saint Anselm College. Her research interests include congressional politics and women and politics, and her research on gender differences in attitudes toward negative advertising has appeared in *American Politics Research*. She teaches courses on American politics, including campaigns and elections, research methods, women and politics, and congressional politics.

Steven Lyttle, PhD, is a principal lecturer in psychology and head of the Division of Psychology at De Montfort University in Leicester, United Kingdom. He is a developmental psychologist with an interest in infancy and childhood. His research includes studies of the development of very low birth weight children, young people's images of a range of legal and illegal substances, and the lived experience of breastfeeding in first-time mothers. Steven is a graduate member of the British Psychological Society and the Society's Graduate Education Committee.

Deborah McCarter-Spaulding, PhD, is an associate professor of nursing at Saint Anselm College in Manchester, New Hampshire. She teaches childbearing in both the classroom and in the clinical setting. She has been an International Board Certified Lactation Consultant (IBCLC) for over twenty years and uses her breastfeeding knowledge both for teaching and research and in her clinical practice as a per diem nurse at Catholic Medical Center. Her most current research addresses breastfeeding self-efficacy in African American women.

Chris Mulford, IBCLC and mother of two grown children, was a breastfeeding activist from 1970 to 2011. She retired from work as a nurse and international board-certified lactation consultant in a hospital setting, private practice, and the WIC program. Her volunteer experience included La Leche League, state breastfeeding coalitions, the U.S. Breastfeeding Committee, and the Women and Work Task Force at WABA (World Alliance for Breastfeeding Action). She died suddenly in fall 2011.

Jennie Naidoo, PhD, is principal lecturer in Health Promotion and Public Health at the University of the West of England, Bristol. A sociologist, she was employed as a researcher and health promotion officer with the NHS before joining UWE. Her research interests include the evaluation of health promotion interventions designed to address socioeconomic inequalities, and she is a best-selling author of health promotion textbooks.

Mary C. Noonan, PhD, is an associate professor of sociology at the University of Iowa. Her current research focuses on the sex-based earnings and promotion gaps among lawyers. Other work examines the relationship between work-family policies and earnings. She teaches courses on gender, family, and quantitative methods.

David Pontin, PhD, holds the Aneurin Bevan Chair in Community Health at the University of Glamorgan, in partnership with the Aneurin Bevan Health Board, Wales. His research interests include child health and community nursing. He is an associate of the ALSPAC (Avon Longitudinal Survey of Parents and Children) project based in Bristol and has published work on breastfeeding based on ALSPAC data. He has been a Public Health Nurse in the United Kingdom and has worked with mothers and local communities to support breastfeeding.

Phyllis L. F. Rippeyoung, PhD, is an associate professor in the Department of Sociology and Anthropology at the University of Ottawa. Her research is in the area of social stratification, with a particular interest in the relationships between work, education, and politics on gender and racial inequality. Her current focus is on the complex relationship between breastfeeding and women's paid and unpaid labor. She teaches courses on research methods, work, and gender.

Louise Marie Roth, PhD, is an associate professor of sociology at the University of Arizona. Her primary research interests are gender, family, organizations, and law. Her earlier work analyzed gender inequality on Wall Street, and her publications include *Selling Women Short: Gender Inequality on Wall Street*. Her current research analyzes American medicine, with a focus on birth.

Lindiwe Sibeko, PhD, is currently a Canadian Institutes of Health Research postdoctoral fellow in social and transcultural psychiatry at McGill University, as well as a dietitian-nutritionist and an international board certified lactation consultant. Her research interests center on the health of vulnerable populations, with a focus on understanding the impact of poverty on the health of women and children, their family structures, and social networks. Her fieldwork has taken place in peri-urban and settlement communities in South Africa, with marginalized HIV-infected and affected women.

Paige Hall Smith, MSPH, PhD, is the director of the Center for Women's Health and Wellness, and associate professor of public health education at the University of North Carolina at Greensboro, where she also has a faculty appointment in the Women's and Gender Studies Program. In 2004 she was the recipient of the Linda Arnold Carlisle Professorship in Women's and Gender Studies at UNCG. She codirects the Breastfeeding and Feminism Symposia and is also the cochair of the Gender Working Group of the World Alliance for Breastfeeding Action. She has received federal, state, and local funding for her research on breastfeeding, violence against women, and women's reproductive health.

Emily C. Taylor, MPH, is the senior programs director at the Carolina Global Breastfeeding Institute, in the Department of Maternal and Child Health, Gillings School of Global Public Health, University of North Carolina at Chapel Hill, and has been a principal organizer for the Breastfeeding and Feminism Symposia series.

Erin N. Taylor, PhD, is an assistant professor of political science at Western Illinois University. Her early research used feminist analyses of caretaking and liberal theory to examine the ideology and rhetoric of the childfree movement. More recently, she has turned to feminist moral philosophy for insight into guilt as it relates to breastfeeding advocacy. She teaches courses in American government, political thought, and citizenship.

Penny Van Esterik, PhD, is professor of anthropology at York University, Toronto, where she teaches nutritional anthropology, advocacy anthropology, and feminist theory. Past books include *Beyond the Breast-Bottle Controversy*, *Materializing Thailand*, *Taking Refuge: Lao Buddhists in North America*, and *Food and Culture: A Reader*, edited with Carole Counihan. She is a founding member of World Alliance for Breastfeeding Action and has been active in developing articles and advocacy materials on breastfeeding and women's work, breastfeeding and feminism, and contemporary challenges to infant feeding.

Lora Ebert Wallace, PhD, is an associate professor of sociology at Western Illinois University. Her recent research has focused on the medicalization of infant feeding and feminist approaches to understanding changes in the medical institution and health behaviors. She teaches classes in medical sociology, sociology of mental health, sociology of women's health, sociology of family, introductory sociology, and sociological research methods.

Iain Williamson, PhD, is a chartered psychologist and registered practitioner psychologist and works at De Montfort University, Leicester, United Kingdom, where he is the program director for the MSc Health Psychology. His interests are primarily in the areas of health representations and experiences among minority and marginalized communities, with a focus on infant feeding and maternal well-being, eating difficulties across the lifespan, and various aspects of lesbian and gay health. He is a member of the International Society for Critical Health Psychology and also acts as an expert member of a regional National Health Service Research Committee.

Jacqueline H. Wolf, PhD, is professor of the history of medicine and chair of the Department of Social Medicine at Ohio University. She specializes in the history of women's health, children's health, and public health. She is the author of many articles on the history of breastfeeding practices and the effect of those practices on public health. She is also the author of two books: *Don't Kill Your Baby: Public Health and the Decline of Breastfeeding in the 19th and 20th Centuries* and *Deliver Me from Pain: Anesthesia and Birth in America.*

Index

Abbott Labs, 172
Abt, Isaac, 88
Ad Council, 227
African American: culture, 75; women, 10, 64, 76, 79, 170
American Academy of Pediatrics (AAP), 125, 170, 172, 173, 193, 226, 266
American Association for the Study and Prevention of Infant Mortality, 89
American Association of Obstetricians and Gynecologists, 93
American Board of Obstetrics and Gynecology, 94; formed, 93
American Gynecological Society, 92, 93
American Medical Association Council of Medical Education, 93
American Pediatric Society, 91
Arendt, Hannah, 264
Arora, Samir, 227
Artis, Julie, 15
Asian women, 56, 145
Assess, Act, and Adapt Model, 43
Association of Schools of Public Health, 40
Auerbach, Kathleen, 54, 56
Augustine, 262
Australian Breastfeeding Association, 216
Australian National Breastfeeding Strategy, 215

Baby-Friendly Hospital Initiative (BFHI), 111, 174
Badinter, Elisabeth, 140
Baer, Edward, 196
Bartky, Sandra, 197, 198
Bartlett, Alison, 183
Bateson, Gregory, 59
behavior change, individual, 1, 25, 39, 43, 44, 227
Benjamin, Regina M., 8, 48
Berkeley Media Studies Group, 149
Best for Babes, 266, 267

Best Start, 81
biomedical system, 99, 102, 103, 107
biomedicine, 62; culture of, 61
black women, 5, 6, 70, 145, 158. *See also under* African American
Blum, Linda, 16, 185
bonding, 60, 135, 136, 139, 182, 185, 186, 199, 200, 206, 223, 230, 256, 261, 273
bottle-feeding culture, 7
Bottorf, Joan, 182
Bourdieu, Pierre, 203, 204
boxification, 56, 57
breast cancer, 95, 227
breastfeeding, benefits of, 8, 16, 21, 72, 89, 204, 205, 131, 133, 135, 140, 145, 148, 170, 175, 177, 186, 195, 205, 216–220, 226, 227, 233, 240–243
Breastfeeding Best Start (UK), 111
breastfeeding disparities, 74, 78, 81, 82; ethnic, 157, 159; racial, 145, 157, 158, 159; socioeconomic, 157, 159
"breastfeeding Nazis," 4
breastfeeding practices, 4, 22, 25, 26, 31, 34, 82, 208, 210, 211n28, 256
Breastfeeding Promotion Act, 151
breastfeeding style, 54, 55
"breast is best," 8, 62, 68, 72, 117, 170, 182, 249, 281
breast pump, 66, 70–72, 98, 104, 106, 125, 134, 147, 150, 152, 164, 183, 186, 205, 228, 231, 284
Brown, Jane, 228, 229, 232
Business Case for Breastfeeding, 8, 147

Cahn, Naomi, 238, 243
caregivers, 123, 128, 129
caregiving, 123, 124, 126, 128, 129
carework, 28–30, 123, 124, 127, 128, 130, 131; in Canada, measured, 127, 128
Carter, Pam, 16, 198
Cartesian duality, 80
cathexis, 31–33

Cesarean birth, 46, 47, 59, 182, 271, 275
Childbirth Education Association
   (CEA), 127
child care, 27, 28, 30, 125, 154, 163, 164,
   200, 241; as gendered activity, 125,
   133; father involvement in, 135–141;
   policy, 153
Child Care Development Fund, 153
childhood sexual abuse, 10, 269–279
child rearing, 124–126
choice, xi, 5, 6, 18, 19, 64, 149, 158, 169,
   195, 206, 239, 260, 281, 284; informed,
   110, 112, 116, 141, 149, 153; rhetoric
   of, 148
Civil Rights Act, Title VII, 151
class, social, 4, 9, 37, 81, 144, 150, 154, 159,
   208, 238; defined, 237
Clinton, Bill and Hillary, 263
Coalition for Improving Maternity
   Services, 47
Collette, Toni, 215
Collins, Patricia Hill, 151
commodification, 174, 175
Connell, R. W., 26, 28–32
Convention on the Elimination of All
   Forms of Discrimination Against
   Women (CEDAW), 42
Convention on the Rights of the
   Child, 48
Crenshaw, Kimberlé Williams, 81
critical race scholarship, 175
cultivation theory, 228

Daly, Mary, 128
Deigh, John, 197
DeLee, Joseph, 87, 92, 95
Department of Health and Aging,
   Australia, 215
depression, 69–71
Descartes, 262
Determinants of Health Models, 43, 44
difference framework, 149
disability, 5, 32, 150, 152
Discovery Health Channel, 229
domestic violence, 69
Doucet, Andrea, 139
Draper, Susan B., 136
Dykes, Fiona, 183

Early Childhood Longitudinal study—Birth
   Cohort survey, 137; described, 142n14
Edwards, John and Elizabeth, 263
Elson, Diane, 130
employment, xii, 10, 42, 43, 71, 72, 128,
   132, 142n17, 145, 161, 251, 264, 265,
   285; characteristics, 154; gendered, 125;
   mothers and, xiii, 27, 31, 144, 243, 282,
   283, 284
England, Paula, 128
equality framework, 149, 158
equality vs. difference debate, xiii
Ertman, Martha, 174
ethnography, 57, 61, 63; defined 55, 56
exclusive breastfeeding, xii, 36, 37, 42, 111,
   129, 131, 145, 146, 208, 209

Facebook, 260, 266
Family and Medical Leave Act (FMLA),
   153, 158
feeding schedules, 90
femininity, 29, 34, 54, 175, 198, 219
feminism: defined, 2, 53, 55;
   standpoint, 2
FirstRight, 266
Fitoussi, Jean-Paul, 123, 131
Fletcher, Joyce, 29
Folbre, Nancy, 128
Forbes, Bettina, 266
formula: history of the word, 91; as norm,
   xii, 39, 100, 226–228, 232, 250, 252; risks
   of, 38, 65, 67, 72, 195, 227, 283
Foucault, Michel, 6, 203, 208, 210, 217,
   218; power/knowledge, 207; scholarship
   influenced by, 21

Galtung, Johan, 65
gender, xi, 4, 5, 7, 9, 23, 26, 75, 81, 125, 133,
   150, 252; beliefs, 124; domestic labor
   and, 133, 141; equality, 23, 24n27, 124;
   equity, 25, 48, 141, 283, 285; gap, 133;
   inequality, 25, 31, 33, 53, 61, 134;
   inequity, 74, 283; roles, 134, 136,
   282, 283; theory of gendered
   organizations, 157
Gerbner, George, 228
Global Strategy for Infant and Young Child
   Feeding, 48

good mother, concept of, 15, 19–22, 32, 33, 181, 185, 187, 200, 201, 204, 208, 209, 266, 281, 283
Goodwin, Michelle, 175
Greer, Germaine, 283
Greiner, Ted, 25
guilt, 2, 193, 194–199, 206, 254
gynecology, 93–95

Haraway, Donna, 2, 186
Hausman, Bernice, 141, 196, 200, 239
Healthy People 2010, goals for breastfeeding, 42, 260
Healthy People 2020, 106
Himmelweit, Susan, 125
Hispanics, 56, 79, 145. See also Latinas
HIV, 37, 65, 106, 171, 209, 227
Huber, Joan, 134

ideal worker, 29, 30, 32, 149, 157, 158
ideology, 2–4, 6, 9, 11n4, 15–23, 54, 140, 195, 208, 259, 262, 263, 282; of masculinity, 34
individualism, 206, 207
inequality, xi, 3, 25, 29, 30, 32, 53, 74, 81, 141, 142, 244; racial and socioeconomic, 150
Infant Feeding Practices Study II (IFPS II), 160, 162
Innocenti Declaration, 48, 252
insufficient milk, 90
intensive mothering, 208
International Board Certified Lactation Consultant (IBCLC), 99, 100, 101, 106
International Board of Lactation Consultant Examiners (IBLCE), 100, 105
International Breast Milk Project, 172
International Code of Marketing of Breast-milk Substitutes, 48, 215, 252
International Labor Organization (ILO), 26, 125, 128, 129
International Lactation Consultant Association (ILCA), 98, 101, 104
International MotherBaby Childbirth Organization, 47
Internet, 140
intersectionality, 5, 74, 80, 81, 150

Jacknowitz, Alison, 159
jaundice, 231
Jones, Camara P., 75
Jordan, Pamela L., 135, 136
Journal of Human Lactation, 101

Kahn, Robbie, 220
Kaiser Family Foundation, 226
Kama Sutra, 218
Kedrowski, Karen, 197, 198
Kelleher, Christa, 198
Kitzinger, Sheila, 54
Klaus, Marshall, 186
Kleinman, Arthur, 128
Kuznets, Simon, 123

lactation consultant, 9, 98–107, 161, 232, 263, 275, 284
lactation failure, 4, 19, 20, 90
Lactational Amenorrhea Method, 38
lactivism, 2, 207, 264
lactivists, 170, 265
Ladd-Taylor, Molly, 21
La Leche League, 21, 58, 99–101, 127, 171, 194, 236
latch: painful, 115, 231; poor, 272; problems with, 182, 184, 232, 242, 271; proper, 115, 117, 118
Latinas, 75, 164. See also Hispanics
Law, Jules, 16
Lawless, Lucy, 216
Learning Channel, The, 229
let-down, 114, 115
Life Cycle Reproductive Health Model, 43, 45
Lipscomb, Michael, 197
Locke, Jill, 199
low-income mothers, 64, 67, 68, 71, 72, 73n1, 153, 211n16, 267n10
low-income women, 67–69, 72, 146, 151, 152, 154, 157, 159, 160, 163, 251. See also working-class women
Lucas, Jennifer, 157
Lunt, Paul, 237
Lupton, Deborah, 218, 219

Madonna, 21, 223, 259, 263
Maher, Vanessa, 135, 136

male supremacy, 30
Maloney, Carolyn, xii, 151
Manion, Jennifer, 195, 196, 198, 199
Marmet, Chele, 100
masculinity, 28–30, 32, 34, 54
Maternal and Child Health Pyramid, 43
maternalism, 103, 104, 107, 205, 206
maternity leave, xiii, 2, 3, 28, 30, 146, 147,
    149, 153, 154, 158, 162, 164, 165, 187, 216
McCarter-Spaulding, Deborah, 157
McLeod, Carolyn, 238, 243
Mead, Margaret, 59
Mead Johnson, 172
Medela, 228, 233
Medicaid, 152
medicalization, 9, 58, 187; of breastfeeding,
    98, 99, 102, 103, 105–107, 117, 180; of
    childbirth, 87, 104, 107; defined, 101; of
    family life, 6; of infant feeding, 6, 87, 99,
    102, 116; of women's reproductive
    health, 99
medical model, of breastfeeding, 205
Michie, Helena, 238, 243
midwifery, 102, 111
midwives, 93, 94, 100–102, 109n35, 111,
    260, 264
milk banks, 126, 171, 172, 175, 176,
    178n23, 215
milk expression, 10, 125, 147, 161–165,
    180, 183–186, 231, 284, 285; pumping,
    19, 33, 67, 72, 125, 146, 150, 151, 160,
    164, 166n21, 174, 179n12, 181, 183–187,
    188n5, 219, 240, 265, 284; exclusive,
    130, 181, 278
milk sharing, 171
Millennium Development Project, 48
Mommy Wars, xiii
Morse, Janice, 182
mother/infant dyad, 38, 45–47, 99, 100, 136,
    205, 210
Murphy, Elizabeth, 181
Muslim societies, milk siblingship in, 60
My Brest Friend, 233

National Alliance of Breastfeeding
    Advocacy (NABA), 266
National Breastfeeding Awareness
    Campaign (NBAC), 7, 11n5, 17, 18, 21,
    22, 150, 174, 175, 193, 227, 228

National Nutrition Council of Norway, 129
National Organization for Women (NOW),
    125, 126, 150
neoliberal contexts, 18
neoliberalism, defined, 24n11
Nestlé, 172
New Mothers' Breastfeeding Protection and
    Promotion Bill, xii
nipple confusion, 185
Nordegren, Elin, 263
norms, 184, 201, 255, 257; authoritative, 30;
    behavioral, 16; biological, 144;
    biomedical, 103; as cathexis, 31, 33;
    childbirth, 94; community, 20, 203;
    cultural, 6–8, 44, 71, 106, 204, 209, 222,
    256, 260; ideal worker, 158, 161; infant
    feeding, 205; labor-related, 29; male, 158,
    284; of medical monitoring, 91; of
    mothering, 223; organizational, 153;
    public health, 207, 208; social, 26, 30, 39,
    44, 154, 223, 251, 256, 282; workplace,
    30, 162
Nutrition Model, 44

obesity, 38, 39
obstetrics, 9, 45–47, 87, 88, 92–96, 99, 229,
    236, 239
"one best way, the," 62
Oppong, Christine, 26–28, 30, 31, 124
Orbach, Suzie, 236, 237
Ott, Brian, 221

pain, 112, 114–118, 184, 231, 242;
    management, 181
participatory action, 210
Patient Protection and Affordable Care Act
    (PPACA), xii, 8, 125, 151, 157, 164, 174,
    264, 285
pay equity, 28
pediatricians, 87–92, 95, 96, 99, 127,
    175, 195
pediatrics, 9, 10, 46, 87, 88, 91–93, 96, 99,
    172, 239
Peuchaud, Sheila Rose, 228, 229, 232
Pinkston, Ashley, 186
Plato, 262
positioning, 113; poor, 112, 114, 115
poverty, 5, 9, 25, 32, 61, 63, 68, 79, 80, 127,
    153, 203, 206–208, 267n10

praxis, 54
pregnancy discrimination, 149
Pregnancy Discrimination Act, xii, 152
Prolacta Bioscience, 170–171, 172, 175, 176
public breastfeeding, 2, 67, 71, 181, 240,
    249–256, 259, 260, 263, 265, 267
public health: constructs, 41, 42, 49;
    defined, 39, 40, 55; messaging, 1, 8, 10,
    105, 106, 205, 227; planning, 9, 42–44;
    policy, 1, 9, 15, 16, 23, 37, 47, 57, 60, 61;
    practice, 4, 25, 60; prevention, 39, 40,
    270; programming, 9, 36, 37; promotion,
    1, 4, 5, 112, 184, 203

Qualitative Comparative Analysis: defined,
    166n21; fuzzy set, 166n21
queer theory, 53

race, 4, 5, 6, 9, 10, 17, 57, 74, 77, 80, 81,
    144, 145, 150, 153, 154, 160, 164, 238,
    261; categories, 75, 79; as a social
    construct, 78
racism, 4–6, 61, 74–82, 83n17, 283;
    institutionalized, 75, 76, 83n17;
    internalized, 75, 77; personally mediated,
    75, 76; racial discrimination, 147
randomized controlled trial (RCT), 22, 37
Reagan, Nancy, 227
repressive hypothesis, 217
Reskin, Barbara, 146
Reye's syndrome, 227
rhetoric, 15, 16; defined, 17, 22, 23, 40, 148,
    194; reproductive, 149
Riggs, Danielle, 266
rights discourse, 148
rights framework, 15, 18–20, 45, 148
Riordan, Jan, 54, 56, 110
rites of passage, 203, 204
role strain, 27, 28, 34
roles, xii, 3, 9, 26, 27, 30, 32, 41, 124, 126,
    127, 129, 205, 236
Rosin, Hanna, 3, 15, 134, 135, 140
Rotch, Thomas, 91

Sanford, Mark and Jenny, 263
Sarkozy, Nicolas, 123, 131
Scientific Advisory Committee on
    Television and Social Behavior, 232
Scott, JoAnne, 100

Sen, Amartya, 123, 131
sex discrimination, xiii, 28, 152
sex inequity, 23
sexual division of labor, 28, 30–32, 34, 53
sexual harassment, 28
sexualization: of breastfeeding, 272; of
    breasts, 181, 229, 249, 259, 271, 283; of
    women's bodies, 32, 33, 283
sexual objectification, of women, 34
shame, 22, 59, 60, 193, 196, 198–201, 254
Sharia law, 60
Shell, Ellen, 100
Sherman Antitrust Act, 172
Silbaugh, Katharine, 174
Similac, 231
situated knowledge, 2
Smith, Julie, 130
Smith, Linda, 100
Smith, Paige Hall, 154
social change, xii, 81, 141, 216, 257,
    265, 270
Social-Ecological Model (SEM), 7, 44, 45,
    47, 65, 68, 72, 74, 75, 144, 232, 249,
    250, 257
social-ecological spectrum, 38
social ecology, 64, 65, 67
social justice, 10, 74, 81
social marketing, 7, 220, 222, 224,
    255–257
socioeconomic status, 17, 79, 145, 147,
    153, 154
Sparks, Johnelle, 79
Spitzer, Elliot and Silda, 263
Standing, Guy, 128
Stearns, Cindy, 181, 251, 252
Stefani, Gwen, 240
Stiglitz, Joseph, 123, 131
Stockholm syndrome, 77
structural violence, 64, 65, 68–72
Sudden Infant Death Syndrome (SIDS), 39
Surgeon General's *Blueprint for Action on
    Breastfeeding*, 48
Surgeon General's *Call to Action to Support
    Breastfeeding*, 48, 285
symbolic capital, 204, 209

Ten Essential Public Health Services, 43
Ten Steps of the Mother-Friendly Childbirth
    Initiative, 47

Ten Steps to Optimal MotherBaby Maternity Services, 47
Ten Steps to Successful Breastfeeding, 110
total motherhood, 198, 200, 201
Traina, Christina, 222, 223
twilight sleep, 93

Umansky, Lauri, 21
United Nations Children's Fund (UNICEF), 37, 44, 48, 106
United Nations Fourth World Conference on Women, 128
United Nations Systems of National Accounts (UNSNA), 123, 128, 130
United States Centers for Disease Control and Prevention (CDC), 44
United States Department of Agriculture (USDA), 8, 174
United States Department of Health and Human Services (DHHS), 8, 37, 147, 174, 175
United States national breastfeeding committee, 106
United States Office of Global Women's Issues, 42

Van Esterik, Penny, 102, 141
Van Gennep, Arnold, 203
Virgin Mary, 263. *See also* Madonna

Wall, Virginia R., 135, 136
Wallace, Louise M., 111

Walters, Barbara, 265
Waring, Marilyn, 123
Warner, W. Lloyd, 237
weaning, 89, 117, 146, 147, 162, 200, 278; early, 17, 18, 110, 112, 118, 130, 197, 240
Weisskopf, Susan, 223
wet nurses, 88, 126, 129, 170, 171, 175, 228
Whitehead, Dean, 219, 220
Wiessinger, Dianne, 194
Wight, Nancy, 195
Williams, Joan, 28, 149
Wolf, Joan, 3, 15, 196, 198, 200
Women, Infants, and Children program (WIC), 8, 64, 69–71, 76, 106, 152, 172–174
women of color, 76, 146, 154, 157–159, 163, 177
women's rights, 2, 16, 17, 19, 37,116, 148
Woods, Tiger, 263
working-class women, 10, 237, 241–242, 243, 244. *See also* low-income women
workplace, 10, 34, 39, 127, 147, 150, 157–160, 162–164, 169, 251, 283
World Food Conference (1973), 129
World Health Organization (WHO), 19, 37, 44, 59, 106, 185, 215

Young, Iris, Marion, 222

Available titles in the Critical Issues in Health and Medicine series:

Emily K. Abel, *Suffering in the Land of Sunshine: A Los Angeles Illness Narrative*

Emily K. Abel, *Tuberculosis and the Politics of Exclusion: A History of Public Health and Migration to Los Angeles*

Marilyn Aguirre-Molina, Luisa N. Borrell, and William Vega, eds. *Health Issues in Latino Males: A Social and Structural Approach*

Susan M. Chambré, *Fighting for Our Lives: New York's AIDS Community and the Politics of Disease*

James Colgrove, Gerald Markowitz, and David Rosner, eds., *The Contested Boundaries of American Public Health*

Cynthia A. Connolly, *Saving Sickly Children: The Tuberculosis Preventorium in American Life, 1909–1970*

Tasha N. Dubriwny, *The Vulnerable Empowered Woman: Feminism, Postfeminism, and Women's Health*

Edward J. Eckenfels, *Doctors Serving People: Restoring Humanism to Medicine through Student Community Service*

Julie Fairman, *Making Room in the Clinic: Nurse Practitioners and the Evolution of Modern Health Care*

Jill A. Fisher, *Medical Research for Hire: The Political Economy of Pharmaceutical Clinical Trials*

Alyshia Gálvez, *Patient Citizens, Immigrant Mothers: Mexican Women, Public Prenatal Care and the Birth Weight Paradox*

Gerald N. Grob and Howard H. Goldman, *The Dilemma of Federal Mental Health Policy: Radical Reform or Incremental Change?*

Gerald N. Grob and Allan V. Horwitz, *Diagnosis, Therapy, and Evidence: Conundrums in Modern American Medicine*

Rachel Grob, *Testing Baby: The Transformation of Newborn Screening, Parenting, and Policymaking*

Mark A. Hall and Sara Rosenbaum, eds., *The Health Care "Safety Net" in a Post-Reform World*

Laura D. Hirshbein, *American Melancholy: Constructions of Depression in the Twentieth Century*

Timothy Hoff, *Practice under Pressure: Primary Care Physicians and Their Medicine in the Twenty-first Century*

Beatrix Hoffman, Nancy Tomes, Rachel N. Grob, and Mark Schlesinger, eds., *Patients as Policy Actors*

Ruth Horowitz, *Deciding the Public Interest: Medical Licensing and Discipline*

Rebecca M. Kluchin, *Fit to Be Tied: Sterilization and Reproductive Rights in America, 1950–1980*

Jennifer Lisa Koslow, *Cultivating Health: Los Angeles Women and Public Health Reform*

Bonnie Lefkowitz, *Community Health Centers: A Movement and the People Who Made It Happen*

Ellen Leopold, *Under the Radar: Cancer and the Cold War*

Barbara L. Ley, *From Pink to Green: Disease Prevention and the Environmental Breast Cancer Movement*

David Mechanic, *The Truth about Health Care: Why Reform Is Not Working in America*

Alyssa Picard, *Making the American Mouth: Dentists and Public Health in the Twentieth Century*

Heather Munro Prescott, *The Morning After: A History of Emergency Contraception in the United States*

David G. Schuster, *Neurasthenic Nation: America's Search for Health, Happiness, and Comfort, 1869–1920*

Karen Seccombe and Kim A. Hoffman, *Just Don't Get Sick: Access to Health Care in the Aftermath of Welfare Reform*

Leo B. Slater, *War and Disease: Biomedical Research on Malaria in the Twentieth Century*

Matthew Smith, *An Alternative History of Hyperactivity: Food Additives and the Feingold Diet*

Paige Hall Smith, Bernice L. Hausman, and Miriam Labbok, *Beyond Health, Beyond Choice: Breastfeeding Constraints and Realities*

Rosemary A. Stevens, Charles E. Rosenberg, and Lawton R. Burns, eds., *History and Health Policy in the United States: Putting the Past Back In*

Barbra Mann Wall, *American Catholic Hospitals: A Century of Changing Markets and Missions*

CPSIA information can be obtained at www.ICGtesting.com
Printed in the USA
BVOW080029240712

296010BV00001B/1/P

9 780813 553030